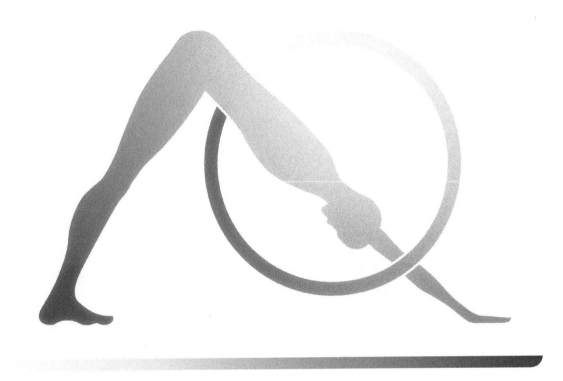

Yoga: Point + Process

Volume 1

Michael Bridge-Dickson

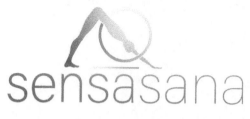

sensāsana
āsana that makes sense

Yoga: Point + Process, Volume 1
A detailed study of 36 Basic Yoga Poses for teachers and practitioners

Text, illustrations, layout, and design copyright © Michael Bridge-Dickson.

First Edition, 2017

Bridge-Dickson, Michael, 1978~

ISBN 978-1-7751054-0-4

Publisher's Note:

The practices described in this book are not intended to replace professional medical advice or the guidance of a skilled teacher. Always consult with a health care provider before embarking on any physical practice.
The reader assumes all risks in practicing the exercises described in this book.

Published and distributed by:

sensâsana | âsana that makes sense
yoga@sensasana.com
www.sensasana.com
Montreal, QC
Canada

The flame of intelligence resides within us all.
I am fortunate to have sat at the hearth of
some truly brilliant yogic flames.

Yoga: Point + Process

is dedicated to those yogis,
their teachers, and theirs before them.

May this book serve as a bridge between us and you,
sparking your inner intelligence through
embodied consciousness.

Yoga: Point + Process

Foreword

Preface

Introduction

Poses

Contents

Yoga: Point + Process

Contents

"Form can provide a context for deeper explorations,
and most importantly, for freedom."

~ Carrie Owerko

from Carrie Owerko

I met Michael in an Iyengar Yoga workshop that I was teaching in Montreal.

From the get-go, I could see that he was bright, keen, curious, and full of enthusiasm for the subject of yoga. He listened attentively and was a cheerful, open-hearted presence throughout the workshop.

He gave me a copy of the book he was working on and asked if I would mind taking a look at it.

As I turned the pages, I was immediately delighted by the beautiful illustrations (Michael's own) and the care that he had taken with each and every page.

It was evident from that first glance that he had spent countless hours poring over the content. His illustrations are simple, clear, and elegant; and he has taken the same care, attention to detail and pursuit of clarity in the instructions that accompany the illustrations. The whole book is filled with intelligence and elegance.

Micheal is a very creative and positive person, and that creativity and positivity is evident in his teaching and everything that he makes.

This beautiful book is no exception.

It will be a wonderful practice companion for students who are hoping to establish a home practice, and for teachers of yoga who are interested in learning how to simply and effectively incorporate the use of props into their classes.

His illustrations are also helpful aids for both students and teachers as they explore the sense of direction within the poses.

Michael has provided the type of practice explorations that will inspire students to look around their homes and apartments for inspiration and possibility, and begin to use what is readily available in their environment to make their practice more accessible, effective, and even therapeutic.

I know that this project was a labor of love for Michael. I think that is what shines out from its pages. **Yoga**: Point + Process is a unique and wonderful contribution to the diversity of yoga books available.

New York, New York
October, 2017

Yoga: Point + Process

This book's process began in 2010, its aim being a unique and comprehensive, yet practical tool that supports learning, practicing, and teaching āsana with precision and detail.

Despite an emphasis on precision and detail, it is important to remember that the point of yogāsana is not reaching perfection of an arbitrary ideal — though this is a logical conclusion when studying such a technical manual.

Rather, yogāsana is about function and resilience, while gathering action and energy in an efficient way.

When approached from this perspective, yogāsana is no longer a goal of physical achievement, but a continual process in which consciousness seeps through the physical, mental and emotional layers to the spiritual, constantly changing us both within and without.

Practicing alignment principles and bringing precision to the body's movements are an endeavor in sharpening the mind and refining consciousness as it pervades the entire being.

To this end, **Yoga:** Point + Process serves as a supplement to sensāsana Teacher Training programs, but is also structured in a way that is accessible to any student of yogāsana, at every level of experience, whether purely for self-practice or to help teachers hone their practice and teaching.

Throughout, this manual is intended to:

· *Simplify* your practice in the pose's most basic form
· *Explore* your sensations as the pose develops
· *Nourish* your awareness by learning to rest
· *Synthesize* your āsana experience and awaken within

This method extends beyond the āsanas in this manual as you begin to see how āsanas break down to the elements they are built upon, and as common threads and principles become evident through the *Simplify, Explore, Nourish,* and *Synthesize* pattern.

Newer practitioners will find in this manual a methodical practice that constructs each pose from its most rudimentary aspect, appropriate for the very first time you ever do the pose, and then guides practitioners through a logical development to the more classic forms.

Seasoned practitioners already familiar with the poses described will find opportunities to study basic principles and refine their practice, while filling in many gaps that may exist between the familiar forms and their finer details.

Within the *Simplify*, *Explore*, *Nourish*, and *Synthesize* structure, each stage is a complete description of practicing that pose's variation: from when to learn and practice, what may be gained and what cautions to consider, to what you'll need prior to practicing.

The descriptions continue through complete point · by · point instructions that take you from preparation, entering and exiting the pose safely, to what to do while sustaining the poses themselves, and finally some tips on responding to challenges as they arise.

Hundreds of original illustrations accompany this text. These illustrations clarify the instructions to help you follow along — emphasizing important details such as props, lines of movement or action, guides for correct placement, and occasionally what to watch out for or avoid when potentially damaging or harmful.

I've worked hard at creating a valuable, top-notch resource that supports your practice and study.

These pages represent countless hours of practice and research put into writing, illustration, and design. Please respect my efforts by not copying and distributing this content, in part or in full, digitally or physically, whether freely or profitably without express permission.

Yoga: Point + Process is part of a larger vision at sensāsana to provide an array of reference tools and study aids that I hope will help your yogāsana experience make sense — from your physical practice through to your deeper understanding of the poses and their expression.

May these efforts benefit you and those you come into contact with.

Michael Bridge-Dickson
Montreal, Canada
July, 2017

ॐ This material is meant to supplement yogāsana study and is in no way intended to replace instruction from a live teacher.
Consult with a physician before embarking on any exercise routine, including yogāsana practice.
Please read and observe the cautions outlined at each stage of every pose.
The reader practices the poses in this manual at his or her own risk.

"The beautiful thing about learning is that nobody can take it away from you."

~ BB King

*"Absorb what is useful,
Discard what is not,
Add what is uniquely your own."*

~ Bruce Lee

How to Use This Book

Any useful reference should ideally have information organized in a way that is easy to find, and presented in some logical fashion. I've tried my best to achieve this end from the more general outline of the book to how more specific kinds of information unfold.

This book's main content is the step-by-step instructions for individual âsanas, and these instructions are given in succinct, point form, leading practitioners logically through practice process, from instruction to instruction, stage to stage, and pose to pose — hence the name, **Yoga**: Point + Process.

The poses outlined in this book are, for the most part, organized from most fundamental to those that require more foundation. This is not necessarily the order in which poses are practiced in a given sequence, but are instead the order in which they should be learned and introduced over time.

For instance, *Viparita Karani* is usually practiced after *Sarvangasana* in a daily sequence, but is best learned before even considering *Sarvangasana*. Therefore, *Viparita Karani* appears before *Sarvangasana* rather

than after. This is also the case for many Standing and Seated Poses as they are presented here.

Within that overall structure, every pose is dissected into four stages: *Simplify*, *Explore*, *Nourish*, and *Synthesize*. Each of these stages is dedicated a 2-page spread.

On each stage's 2-page spread, information is organized in the same format for every pose at every stage to ensure clarity and consistent ease of use.

Knowing this format in advance will help you navigate your way as you practice with this companion — instructions appear on the left-facing page, and the illustrations are on the right-facing page.

I'd recommend glancing at the title bar and the information directly below it before practicing the pose, as this information is useful to know before practicing that stage of that pose, letting you know what the pose does, when it should and should not be practiced, what you'll need, and some notes on its general form.

When considering poses to practice, it is usually reasonable to work through the entire book

practicing only the *Simplify* stages of each pose, then work through again at the *Explore* stage, and so on to *Synthesize*. There are a few exceptions, where you may need to practice the *Explore* or *Nourish* stage of a foundational pose before practicing the *Simplify* stage of subsequent poses.

You may also choose to delve deeply into each pose and practice all four stages sequentially, working on the same pose from *Simplify* to *Synthesize*. Dedicating one practice to this process for only one pose per day (and if time allows, continue with your regular yoga practice) will develop your understanding of that pose and may help you connect finer aspects of that pose to others you are practicing that day.

Note too that the variations presented here are by no means exhaustive. Principles from one pose can often be transferred to others. When investigating the poses, their principles, and prop use, consider how what you are experiencing can be applied in other ways. The precise approach is intended to provide a structural framework for experimentation and increase the possible options.

Below is a more specific breakdown of the 2-page format that every pose variation follows, outlining where you will find each piece of information.

Title Bar

Across the top of each spread is a title bar displaying the which stage of the pose you are on. This title bar is color-coded: the lightest blue signifies the *Simplify* stage, and the darkest blue the *Synthesize* stage.

The pose's name appears first on this title bar in Sanskrit, and then below in English.

On the right-facing page, the title bar has a short overview of that pose stage, with some common benefits and uses for that variation. This is merely a snapshot of the pose's value and characteristics, which will extend beyond this brief overview.

Note that any pose's uses and benefits may vary from individual to individual.

Each stage builds upon the stage before, and may also build upon a previous pose as its foundation.

The four stages are:

Simplify

· The pose's entry level variation, appropriate for almost anyone, at any practice or experience level

Explore

· Also appropriate for most levels, a slightly more complex variation that requires some basic understanding

Nourish

· A variation that enables practitioners to explore deeper layers of the pose; often the Restorative or supported variation

Synthesize

· The classic expression of the pose, unifying aspects from the previous three stages, along with instructions that build upon and refine those prior

When the pose's name changes within the four-stage format, understand that the first pose is foundational to the second in exactly the same way that the *Simplify* is foundational to *Explore*, and *Explore* is foundational to *Nourish*, and so on. Only the name and specific description changes as the pose progresses.

Nonetheless, view these differently named poses as being on the same continuum as those with a consistent name throughout. The different names can sometimes give more insight into that pose stage's effects uses, which can be valuable information for both study and practice.

How to Use This Book

Before Practicing

Below the Title Bar, the top section for each stage includes some preliminary information — useful things to know while considering the pose and before practicing it, such as:

Learn + Practice

- When to place this variation in a given sequence: either near the beginning, middle, end, or at any point
- Prerequisite and recommended poses to practice before this variation
- Poses that should be practiced only after this variation

Related Poses

- The most directly related poses, additional to those mentioned in reference to *Learn + Practice*

Safety Factors

- Major and minor contraindications
- In most cases, only things to watch out for, or recommended sub-variations for particular consideration

Contact Points

- Parts of the body that are foundational contacts
- Contacts may be with the floor, the wall, props, or other body parts, if foundational to the pose
- When there are numerous contact points, only the most important are listed

External Supports

- All props necessary for the stage and its variations
- When additional props are required for *Responses* to *Challenges*, these props are listed on the next line

Essence of Form

- The primary actions of the pose: flexions, extensions, abductions, adductions, leg and arm rotations, etc
- Note that rotations, though often fundamental, are actions and therefore considered secondary within the form's essence

Consider these aspects before practicing the pose, either in general or that particular variation. Obtain the necessary props and practice prerequisite and foundational poses before setting up.

Instructions

The main content on the left-facing pages are the instructions themselves, outlining:

Prepare

· How to set up the listed props before starting

Enter

· What poses, if any, to begin in before entering the actual pose
· Step-by-step instructions on how to move into the pose safely
· Each instruction builds on the last

Sustain

· What to do while in the pose
· How to get the most out of the pose while you are there
· Actions generally do not change the shape of the pose itself, being more subtle and experiential rather than outwardly visible

Exit

· How to come out of the pose safely
· How long to hold the pose (if appropriate)
· What to do once out of the pose, if anything
· Whether or not to repeat the pose, and how many times

Challenge

· Problems typically encountered in that pose's variation and at that level of experience

Response

· How to address these challenges with props, modifications, and which actions to emphasize

These *Challenges* and their *Responses* may relate to the *Safety Considerations*, and/or to several poses or several stages of the same pose, so read these *Challenges* and their *Responses* for every stage of the pose, even if you are not practicing that variation.

Text for *Challenges* and their *Responses* is usually written in full sentences, rather than bulleted point form, but are still succinct. They are also numbered so that each *Response* corresponds to its same numbered *Challenge*.

Illustrations, as well as other sections, stages, and poses are referenced in *italics*.

Additional, but not essential details about the pose and alternative instructions will occasionally appear within the appropriate sub-category with an ☸ instead of a standard bullet · and the instruction will be *italicized*.

Illustrations

Illustrations are all numbered in reference to instructions on the facing page. They are referenced throughout the corresponding text.

Numbering is by pose stage first (*I* for *Simplify*, *II* for *Explore*, *III* for *Nourish*, and *IV* for *Synthesize*), then lower-case letter numbering.

The Illustrations support and clarify the text, featuring directional arrows, highlighting props, actions, movements, and showing the general forms.

Guidelines

Organized in this way, maximum information is packed in a concise and consistent manner, with instructions reduced to their essence, and presented logically and practically: each instruction continues from the last.

Nonetheless, there are some additional practice principles and guidelines to consider before delving into any specific poses.

First and foremost, do not exceed your personal capacity. Ensure your breath is free and that there is no excessive strain in performing each āsana. Āsana practice should be challenging, but also nourishing. If you find that you are fatigued and feel drained well after your practice session, it is likely that you are over-efforting and that the āsana level exceeds your current level of practice.

Conversely, your practice may not be sufficiently energizing if you are not challenged at all. Some challenge develops resilience — a primary practice benefit.

That said, different practitioners have different needs at different times. If you are recovering from illness or injury, a mild, Restorative practice that is not very challenging is

recommended. If you are in good health and relatively free of injury, a more vigorous practice may be appropriate.

Here again, the breath is your most reliable guide: when the breath is held or restricted, effort in the pose is excessive and its benefits are unlikely to continue. When you experience breath restriction, see if it is possible to reduce some effort where you are. If this does not free the breath, back off of the pose and see if the breath settles. If not, carefully *Exit* the pose and consider one of the variations in the *Challenge* and *Response* section for your current stage, or return to a previous stage.

This is why, besides being a useful learning structure, this four-stage approach to āsana practice is presented where you can fine-tune your practice not only according to your level of overall physical and intellectual study of these poses individually and as a whole, but also your current state from day to day, week to week, and year to year.

What is appropriate practice for you today may not be appropriate tomorrow, and I hope that this book gives you the tools to adjust your practice accordingly as

you develop sensitivity to your needs through understanding.

For this reason, it is also recommended that you learn each stage well before progressing to the next — even if you are a seasoned practitioner — as the fundamental steps, principles, and actions presented in *Simplify* are built upon in *Explore*, which are then further built on in *Nourish* and *Synthesize*. When working on a particular pose, practice each stage in its entirety.

For more general practice, master the *Simplify* stage of several poses for a few weeks or months, then go back and revisit the same poses at the *Explore* stage, and continue the process through *Nourish* and *Synthesize*.

Working in this way can circumvent problems you may encounter by progressing too quickly. Additionally, whenever you encounter difficulty in later stages of a pose, practicing the *Simplify* and *Explore* stages are where you can address and work with these *Challenges* in a way that is more sustainably integrated, especially if you are recovering from injury or trauma.

No matter which of the four

variations you practice, it may be useful to read the instructions for the other stages as well. While the instructions are often similar, they are also progressive, and many are universal — being applicable to any stage. This means that you may apply certain instructions from all stages while still practicing the *Simplify* variation; and conversely, some practitioners may need to refer back to previous instructions while practicing your current variation.

To ensure the breath remains free, instructions follow the following formula whenever possible:

Foundation ➤ Breath ➤ Movement

That is, each instruction contains a foundation, a point to establish or maintain before moving, then a breath and subsequent movement. For example, an instruction about pressing the big toe mounds into the floor establishes a foundation, and so the next instruction would be to keep the big toe mounds pressing into the floor before performing the next movement or action along with a breath instruction.

In this book, due to space considerations, this formula is not always followed but it is nonetheless assumed that the previous instruction be kept unless specified.

Ideally, the movement and breath should coordinate to a nearly inseparable extent — even if they must be differentiated linguistically. Because breath and movement coincide, the breath phase of an instruction may follow the movement phase instead of preceding it.

Again, due to the space and layout considerations, breath instructions are often omitted unless crucial.

This does not make the breath any less important, so whenever breath instructions are absent, link each movement or action with the breath.

In general, lifting, lengthening, and widening actions are done on inhalations; descending, squeezing, pushing, and releasing actions are done on exhalation. Muscular invigoration is typical of inhalations, creating stability and therefore inhalations are ideal for establishing and affirming foundations before movement.

Since tensions and excess activity are often released while exhaling, movements are usually better done on exhalations.

When in doubt, stabilize the previous movement or action on inhalations and initiate new movements and actions during exhalations, even if this requires a little extra attention.

In essence:

Inhale — stabilize the foundation

Exhale — keeping foundation, create movement or action

Except when otherwise indicated, follow these additional breath guidelines:

· Breathe in and out through the nose and as naturally as possible without force, holding, or exaggeration
· Let Ujjayi breath show itself naturally rather than creating it artificially (if you do not know what Ujjayi breath is, breathing naturally is your best option)
· Keep your breath soft, smooth, and natural during practice, with any associated sound subtle and nearly imperceptible
· Release the throat, jaw, and tongue, and allow the belly to move freely with your breath

Putting a Practice Together

Beyond the breath and specific individual poses, an important consideration in practice is sequencing.

Structuring your own sequences is a vast subject beyond the scope of this book, but there are many helpful hints throughout regarding sequencing.

Most poses suggest prerequisites under *Learn + Practice,* and the *Related Poses* give helpful clues as to what other poses might go well together. The *Challenge* and *Response* sections often also suggest poses that, though not always prerequisite, are helpful in addressing potential problems and are therefore wise additions to sequences.

One general practice is to select a few poses from each pose category. Like the template that follows, practice a few warm up and centering poses first, then some Standing Poses.

Two common progressions after the Standing Poses are to start with Back Bends, Twists, then Forward Bends, -or- follow the progression of this book after the Standing Poses: Seated and Forward Bends, Twists, then Back Bends. The former is better suited to sequences structured for afternoon or evening practice, the latter is better suited to morning or earlier in the day.

Finish with *Sarvangasana, Setu Bandha Sarvangasana, Viparita Karani,* and/or *Savasana* or other settling, Restorative finishing poses.

However you structure your practice, it is not advised to alternate between pose categories, especially in extremes. When practicing a few poses from each category, also avoid extremes and deep poses.

When you do want to work more deeply, I suggest working only with that pose category and its relatives so that your body is well prepared and willing to go deeper without shocking the nervous system.

A generic, standard sequence pattern that most would do well to follow is of a gradual arc of five sections:

First:
Warm-up and centering.

This stage prepares mind and body for the practice to come, by demarcating space and time dedicated to practice. It is your chance to check in with your body, your breath, and establish focus. This phase is around one to three poses, but can include more. These are mild poses that prepare your body for the practice to come.

Supta Tadasana, Virasana, Baddha Konasana, and *Supta Padangusthasana* are excellent starting points that lead well into any emphasis.

Second:
Development or intensity.

This phase makes up the largest portion of the practice, and is the most intense. It should generally be structured from mildest poses to those that require more effort, mobility, or coordination of various elements, each one building on the last.

In a short and simple sequence, you could choose any of the poses in this book and practice each stage in order from *Simplify* to *Synthesize*. Since this book is essentially organized from most basic to most advanced, not only within each pose and its four stages, but also from pose to pose, you could also choose a section of the book and practice all the poses at a given stage from that section. For example, you could practice the *Explore* stage of every Standing Pose.

Third:
Dénouement or Apex.

The apex (sometimes also called the peak pose) pulls together everything practiced so far, and is the deepest and/or most intense pose that will be practiced. This may or may not be a pose that is generally considered "deep" or "advanced" but it will be the deepest, most advanced pose you will practice for the day.

Fourth:
Tempering or counterbalance.

Often where a counter-pose would be practiced, there are differing opinions on this. While it can be beneficial to counterbalance with a pose that is oppositional to the apex, it may be just as beneficial if not more so to temper the apex with a milder, but related pose, or a neutral pose first.

If practicing a direct counter-pose, a mild, but long-held pose is usually a safer counterbalance than a deeper pose that directly opposes the apex.

Fifth:
Closing or quieting.

Here, practice poses that are soothing to the nervous system, and quiet the mind such as *Sarvangasana* and its relatives, neutral poses, and mild Restoratives.

Close with *Savasana*.

It is often tempting to skip this phase of practice, especially when time allocated to practice is limited.

Even if your practice was relatively mild, finish with a symmetrical and passive pose — *Savasana* is ideal, though other poses may be adequate substitutes, provided they are passive, symmetrical, and soothing to your brain, body, and being.

This is the phase in which your body adapts to the changes you instigated through your practice, and your nervous system needs time to re-pattern itself.

If you find you are practicing ardently, but not experiencing the fruits of your efforts, you may need to allot more time to closing postures, especially *Savasana*.

Practicing with Preconditions

Each pose has a set of *Safety Factors*, listed on that pose's pages. These are not necessarily contraindications, but they are warnings of potential risk. When specifically contraindicated, the *Safety Factors* section will say: "Do not practice if ..." Additional cautions mentioned are there to raise awareness of conditions to watch out for, as there may be increased risk.

If unsure, avoid that pose or variation until you consult with your health care provider and a teacher well versed in yoga's therapeutic uses and effects.

These guidelines do not — and can not — address major health issues. Consult with your doctor and a qualified yoga therapeutics teacher if you suffer from any major health issues before practicing the poses outlined in this book.

Specific precautions for women's health such as practicing during pregnancy and menstruation are based on the advice of seasoned female teachers and practitioners such as Geeta Iyengar, Bobby Clennell, and Lois Steinberg, as well as the accumulated anecdotal evidence observed among female students and

fellow teachers. Nonetheless, it is recommended that female students take ownership and responsibility for their own bodies, investigating potential health risks and benefits through research, individual observation, and when available, consult with an experienced teacher familiar with yoga's short- and long-term effects on female health.

Here is a brief overview of common precautions that you can be cognizant of during your practice:

High Blood Pressure/ Hypertension — do not raise the arms overhead, particularly in Seated and Standing Poses where the spine is vertical, as this raises blood pressure.

Be careful of poses where the head is below the heart, such as *Adho Mukha Svanasana*, *Uttanasana*, and *Sarvangasana*, that pressure within the skull and behind the eyes is minimal. Supporting the head will usually help, but if it doesn't, practice only short, mild holds in these poses or avoid these poses altogether.

Practice poses like the *Simplify* and *Explore* stages of *Adho*

Mukha Svanasana, and keep the hands on hips or extended laterally for *Urdhva Hastasana*, *Utkatasana*, *Virabhadrasana A*, and other poses where the arms would typically be raised overhead.

Twists may also raise blood pressure, even if only temporarily, so practice only open Twists such as *Trikonasana*, *Parsvakonasana*, *Janu Sirsasana*, and *Marichyasana A* and avoid closed Twists such as *Bharadvajasana* and *Marichyasana C*.

Low Blood Pressure — use care when coming out of all Forward Bends, especially Standing Forward Bends, such as *Adho Mukha Svanasana*, *Uttanasana*, and *Prasarita Padottanasana*.

When coming out of these poses, exhale instead of inhaling as this will disturb blood pressure less.

Emphasize Standing Poses and Back Bends at a moderately vigorous level of practice. Avoid over-exertion, however, as this can have a detrimental after-effect.

Circulatory Problems

Introduction

— provided no other contraindications are present, Standing Poses, Back Bends, Twists, and Inversions are all helpful.

Gradually introduce Inversions, however, both long-term and within each practice session.

Emphasize expansive action and ensure venous return. Do not tolerate limb tingling or numbness to any degree — *Exit* any pose you experience tingling or numbness in, as this may indicate blood flow restriction.

Diabetes — moderate to vigorous practice is advised, but start slowly and increase intensity gradually over weeks or months. Sustained, moderate practice is favored over sporadic, vigorous practice.

Ensure core temperature is kept moderate — not too high, and not too low. Check in with your health-care provider periodically. Avoid all full Inversions unless cleared by your doctor, and ensure that eye pressure does not increase in partial Inversions such as *Adho Mukha Svanasana* and *Uttanasana*.

As for blood pressure and

circulatory issues, introduce full Inversions gradually, being cautious that eye pressure does not increase.

Glaucoma, Detached Retina, and Eye Strain — avoid all full Inversions. In partial Inversions, such as *Adho Mukha Svanasana* and *Uttanasana*, ensure that eye pressure does not increase. Introduce partial Inversions gradually.

Keep the breath smooth and steady, and gently increase the length of exhalations, especially in vigorous poses such as Standing Poses, Back Bends, and Twists.

Do not hold the breath and observe and reduce any tendency to suspend the breath at the end of inhalation in particular.

Depression — practice moderately vigorous Standing Poses followed by Restorative Back Bends. Unless otherwise contraindicated, poses with arms extended overhead (*Urdhva Hastasana*) are helpful.

Avoid deep and/or long-held Forward Bends, especially seated, but practice *Supta*

Padangusthasana and *Urdhva Prasarita Padasana* to lengthen the hamstrings. Partial and full Inversions may also be helpful if not contraindicated for other reasons.

Disc Herniation — do not jump or bounce into, out of, or while in any pose.

For posterior herniations, avoid Forward Bends that involve spinal rounding. Ensure the hamstrings are well prepared with *Supta Padangusthasana* and *Ardha Uttanasana* (*Wall Push*) before all Forward Bends. For Seated Poses, sit on generous height, or avoid them altogether. Mild Back Bends are advised.

For anterior herniations (which are more rare) avoid Back Bending Poses and Twists. Neutral Standing Poses and Forward Bends are recommended.

Neck Injury — avoid extremes in flexion, extension, and twisting the head and neck. Soften the tongue, throat, and jaw in all poses and before any neck or head movement, even if minor.

Work on opening and lifting

Practicing with Preconditions

the chest, reducing upper back tension including kyphosis.

Do not jump or bounce into, out of, or within any pose. Use caution in poses where the head is supported, ensuring that the head support reduces tension, does not cause neck compression, and if possible, creates traction.

Kyphosis (rounding of the upper back) — supported Back Bends and armpit/chest openers such as *Urdhva Hastasana* and *Ardha Uttanasana* (*Wall Push*) are ideal.

Support the head in supine poses, but ensure support does not exacerbate kyphosis. Do not round the upper back in Forward Bends.

Avoid Seated Poses, especially Twists, until kyphosis is well managed.

Also avoid *Sarvangasana* if kyphosis is severe.

Scoliosis — this is a highly individual structural issue. Generally, Back Bends and Standing Poses are recommended, but individual cases always vary.

Forward Bends should be avoided — but this will depend on the nature and severity of the scoliosis. Twists can be practiced, but be extremely conscious of the tendencies created by the scoliosis and avoid the urge to follow those tendencies, as they will exacerbate the inherent twist. When working against the scoliosis, use great care, as working too severely can cause the structure to react toward the scoliotic twist.

When working deeply, it may be helpful to mildly follow the inherent twist to release the musculature first, then oppose it as long as there is little to no resistance.

Poses specific to scoliosis are beyond the scope of this book, but in general any pose that creates traction will usually be helpful, and do not practice poses that exacerbate your scoliosis or create pain.

SI Joint Pain and Dysfunction — strengthen the transverse abdominus (instructions for doing so are in *Supta Tadasana* and *Tadasana Urdhva Hastasana*, and carried throughout this book, as it

is a common issue among yogāsana practitioners).

Avoid deep Twists, even if they provide temporary relief. Do not pull the torso forward using the arms in Seated Forward Bends, or pull the leg in *Supta Padangusthasana A*.

Be cautious of all asymmetrical Standing Poses, and do not roll the pelvis open laterally in these poses or force it to be "square."

Lateral hip openers (*Supta Padangusthasana B, Baddha Konasana, Upavistha Konasana, Trikonasana, Virabhadrasana B, Parsvakonasana*, etc.) often exacerbate SI joint pain, so refrain from practicing them too often or deeply.

It may be helpful to practice all poses with a strap around the iliums to stabilize the pelvis. In general, poses that create or require internal rotation will be most helpful.

Supta Padangusthasana A + B and *Setu Bandha Sarvangasana* may help reset the sacrum between the iliums.

Shoulder Injury — work to stabilize the shoulder joint

by keeping the head of the humerus drawing toward the shoulder while simultaneously extending the shoulder blades and collarbones away from the mid line.

Avoid weight-bearing in the arms, such as for *Adho Mukha Svanasana* and *Urdhva Mukha Svanasana* until injury is managed.

Do not practice the *Explore*, *Nourish*, or *Synthesize* stages of *Chaturanga Dandasana*, but the *Simplify* stage with arms straight may be practiced when injury is managed.

Do not practice extreme shoulder openers, which includes extreme armpit extension, extreme internal and external arm rotations, and "binding" poses where one arm wraps behind the torso and catches the opposite arm's wrist.

Many suggestions on stabilizing the shoulder joints are given throughout this book where appropriate.

Wrist and Elbow Injuries —
similar to the recommendations for shoulder injuries, particularly with regards to weight bearing and rotations.

Avoid elbow hyperextension and extreme wrist flexion. Practice weight-bearing poses with the hands on a wall or chair instead of the floor.

Wrist flexion can often be reduced by using a slant board or wedge under the heels of hands, and/or turning the hands out slightly. Avoid using the fists as an alternative whenever possible, as while this does prevent wrist flexion, it decreases the helpful stabilizing action in the forearms.

Pulled Hamstring — avoid all
Forward Bends and hamstring openers for at least the first 3-6 months, including *Baddha Konasana*. Strengthen the hamstrings with *Utkatasana*, *Salabhasana*, and *Setu Bandha Sarvangasana*. Release hamstring fibers in *Virasana*, particularly *Explore*.

Support the hamstring(s) whenever possible, and you can tie a strap firmly around the injured hamstring at the point of injury. Use this support as feedback to avoid stretching those fibers, and to draw the hamstring forward, toward the femur and away from the strap.

Hip Replacement — avoid
extreme rotations and abduction, and do not practice poses where the femur crosses the pelvis' mid line.

Reduce the angle the legs open in *Baddha Konasana* and *Upavistha Konasana*, with support under the femurs even when not otherwise indicated.

Use care that lateral Standing Poses and all Forward Bends are not too extreme. Stabilize the pelvis and femurs in Twists by bracing the legs or holding a block between the thighs.

Groin Injury — similar to
the precautions for Hip Replacements and SI joint pain and dysfunction.

In all poses requiring groin extension such as most Standing Poses and Back Bends, ensure the groin flesh does not "puff" toward the skin. Instead, deepen and recede the groin flesh away from the skin. In poses requiring groin (hip) flexion, ensure space between the femurs and front iliums is retained by descending the femurs and lifting the front iliums off the femurs.

Practicing with Preconditions

You may also need to create lateral groin space either by taking a wider stance in narrow-stance poses, or by resisting the heels laterally, or both. Many specific groin instructions and ways to create and retain space in the groins are given throughout this book.

Knee Injury — strengthen the quadriceps by lifting the kneecaps in straight-leg poses, and keeping a pushing action in the feet in bent-leg poses.

Release and lengthen the hamstrings to take strain off the quadriceps and knees.

In bent-leg Standing Poses, keep the tibia vertical, with the knee directly atop the ankle (the one exception to this is *Utkatasana*, but strengthen the quadriceps well before practicing).

Also be mindful that the legs do not hyperextend in straight-leg poses. Avoid this by either supporting the backs of the legs or resisting the tibia heads forward, or both.

Perform all leg rotations by the femur within the hip joint, and be especially careful that the knees do not torque in any way, evidenced by the lower leg rotating independent of the femur, or the knees collapsing in or out in bent-leg poses.

Do not tolerate any pose that causes or exacerbates existing knee pain. Do not "stand" on the knees, where the legs are bent with knees on the floor and pelvis is atop the knees, such as in *Ustrasana* and its preparatory position.

During Menstruation — depending on how you feel, avoid or limit vigorous practice, particularly Standing Poses and deep Back Bends.

Every woman's cycle is different, but in general — and particularly if there are already specific concerns — do not practice full Inversions where the legs and pelvis are both above the heart.

In this book, the only such Inversions are *Viparita Karani* and *Sarvangasana*. If you are already practicing *Sirsasana* (not included in *Volume 1*), substitute *Uttanasana*, *Prasarita Padottanasana*, or *Adho Mukha Svanasana*, all with the head supported.

Mild, Restorative Back Bends and long-held Forward Bends are recommended, with little to no Twists until flow has stopped.

Pregnancy — most poses in this book are safe to do throughout pregnancy.

However, avoid Twists and poses that put direct pressure on the abdomen. Ensure there is adequate space in the lower abdomen by taking a wider stance in narrow poses, and not practicing any poses where one or both legs cross the body's mid line.

Do not jump during Vinyasas or into and out of Standing Poses. Do not practice *Virabhadrasana B* after the second trimester; practice *Parsvakonasana* instead.

In long-held poses, do not tolerate any degree of numbness or tingling — *Exit* of the pose carefully, but immediately.

Vertigo — support the head when supine so that the forehead slopes downward and the cervical arteries are not compressed. In more extreme cases, avoid all unsupported lying down poses, partial and full Inversions, and in Standing Poses, do the supported variations for additional balance.

Avoid poses that create extreme positions in the head, whether extreme flexion, extension, or twisting. Be careful not to create neck extension when turning the head, even in mild degrees. Use care when using props.

❀ *For more severe or complex health concerns and conditions, consult your doctor and a yoga therapist before embarking on a personal practice. Most poses at the Simplify stage will not be harmful, but use good and reasonable judgment when practicing these poses.*

Other general precautions include:

Not practicing when sick or recovering from illness — especially if accompanied by fever. Restorative and mild supported poses may be practiced when recovering, but save active practice for when you are fully recovered.

Not eating or drinking immediately before or during practice. The usual recommendation is not to eat for 2 hours before practice, and to not consume liquids for an hour before practice. When this is not possible, try not to eat for at least an hour before practice, and do not drink liquids, even water, during practice. There is a common trend of sipping water throughout practice, but is better advised to hydrate well before and after practice, so as not to divert digestive energy from the organs of action. Eating after practice can be done nearly immediately, but do not eat heavily until at least an hour or so after practice.

Practice in a comfortable temperature, neither too hot or too cold. An excessively heated room can cause dehydration, heat stress, higher blood pressure, and aggravate the nervous system, as well as reducing sensitivity to potential injury, thereby increasing risk. Similarly, practicing in a room that is too cold can reduce circulation, cause unnecessary tension, and also increase susceptibility to injury.

Reduce distractions at home, by turning off electronic and communication devices, and dedicating a space specifically for practice, even if only for the time you will be practicing.

Try to practice around the same time of day, for the same amount of time each session. This may not always be possible, but the body and mind respond well to regularity, so keep that in mind when practicing irregularly.

Practice invigorating poses if your practice is earlier in the day, and calming, Restorative poses if later in the day. Try not to practice too late in the evening, usually not past 11pm. Different practitioners are affected by practice differently, but even calming poses may be too stimulating if practiced at the very end of the day, causing restless sleep. Practicing too late can also cause a reactionary tightness, leading to greater stiffness upon waking. Morning practice tends to have the opposite effect.

When it's appropriate to challenge yourself, work near the edge between comfort and discomfort, but not past that edge. Explore your relationship with both challenge and discomfort, and sincerely consider what is best for your body, not your desires for achievement. Watch with patience and sensitivity, as this relationship changes over time, your capacity for sensation increases, and as you develop a deeper relationship with yourself.

Enjoy your practice and honor your body — it is a wonderful exploration!

Learn + Practice

Learn early, before Standing Poses, Back Bends, and Inversions

Linked Poses

All poses, particularly neutral and extended-leg poses, Standing Poses and Inversions

Safety Factors

Lower back strain, vertigo; practice over lengthwise bolster if pregnant, 1 l

Prepare

- Set the mat's short end to wall
- Place folded blanket at the head end of mat
- Have a block and 2 straps nearby

Enter

- Sit facing the wall with legs extended, feet against wall, 1 a
- Manually internally rotate thighs
- Place a block narrow and lengthwise between the thighs, close to the perineum, 1 b
- Ensure block does not make contact with the inner knees
- Tie strap around thighs at greater trochanters and lower thighs, 2-3" above knees, 1 c
- Tighten straps such that they help maintain internal rotation
- Pressure from both straps should be equal
- Ensure buckles are not contacting the thigh flesh
- Keeping feet against the wall, bend legs slightly and move pelvis 1-2" closer to wall, 1 d
- Lie back on hands, lowering the torso to the floor, 1 e
- Pressing feet into wall, fully extend legs while lying down
- Rest arms 30-45° beside torso, palms upturned, 1 f

Sustain

- Extend legs evenly away from the back pelvis
- Equalize pressure through both feet into wall
- Push into wall through all 4 corners of each foot, 1 g
- With foot pressure constant, symmetrically squeeze block between both thighs, 1 h
- Roll upper inner thighs toward floor, slightly internally rotating
- Keeping block pressure, resist heels and greater trochanters laterally away from each other, 1 i
- Release front thighs away from strap pressure and descend back thighs into straps
- Rest back ribs toward floor
- Without narrowing the space between the shoulder blades, descend shoulders into floor
- Soften the abdomen and breathe freely

Exit

- Bend the legs, bringing feet flat to the floor, 1 j
- Remove block and loosen straps
- Exhaling, roll to the right
- Press into hands, coming up from the side to seated, 1 k
- Remove straps and sit upright

Challenge

1. Feet lose contact with wall
2. Legs externally rotate
3. Lower back discomfort or compression
4. Lying supine contraindicated due to pregnancy or vertigo

Response

1. Move pelvis closer to wall before lying down. Push wall away from pelvis, rather than pushing pelvis away from feet.
2. Grip upper thighs more firmly, catching thigh bones when internally rotating thighs before tightening straps. Tie straps so that they pull the fronts of both thighs toward each other in slight internal rotation. Maintain foot placement with mid lines parallel.
3. After lying down, bend legs and move buttocks closer to the wall. Use the mat's traction to drag buttocks away from back ribs when re-extending legs.
4. Lie back over a bolster, 1 l, elevating torso so that the head and heart are above pelvis. Support head well so that it does not tilt back. Set bolster 4-6" away from back pelvis.

Tadasana is the root of all Standing Poses. The wall simulates the floor and teaches pushing action. Practicing this pose supine reduces joint compression and differentiates leg extension from weight distribution, creating symmetrical action in the feet, legs, pelvis, and trunk.

Contact Points

Feet, back pelvis, back ribs, shoulder blades, back of skull

External Supports

Mat, block, 2 straps, blanket
Additional blanket, bolster

Essence of Form

Leg and spine extension; legs slightly internally rotated, arms passively external

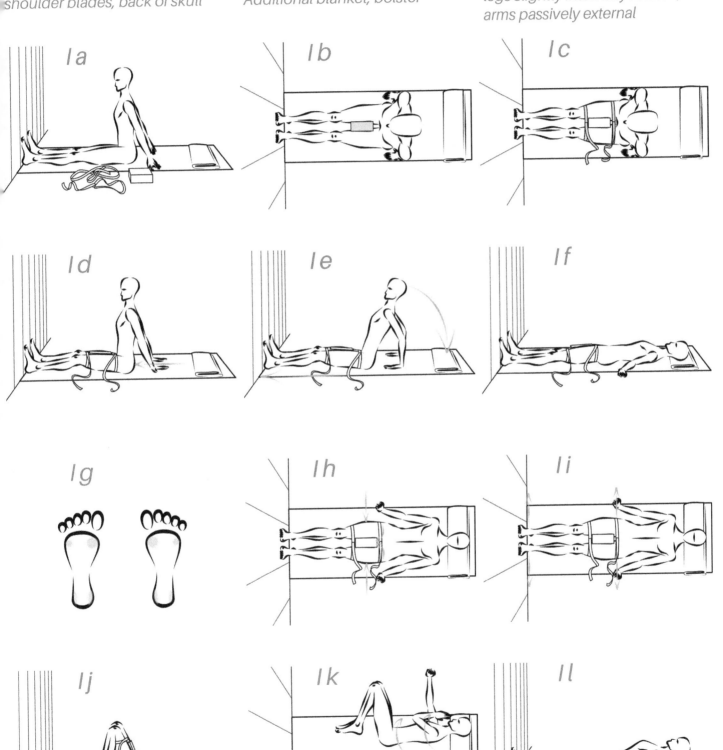

Learn + Practice

In conjunction Simplify, before Standing Poses, Back Bends, and Inversions

Linked Poses

All poses, particularly neutral and extended-leg poses, Standing Poses and Inversions

Safety Factors

Lower back strain, vertigo; Use care with pelvic and abdominal pathologies

Prepare

- Mat away from wall, with room to extend legs
- Place folded blanket on mat to support head

Enter

- Lie down on mat, with legs bent and feet flat on floor, feet and thighs parallel, hip-width apart
- Have a neutral lumbar spine, L4 + L5 lifting away from floor
- Place hands on lower abdomen, between front hip bones and above the pubis, *II a*
- Without using force, soften abdomen and receive hand pressure into abdomen
- Feel changes in tone throughout breath cycle
- Exhaling through the mouth, observe lower abdomen tone under hand contact near the end of exhalation, *II b*
- This is the lower transverse abdominus
- Use this engagement to gather front hip bones toward each other with 10-20% effort, *II c*
- Extend legs and repeat, *II d*
- Without lifting legs, resist heels upward to find lower transverse abdominus, *II e*

Sustain

- Maintain lower transverse abdominal engagement at 10-20% of maximum effort
- Gathering front iliums, resist heels laterally, creating similar action as in *Simplify*
- Keeping tone between and below front iliums, soften middle and upper abdomen
- If tone can be kept in the lower transverse abdominus, breathe naturally through nose and relax the lips and mouth
- Soften pubis skin inward
- Draw the posterior pubis gently toward the rib cage
- Maintain leg and pelvis actions from *Simplify* when legs are extended, pushing 4 corners of feet away from back pelvis
- Neutralize leg rotation, upper inner thighs descending slightly more than outer thighs

Exit

- Engage lower transverse abdominus for 5-10 breaths, gradually increasing hold as capacity allows
- Bend the legs and roll to the right
- Pressing into the hands come to seated

Challenge

1. Difficulty finding and engaging lower transverse abdominus
2. Over-engagement of rectus abdominus once found
3. Lower back pain

Response

1. Exhale through pursed lips. Visualize gathering front iliums as though tying a pants drawstring. Have a partner press downward at ankles or apply weight to tibias when resisting heels upward, *II f*. Legs should not lift; abdominals engage in preparation for lift.
2. Try not to literally move the iliums. Instead, only think of making the movement which will minimally engage the lower transverse abdominals.
3. Press lower back into the floor when legs are bent. Alternately, find lower multifidi: keeping lower transverse abdominals engaged, create similar action with the back iliums, using even less effort. Visualize gathering the back iliums, without actually moving them. The lower multifidi will engage, stabilizing the sacrum and lumbar spine.

Once Tadasana's root leg actions are learned supine, engaging the transverse abdominals help stabilize the pose before standing. Like much of Tadasana, the transverse abdominal actions are applicable to most poses.

Contact Points

Feet, back pelvis, back ribs, shoulder blades, back of skull

External Supports

Mat, blanket
Assistant or weight

Essence of Form

Lower transverse abdominal activation, hip and knee flexion, followed by leg extension

II a

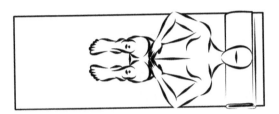

II b

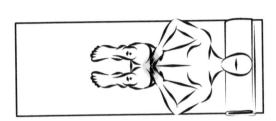

II c

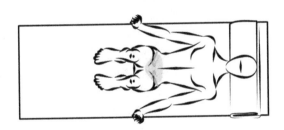

II d

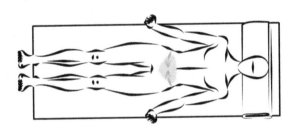

II e

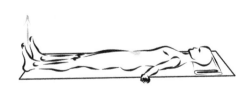

II f

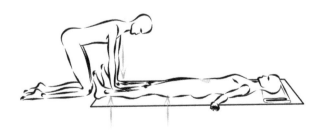

Learn + Practice

Once leg, pelvis, and lower abdominal actions from Explore are integrated

Linked Poses

All poses, but particularly Standing Poses, Back Bends, and Inversions

Safety Factors

As for Explore, be cautious of leg hyperextension

Prepare

· Set mat's short end to wall, with a block and 2 straps nearby

Enter

· Place block between thighs
· Tie two straps as for *Simplify*, one strap at greater trochanters, 2nd just above knees
· Stand with back to wall, heels 1-3" from it, *III a*
· Ensure foot mid lines are parallel
· Engage leg and pelvis actions from *Simplify + Explore*
· Keep pubis and front iliums vertical
· Make contact with buttocks, back ribs, and shoulder blades against wall
· Provided there is no neck strain, keep chin level and rest back of skull against wall
· Rest arms at sides
· Once clear, gradually bring heels to wall, *III b*

🕉 *To deepen femur actions, Enter with block between wall and heels, another block behind upper femurs, below gluteal fold. Press the femurs back while holding the block to wall, III c*

Sustain

· Pushing 4 corners of feet away from back pelvis, squeeze block symmetrically
· Squeezing block, gather front iliums and resist heels laterally, pressing thighs into straps, *III d*
· Soften pubis skin in and up, *III e*
· Anchoring big toe mounds, lift inner arches
· Keeping inner arch lift, draw outer tibias inward
· Engage quadriceps, lifting kneecaps, *III f*
· Press upper femurs back toward wall, *III g*
· Without tucking, descend back pelvis and lift back ribs away from back pelvis, *III h-i*
· Broaden collarbones away from sternum, *III j*
· Hang arms freely from shoulders
· Breathe naturally

Exit

· Come away from wall and rest
· Repeat with heels closer to or against wall
· Remove block and loosen straps
· Can be done without block and straps once *Sustain* actions are integrated

Challenge

1. Inner arch or ankle collapse
2. Knee pain
3. Lumbar discomfort
4. Neck pain

Response

1. Lift inner ankles and roll them toward outer ankles. Place additional block between inner ankles. Lift inner ankles up and draw outer ankles in. Strap big toes together and resist outward.
2. Do not let knees roll in or out. If hyperextending, resist upper tibias forward. Strap around upper tibias to prevent outward roll. *See Response 1.*
3. Widen stance and turn legs slightly inward, outer edges of feet parallel to mat's edge. Strap front iliums toward each other. Practice with block in sacrum, feet a block's distance from wall, *III k.* Lift back ribs away from back pelvis. *See Responses 1 + 2.*
4. Head does not need to touch wall. Extend occiput upward, gently descend chin. Use a foam block to support behind head and provide contact, *III l.*

Standing alert, steady, and balanced is foundational to all Standing Poses. Tadasana establishes a firm and grounded base by teaching foot, leg, pelvis, and trunk actions that foster physical stability and mental stillness.

Contact Points

Feet, back pelvis, back ribs, shoulder blades; back of heels, posterior upper femurs (III c)

External Supports

Wall, block, 2 straps
Additional blocks, strap, foam block

Essence of Form

Leg and trunk extension, posterior femur glide and isometric abduction; arms and legs neutrally rotating

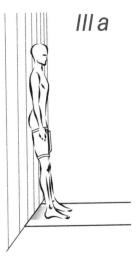

III a

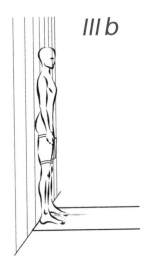

III b

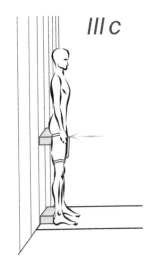

III c

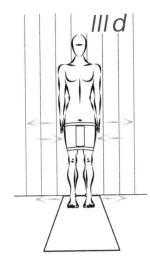

III d

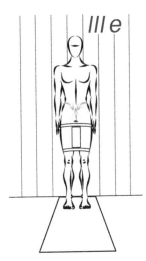

III e

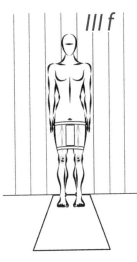

III f

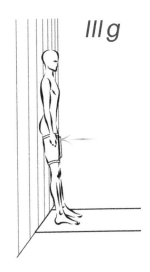

III g

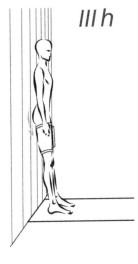

III h

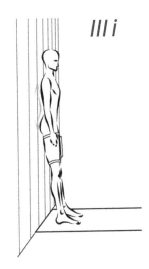

III i

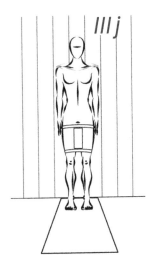

III j

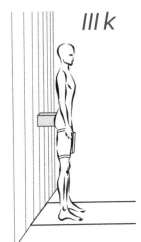

III k

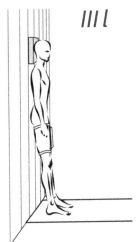

IIl l

Tadasana Samasthiti
Equal Standing

Synthesize

Prepare

- Away from wall, with or without mat

Enter

- Stand with foot mid lines parallel, hip-width apart
- Place hands on hips, middle and ring fingers pressing into front groins, *IV a*
- Feel degree of groin tension under finger contact
- Bend legs slightly, softening and receding front groins, *IV b*
- With legs bent, tilt pelvis until pubis and front iliums align vertically, *IV c*
- Keeping front pelvis vertical, maintain groin softness and move femurs backward, pushing feet away from back pelvis to extend legs, *IV d*
- Once legs are fully extended, keep pelvis vertical with groins soft and release hands to sides
- Vertically stack joint centers — from side: ankle, knee, femur head, hip crest, bottom ribs, shoulder, ear; from front: foot mid line, ankle center, tibia head, thigh center, hip point; pubis, navel, sternum, throat, chin, nose, *IV e-f*

Sustain

- Engage leg, pelvis, and lower transverse abdominus actions from *Simplify*, *Explore*, + *Nourish*
- Keeping front pelvis vertical, press upper femurs back and resist upper tibias forward
- Extend inner legs from groins to big toe mounds
- Drawing outer ankles inward, circularly lift inner ankles toward outer ankles
- Centralize Achilles tendons in each lower leg
- Internally rotate upper femurs and simultaneously externally rotate lower femurs slightly, balancing knee ligaments
- Without bending legs, soften knee pits inward
- Pressing femurs backward, soften sternum inward and lift upper outer chest
- Stacking joint centers vertically, bring diaphragm planes level with floor from front-to-back and side-to-side

Exit

- *Sustain* for between 30 seconds and 3 minutes
- Continue to other poses or rest and repeat

Challenge

1. Uneven weight distribution
2. Hip joint compression
3. Neck and shoulder tension, leg integration lost

Response

1. Differentiate weight from pressure: without lifting left foot, shift weight to right leg and foot. Keeping weight on the right foot, extend left leg out of pelvis, increasing left foot pressure, *IV g*. Repeat, shifting to the left. Return to neutral and balance pushing action through both legs.
2. Stand on a block with pelvis level, hanging the compressed hip's leg, *IV g*. If compression is bilateral, hang left leg first, then right. If unilateral, hang compressed femur first.
3. Practice with shoulder jacket. Pass arms through loop, *IV h*. Add a second strap and hitch to slant board at foot end, *IV i*. Tighten straps with legs bent, then push feet into board to fully extend legs, lifting spine out of shoulder traction, *IV j*. If straps fall off shoulders, twist strap, *IV k*.

Standing equally is often taken for granted. Differences in front and back body ...ction weight distribution, and leg length can all limit the evenness of stance. ...Tadasana Samasthiti balances and neutralizes how the body manages gravitational forces.

Contact Points

Feet
Hands contact the front ...liums and front groins

External Supports

Mat (optional)
Wall (if using for balance)
Block, 2 straps, slant board

Essence of Form

Leg extension, trunk length; legs neutral toward internal rotation, arms neutral

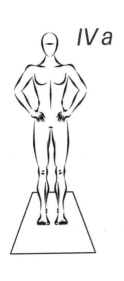
IV a

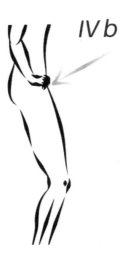
IV b

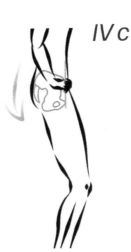
IV c

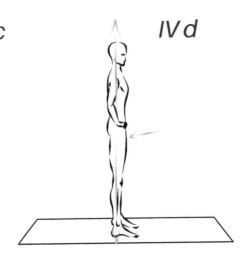
IV d

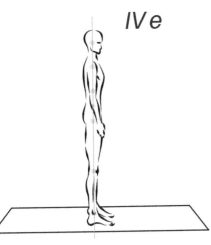
IV e

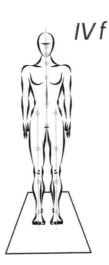
IV f

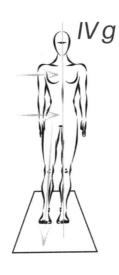
IV g

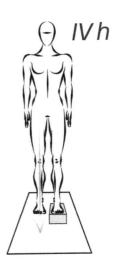
IV h

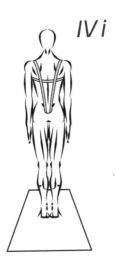
IV i

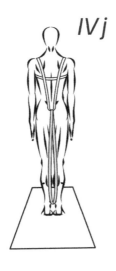
IV j

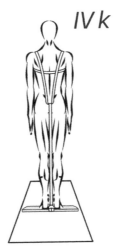
IV k

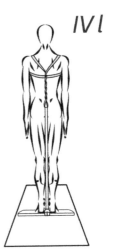
IV l

Learn + Practice

Learn in conjunction with Standing Poses and before Back Bends and Inversions

Linked Poses

Back Bends, Inversions, and raised-arm Forward Bends. Also a Pranayama preparation

Safety Factors

Lower back strain, neck and shoulder injury or restriction May raise blood pressure

Prepare

- Set mat away from wall, with room to extend arms overhead

Enter

- Lie on back, legs bent, feet hip width apart, *I a*
- Establish neutral spinal curves
- Soften hip creases, letting femurs fall into pelvis and away from front iliums
- Evenly descend back pelvis
- Gather front iliums, soften pubis in and up (*Supta Tadasana, Explore*)
- Without flattening lumbar spine, heavily descend bottom back ribs, *I b*
- Extend arms beside pelvis, palms facing downward, *I c*
- Widen between the shoulder blades
- Lengthen inner shoulder blades toward the pelvis
- With arms shoulder-width apart, exhale and raise extended arms toward ceiling, *I d*
- Pin upper outer shoulder blades to floor
- If lost, reset back rib contact
- Keeping back rib contact, exhale and continue moving arms overhead toward floor, *I e*
- Fully lengthen arms throughout

Sustain

- Settle both feet equally
- Pelvis neutral and level, lift L4 + L5 away from floor
- Continuously descend back bottom ribs toward the floor
- Widen the back ribs away from spine
- Extend the bottom ribs and top hip crests away from each other
- Lengthen side body from hips to armpits
- Retract humerus heads into shoulder joints
- Extend backs of arms from shoulder blades to fingertips
- Move arms symmetrically and minimize twisting
- Ensure forehead skin descends toward nose
- Soften the face, throat, and back of neck

Exit

- Hold 10-15 breaths
- Lower the arms and roll to the right
- Press up from the side to sitting

🕉 *Can also be done in movement, exhaling to raise arms, inhaling to lower, 10-30 times*

Challenge

1. Hands do not reach the floor overhead
2. Elbows bend
3. Rotator cuff injury, frozen shoulder
4. Bottom back ribs lift as arms extend
5. Head falls back, throat tension

Response

1. Place bolster laterally to rest back of wrists on, *I f.* Extend backs of arms fully, lengthening from back ribs to fingertips.
2. Tie a strap the elbows and resist wrists outward, *I g. See also Response 1.*
3. Bring arms 45° to the side before raising vertically. Gradually reduce angle. Sweep arms through the lateral plane. *I h.*
4. Place sandbag on lower ribs or *Prepare* with sandbags on floor beyond head at arm's length. Lifting pelvis, slide hands under sandbags. With hands stabilized, lower pelvis and lengthen back ribs and pelvis away from hands, *I i-k.*
5. Support head with folded blanket(s).

Urdhva Hastasana increases shoulder mobility and circulation to the neck and shoulders. Practicing it supine with legs bent isolates the shoulder and makes the movements clearer. It also opens the lungs and ribcage, freeing the breath — especially when raising on exhalation.

Contact Points

Feet, back pelvis, back ribs, shoulder blades, back of skull

External Supports

Mat
Blanket, block, strap, bolster, sandbags

Essence of Form

Arm and shoulder extension, hip and knee flexion; upper arms externally rotated, lower arms internal

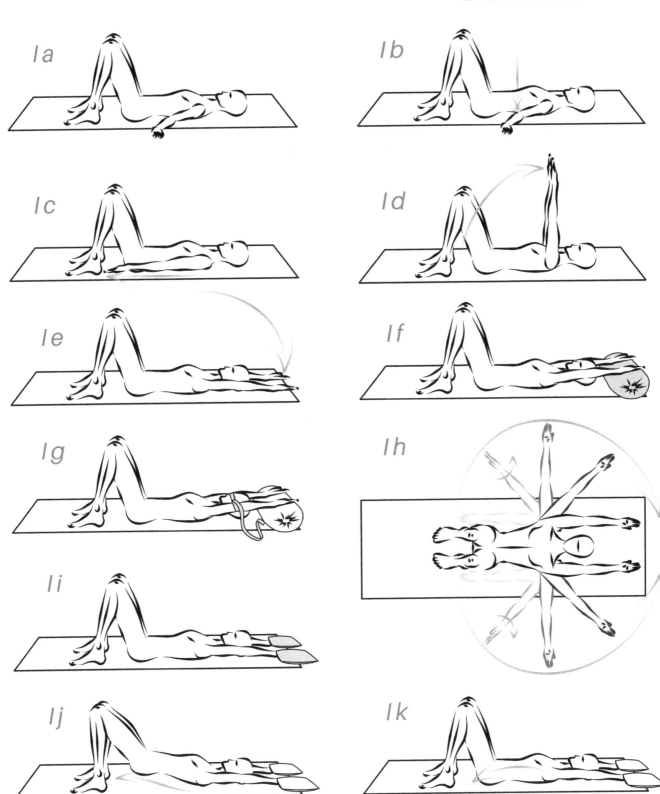

I a

I b

I c

I d

I e

I f

I g

I h

I i

I j

I k

Learn + Practice

Once Simplify is learned well, and arms fully extend with neutral lumbar

Linked Poses

Back Bends and Inversions, particularly raised-arm poses, preparation for Pranayama

Safety Factors

Lower back strain, neck and shoulder injury May raise blood pressure

Prepare

- Mat's short end to wall
- Place a folded blanket at head end, have a second blanket handy

Enter

- Sit facing the wall, legs extended, feet pushing into the wall, *II a*
- Set 2nd blanket behind mid-upper thighs, *II b*
- Strap the thighs at greater trochanters, *II c*
- Pressing into hands, bend the legs and lift the pelvis, scooting it 2-3" closer to wall, *II d*
- Leaning back on hands, lie down on mat, *II e*
- Extend legs away from back pelvis, pressing heels and big toe mounds deeply into wall, *II f*
- Have foot mid lines parallel, whether feet are hip-width or with inner big toes touching
- Press back thighs into blanket and resist laterally into strap
- Ensure L4 + L5 are lifting away from floor
- Rest head on blanket, adjust if necessary to ensure forehead slopes toward nose
- Rest hands beside pelvis with palms upturned

Sustain

- Fully extend legs and resist heels laterally, widening greater trochanters into strap
- Minimally engage lower transverse abdominus by resisting heels toward ceiling and gathering front iliums, *II g*
- Soften pubis skin inward and away from wall
- Without rotating knees inward, descend inner groins and widen inner back femurs
- Pressing into big toe mounds, broaden soles of feet
- With neutral lumbar, descend bottom back ribs
- Maintain leg and torso actions from *Simplify*
- Repeat *Simplify* instructions to raise arms to *Urdhva Hastasana II h*
- Soften neck, throat, and sense organs

Exit

- Hold 5-10 breaths
- Inhaling, raise arms to vertical, then lower them beside pelvis, palms upturned
- Bend the legs and roll to the right
- Pressing into the hands come to seated

Challenge

1. Heel/wall pressure is lost
2. Leg hyperextension
3. Neck tension and shoulder restrictions

Response

1. Initiate arm movement by pushing heels more deeply away from back pelvis before raising arms. Lengthen back body more fully.
2. Resist tibia heads upward as upper femurs descend into blanket. Place a third blanket behind upper calves in *Prepare* to stop the upper tibias from descending.
3. *See Responses 1 through 4* in *Simplify*. Ensure the skull is not actively pressing backward as arms rise. Practice with hands to wall, fingers turned out to the sides, hands 6-12" above wall/floor juncture. Begin with legs and arms bent, hands pushing firmly into the wall, *II i*. Gradually extend the arms, then legs *II j*. As capacity increases, bring hands lower toward wall/floor juncture, *II k*. Maintain external arm rotation and turn fingertips to face floor, *II l*.

Where Supta Tadasana balances leg, pelvis, and trunk actions and Urdhva Hastasana aids neck, shoulder and arm function, practicing them together can help correct minor misalignments from head to toe.

Contact Points

Feet, back pelvis, back ribcage, shoulder blades, back of skull

External Supports

Wall, mat, 2 folded blankets, strap, additional blanket

Essence of Form

Leg and arm extension, legs neutral, upper arms external, lower arms internal

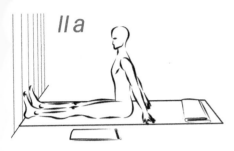

II a

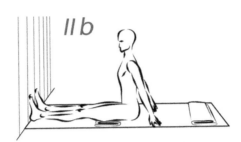

II b

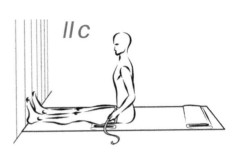

II c

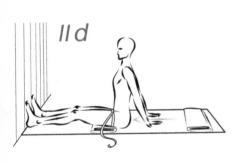

II d

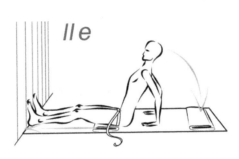

II e

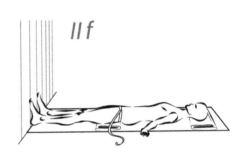

II f

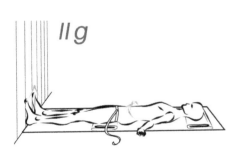

II g

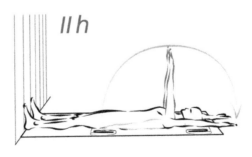

II h

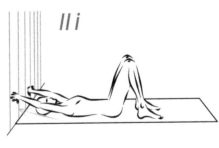

II i

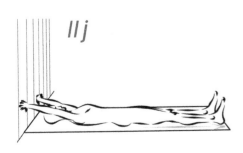

II j

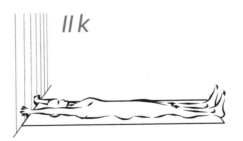

II k

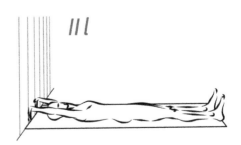

II l

Tadasana Urdhva Hastasana
Mountain Pose with Raised Arms

Nourish

Learn + Practice

Once leg, pelvis, and lower abdominal actions from Explore are integrated

Linked Poses

All poses, but particularly Standing Poses, Back Bends, and Inversions

Safety Factors

As for Explore, do not raise arms overhead if hypertense, be cautious of leg hyperextension

Prepare

- Stand 2-3" from wall with feet hip-width apart, foot mid lines parallel
- Rest back pelvis, back ribs, and shoulder blades on wall, *III a*

Enter

- Fully extend legs, pressing 4 corners of the feet away from back pelvis, into the floor
- Bring pubis and front iliums to vertical
- Engage leg and pelvis actions from *Explore*
- With L4 + L5 moving inward, round forward to move bottom back ribs to wall, *III b*
- Keeping bottom back rib contact, lift collar bones vertically to come upright, *III c*
- Broaden collarbones away from sternum
- Without losing back rib contact, push into feet and raise arms to shoulder level, *III d*
- Retract humerus heads
- Draw bottom shoulder blade tips toward each other and widen upper shoulder blades
- Exhaling, continue arm movement as for *Explore*, raising arms to vertical, *III e*

Sustain

- Engage actions from *Explore*
- Firming thighs, press upper femurs back and upper tibias forward
- Resisting heels laterally, draw lower inner femurs medially
- Lengthen arms from the sides of the trunk to fingertips
- Roll the outer armpits forward while softening and deepening the inner armpits
- Keep arms fully extended throughout
- Lift chest forward away from pubis
- Head neutral, chin neither lifted nor tucked

Exit

- Without losing length from hips to armpits, descend arms beside pelvis
- Keeping side torso length, stay up to an additional minute
- Come away from wall and rest
- Repeat, setting feet closer to wall in *Enter*
- Once heels touch wall, progressively bring feet closer together until inner big toes touch in *Enter*

Challenge

1. Lumbar pain on raising arms
2. Arms widen beyond shoulder width, elbows bend or hyperextend
3. Shoulder compression, neck tension

Response

1. Step feet further away from wall. Keep bottom back rib contact with wall. *See also Response 3.*
2. Strap arms, just above elbows. Only raise arms until just before they cannot remain straight. For hyperextension, resist outward into strap.
3. Practice wall stretch:
- Face the wall, toes 6-8" away from it, *III f*
- Reach hands up wall, arms fully extended and hands shoulder-width apart, *III g*
- Rest forehead on wall, skin sliding toward nose
- Pressing hands into wall, push heels into floor away from back pelvis and bottom ribs, *III h*
- For greater traction, raise heels 1-2" and walk hands also 1-2" up wall, *III i*
- Keeping hands at new height, lower heels, *III j*

In addition to increasing neck and shoulder mobility + circulation, precise articulation of the shoulder and rib cage can reduce kyphosis, reducing tension along the spine's entire length. This may also have a positive effect on breath and thoraco-abdominal organ function.

Contact Points

Feet, back pelvis, back ribs, shoulder blades, Hands (Response 3, III g-j)

External Supports

Wall, mat, Strap

Essence of Form

Arm and leg extension, shoulder flexion, lower thoracic flexion, upper thoracic extension

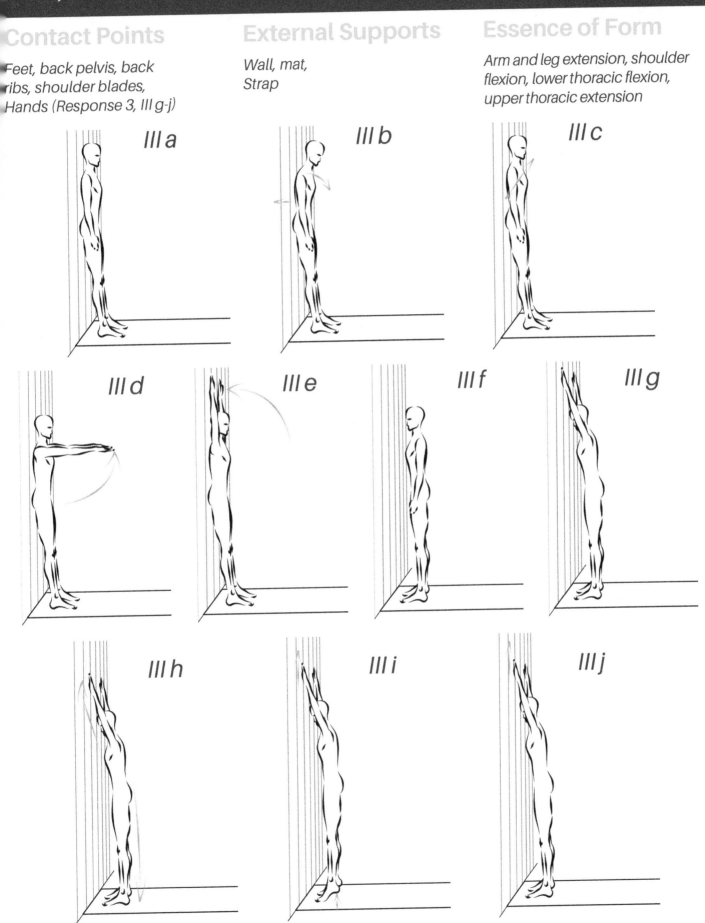

III a

III b

III c

III d

III e

III f

III g

III h

III i

III j

Tadasana Urdhva Hastasana
Mountain Pose with Raised Arms

Synthesize

Learn + Practice

Before Standing Poses and Back Bends, once Nourish is learned well

Linked Poses

All poses, but particularly Standing Poses, Back Bends, and Inversions

Safety Factors

As for Simplify, Explore, and Nourish; do not raise arms overhead if hypertense

Prepare

- Stand with feet hip-width apart or inner big toes touching, foot mid lines parallel

Enter

- Push feet away from back pelvis, pressing upper femurs backward
- Gather front iliums and resist heels laterally, engaging transverse abdominus ≤ 20%
- Soften pubis in and upward
- Neutralize pelvis, front plane vertical and iliums level
- Drawing front ribs inward, lift bottom back ribs
- Keeping femurs pressing back and without protruding front ribs, raise arms vertically, *IV a*

Sustain

- Extend inner groins from pubis to big toe mounds, abducting big toes, *IV b*
- Spread toes and equalize pressure through all 4 corners of each foot

Sustain

- Circularly roll inner ankles toward outer ankles, lifting inner arches, *IV c*
- Resist upper tibias forward
- Press inner upper femurs backward
- Keeping upper inner femurs back, press outer lower femurs backward as well, *IV d*
- Lift the pelvis up away from femur heads
- Lengthen the side torso symmetrically from hips to armpits, *IV e*
- Extending the arms fully, roll outer armpits forward and deepen shoulder creases back
- Descend the bottom sternum and lengthen the upper sternum, *IV f*
- Extend collarbones away from sternum, *IV g*
- Broaden upper shoulder blades and narrow lower shoulder blades, *IV h*

Exit

- Hold for 10-30 breaths
- Keeping torso length, lower arms to sides
- Stay in *Tadasana* a few breaths, then release

Challenge

1. Elbows roll outward
2. Femurs collapse forward
3. Leg and spinal deviations not addressed in *Explore* or *Nourish*

Response

1. Hold block between wrists, strap elbows to gather them, *IV i*.
2. Practice with back to wall, one block between heels and wall, second block behind upper back thighs, under gluteal fold. Without hyperextending knees, press upper femurs backward as arms lift. Do not drop block from behind femurs. Keep back ribs lifted and voluminous, keeping shoulders and back ribs from resting on wall, *IV j*.
3. Practice with back mid line against outer corner where two walls meet, *IV k*. Place a tightly rolled mat between the thighs and bind the legs firmly with 6 straps: 3 around upper leg from greater trochanter to just above knees, 3 around lower leg from top of tibia to ankles, *IV l*. Establish and equalize leg and spine actions before raising arms. Maintain symmetry as arms lift.

Standing evenly on both feet while raising the arms balances both resistance and cooperation with gravity. Full vertical extension from feet to fingertips reduces misalignments as downward and upward forces are opposed.

Contact Points

Feet
Forearms and elbows (IV i), heels and femurs (IV j), legs (IV l)

External Supports

Mat
2 straps, 2 blocks, rolled mat, wall, outer corner

Essence of Form

Arm and leg extension, shoulder flexion, lower thoracic flexion, upper thoracic extension

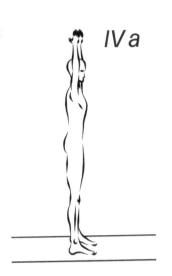
IV a

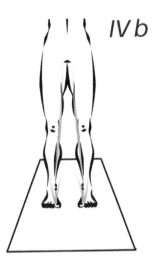
IV b

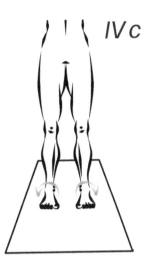
IV c

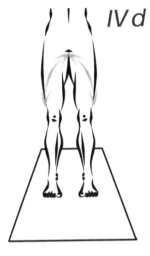
IV d

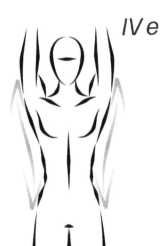
IV e

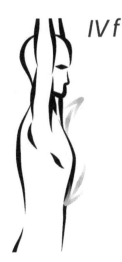
IV f

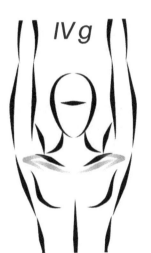
IV g

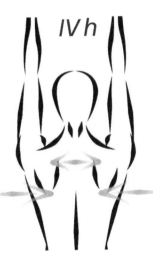
IV h

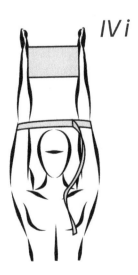
IV i

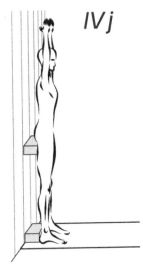
IV j

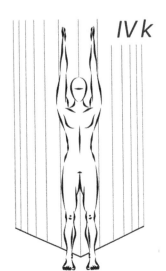
IV k

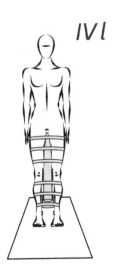
IV l

Mountain Pose with Raised Arms — *Synthesize*

Learn + Practice

Learn early, practice at start of sequences where hip flexion or spinal release is required

Linked Poses

All poses with hip flexion, Forward Bends, Standing Poses, and hip-opening poses

Safety Factors

Use care with knee pain, foot or ankle pain, hip injuries, and posterior disc herniation

Prepare

- Mat's short end to wall
- Set chair on mat, chair back against wall

Enter

- Kneel in front of chair, *I a*
- Rest buttocks on heels
- Have the feet together with big toes touching
- Keeping big toes together, separate legs so that knees are mat-width apart, *I b*
- If buttocks do not easily reach heels, use folded blankets or a bolster between heels and buttocks so that sitting bones settle, *I c*
- Lift one knee and manually drag skin forward and out from under knee, repeat adjustment on second side
- Press hands into thighs and descend femurs
- Gather front iliums and soften pubis in and up
- Keeping buttocks and femurs descending, lift pelvis up and over femurs, exhaling to fold torso forward, *I d*
- Extending arms, catch chair back with hands
- Rest forehead on chair seat, *I e*

Sustain

- Spread toes and draw outer ankles inward
- Release buttock flesh toward heels and away from mid line, *I f*
- Descend inner thighs and outer buttocks
- Soften and deepen inner groins
- Gently draw lower femurs toward each other, broaden upper femurs away from each other
- Lengthen side torso, lifting ribcage off pelvis
- Slide forehead skin down face toward nose
- Release throat and jaw
- Soften abdomen and breathe freely

Exit

- Release hands from chair, press hands into floor or chair seat, *I g*
- Pushing into hands, inhale and lift to seated
- Lift knees and draw them toward each other
- Press to standing, or place hands to floor and extend legs back one at a time, *I h*
- Exhaling, press hands into chair seat and step legs back to *Adho Mukha Svanasana, I i*

Challenge

1. Ankle discomfort
2. Knee pain
3. Front ribs collapse
4. Shoulder strain

Response

1. Drag front ankle skin laterally out form under foot and ankle before folding forward. *Enter* with rolled blanket under ankles or stack blankets under tibias, folded edges at ankle crease, feet hanging off, *I j-k.*
2. Support tibias as for *Response 1.* Place folded straps or rolled cloths behind knee joints to create space, *I l.* Elevate pelvis as in *I c.*
3. Place bolster on top of thighs laterally to support upper abdomen and lower ribs in *Enter, I m.* Press hands into bolster and lift torso over bolster while folding forward. Without moving chair, pull chair with hands to lift side ribs more fully.
4. Instead of catching chair back, catch chair sides or legs or rest hands on chair seat, *I n-o. See arm actions in Nourish.*

Calming and nourishing, this pose gently warms and creates space in the hips, groins, buttocks, and lower back. Extending the arms frees the breath and resting the head equalizes blood pressure. A chair ensures maximum torso extension without strain when the hips are restricted.

Contact Points

Tops of feet and tibias, buttocks, forehead, hands

External Supports

Mat, chair (against wall)
Blankets, bolster, rolled cloths

Essence of Form

Hip and knee flexion, leg abduction, arm and torso extension; external arm rotation

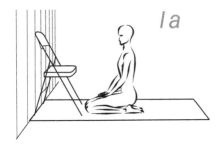
Ia

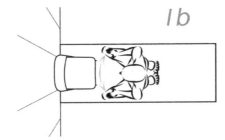
Ib

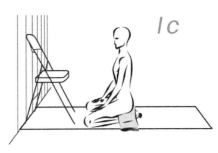
Ic

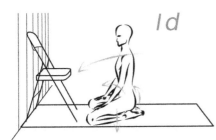
Id

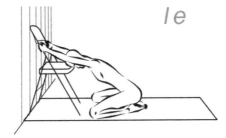
Ie

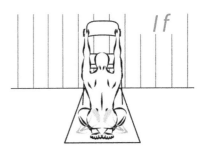
If

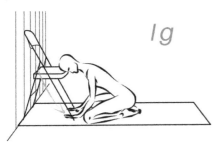
Ig

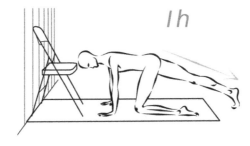
Ih

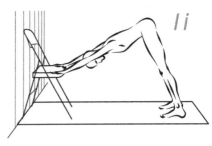
Ii

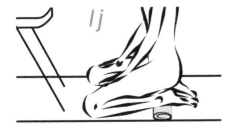
Ij

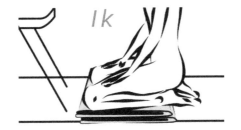
Ik

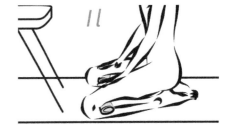
Il

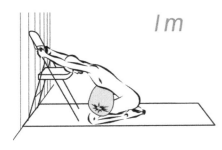
Im

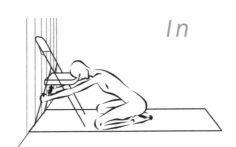
In

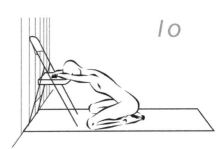
Io

Learn + Practice

Learn early, before Adho Mukha Svanasana; practice before and after Inversions

Linked Poses

Forward Bends and all hip flexion poses, Adho Mukha Svanasana, Inversions

Safety Factors

Same as Simplify, groin injury, be cautious when abdominal compression is contraindicated

Prepare

- Wall not required, mat can be against wall or not, depending on what pose(s) follow

Enter

- Kneeling on mat, sit on heels with big toes together and knees mat-width apart, *ll a*
- Manually adjust knee skin forward and top of ankle skin outward
- Descending femurs, gather front iliums and soften pubis skin inward and upward, *ll b*
- Place hands on floor between knees
- Pressing into hands, drag hands slightly backward to lift and lengthen side torso, *ll c*
- Inhaling, lift front iliums up and over femurs
- With femurs descending and front iliums lifting, exhale and walk hands forward, folding torso toward floor, *ll d*
- Fully extend arms with elbows and forearms lifting away from floor, *ll e*
- Rest forehead on floor, or support forehead on block or folded blanket, *ll f*

Sustain

- Descend buttocks and soften inner groins
- Laterally release lower back muscles
- Lengthen side torso and fully extend arms
- With arms extended, externally rotate arms from shoulder joint, rolling across outer hand and turning palms upward, *ll g*
- Roll outer armpits and upper outer arms toward floor as completely as possible
- Keeping external rotation at upper arms, slowly internally rotate forearms, bringing palms flat to floor, *ll h*
- Spread fingertips and descend index finger roots and base of thumbs

Exit

- Exhaling, walk hands under shoulders
- Pressing into hands, inhale and lift torso to seated, bringing the head up last
- Draw legs together
- Pressing into hands, extend legs back one at a time to open backs of knees

Challenge

1. Ankle or knee discomfort
2. Shoulder discomfort
3. Groins and/or buttocks bind
4. Lower back tension

Response

1. Fold mat to pad under knees and reduce pressure.
   See Responses from Simplify.
2. Increase head support and reduce forward fold to reduce armpit opening. Place hands wider than shoulders in *Enter*. Repeat *Sustain* actions. If external rotation cannot be maintained in upper arms, keep palms upturned.
3. Place sticks across upper femurs, *ll i.* Press sticks down and lift iliums up and over sticks when folding forward. Have an assistant press thumbs into upper groins before and while folding forward, *ll j.*
4. Weight back pelvis with sandbag, partially supported by blocks. Fold mat end or extra mat over pelvis for better traction, *ll k.* Have assistant press upper sacrum and mid-thoracic spine away from each other, *ll l.*

Uttana Balasana is an excellent start to active practice. It is soothing and settling, releases the lower back, and prepares the hips and shoulders for many typical yoga movements. Practice it to establish a calm state prior to or throughout your practice.

Contact Points

Tops of feet and tibias, buttocks, forehead, hands

External Supports

Mat, block, blanket
2 sticks, additional mat, sandbag, assistant

Essence of Form

Hip and knee flexion, leg abduction, arm and torso extension; external arm rotation

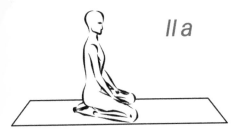

II a

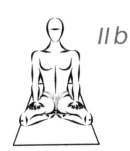

II b

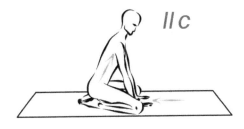

II c

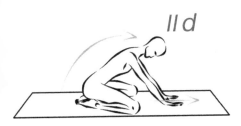

II d

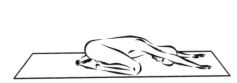

II e

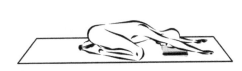

II f

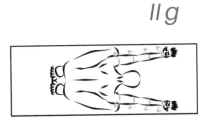

II g

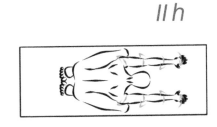

II h

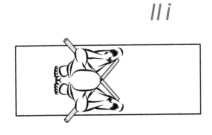

II i

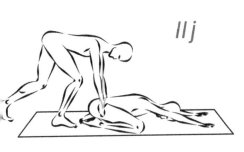

II j

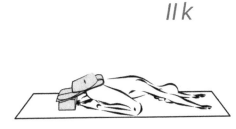

II k

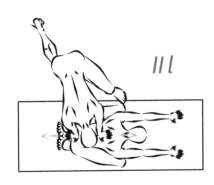

II l

Learn + Practice

Can be learned before or after Simplify + Nourish; practice at start or end of sequences

Linked Poses

Restorative Forward Bending poses, hip openers

Safety Factors

Avoid abdominal compression for cysts, endometriosis, ulcers, etc. and while pregnant

Prepare

- Set bolster lengthwise on mat, with folded blanket across head end

Enter

- Kneel on mat with big toes touching and knees mat width, bolster between thighs, *III a*
- Manually adjust knee skin forward and top of ankle skin outward
- Gather front iliums and soften pubis skin inward
- With pelvis heavy, lift front pelvis and lower abdomen, lengthening front torso, *III b*
- Keeping pelvic lift and torso length, lower torso to bolster
- Bolster should support mid to lower abdomen and front torso
- Avoid turning head, forehead supported on folded blanket
- Rest elbows and forearms on floor beside bolster, *III c*, or cross hands beyond head

ॐ *Set bolster further forward, supporting only chest and head if abdominal pressure is contraindicated, III d*

Sustain

- Descend back pelvis and release lower back and buttock muscles toward heels, away from mid line
- Soften and deepen inner groins
- Rest weight into bolster, keeping arms passive
- Receive bolster support into front torso, using pressure as feedback to indicate tension
- Breathing naturally, let breath shift toward back body as abdomen softens
- Broaden and lengthen back body with each inhalation, *III e*
- On exhalations, receive bolster more deeply into abdomen and front torso

Exit

- Exhaling, place hands under shoulders
- Pushing hands into floor, press to seated on inhalation and sit upright, *III f*
- Pressing hands to floor, extend legs back one at a time to release backs of knees
- Lift into *Adho Mukha Svanasana*, supporting head on bolster, *III g*

Challenge

1. Restricted forward bending capacity
2. Neck compression or tension
3. Shoulder strain
4. Diaphragm restriction

Response

1. Increase bolster height, either with folded blankets on top of bolster or blocks underneath bolster, *III h-i*. Angle bolster upward from pelvis to head rather than just increasing overall height.
2. Try not to turn head. Instead, place additional folded blanket under ribcage as well as forehead to change neck and head angle, *III j*.
3. Increase torso support to reduce armpit opening, *see Responses 1 + 2*. Bend elbows more and bring arms more laterally, *III k*.
4. Place rolled mat or blanket across bolster just below bottom sternum, near solar plexus. Adjust roll position in small increments until diaphragm pressure releases tension, *III l*.

Abdominal pressure encourages the breath to move into the back body and can be soothing. Supporting the torso maximizes the calming, nourishing, and settling aspects of this pose. Using head support so that is does not turn ensures this effect is complete.

Contact Points

Tops of feet and tibias, buttocks, front torso, forehead, forearms, hands

External Supports

Mat, bolster, blanket
Additional blankets, rolled mat, blocks

Essence of Form

Hip and knee flexion, leg abduction, arm and torso extension, abdominal compression

III a
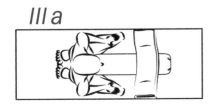

III b
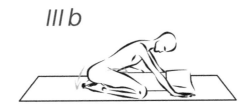

III c
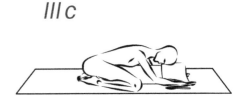

III d
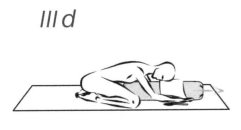

III e
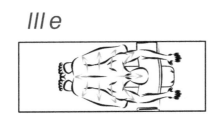

III f
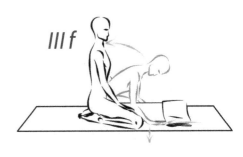

III g
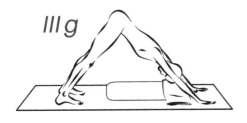

III h
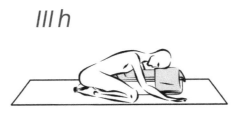

III i
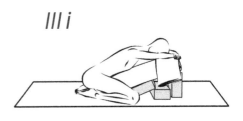

III j
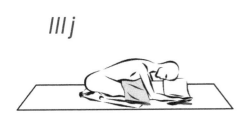

III k
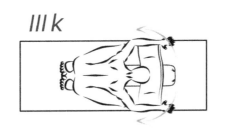

III l
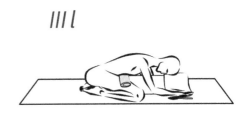

Parsva Uttana Balasana
Side-Bending Wide-Legged Child's Pose

Learn + Practice

Learn and practice before hip-opening poses, Twists, and Side Bends

Linked Poses

Lateral Standing Poses, Twists, Side Bends, and asymmetrical postures

Safety Factors

As for *Explore*, use caution with shoulder, elbow, or groin injury, abdominal pain

Prepare

· As for *Explore*

Enter

· As for *Explore*
· Keeping torso position, walk hands 1/2" closer toward body, bending elbows slightly, *IV a*
· With new hand position, push heavily into index finger and thumb mounds to re-extend arms, pressing groins further backward, *IV b*
· As groins deepen backward, descend buttock flesh more heavily

Sustain

· Continue *Sustain* actions from *Explore*
· Draw outer forearms inward, increasing pressure through index finger mounds
· With index finger mounds heavy, extend inner arms maximally, drawing shoulder creases away from index finger mounds, *IV c*
· Resist upper humeri away from each other

Sustain

· Broaden between shoulder blades and roll outer armpits toward floor, *IV d*
· Equalize side torso length, extending shorter feeling side without shortening longer side
· To further increase side torso length, walk hands and torso toward the right in a side bend, *IV e*
· Receive length along left side torso
· Pressing into right hand, extend right groin away from right hand to reduce right side compression (length will not be symmetrical)
· Walk hands and torso back to center and observe changes
· Repeat, side-bending to the left and pressing left groin away from left hand

Exit

· As for *Explore*
· Alternatively, keep hands forward and tuck toes, *IV f*
· Lifting torso minimally, press into hands and exhale to *Adho Mukha Svanasana*, and step feet further back, *IV g*

Challenge

1. Elbows bend or sag, index finger mounds lift
2. Elbow hyperextension
3. Shoulder compression
4. Front ribs collapse, armpit opening not felt

Response

1. Hold a block between forearms and squeeze inward, *IV h*. Squeezing action usually also lifts forearms and increases index finger mound pressure.
2. Strap around upper forearms, just below elbows, and resist outward, *IV i*.
3. *See Responses 1 + 2*. Strap upper humeri and resist outward, *IV j*. Without moving hands, engage a pulling action instead of pushing action to lift humeri away from armpits, *IV k*. Bring hands wider than shoulder width.
4. Pull hands toward torso as in *Response 3*. Elevate hands on blocks, *IV l*, and alternate between pushing and pulling actions, 5-10 breaths for each direction up to 3 times.

Parsva Uttana Balasana increases the torso length developed in Explore.
Lengthening the side torso unilaterally can more precisely address asymmetries.
Practice this variation in preparation for Side Bends and Twists.

Contact Points

Tops of feet and tibias,
buttocks, forehead, hands

External Supports

Mat
2 blocks, strap

Essence of Form

Leg and hip flexion, leg
abduction, arm and torso
extension, lateral torso extension

IV a
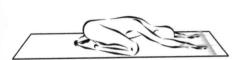

IV b
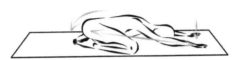

IV c
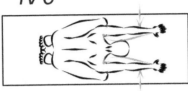

IV d
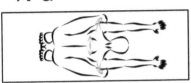

IV e
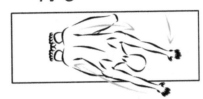

IV f
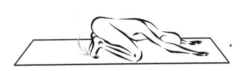

IV g
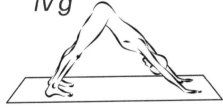

IV h
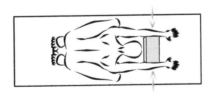

IV i
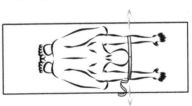

IV i
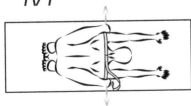

IV k
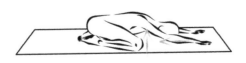

IV l
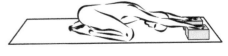

Supta Padangusthasana A
Lying Down Leg Stretch

Simplify

Learn + Practice

*Learn before Standing Poses.
Practice before Standing
Poses and Forward Bends*

Linked Poses

*Standing Poses, Forward
Bends, Supta Tadasana*

Safety Factors

*May aggravate some lower
back and hip injuries; do not
practice with hamstring injury*

Prepare

- Set the mat's short end to wall
- Have a strap nearby, within reach

Enter

- Lie in *Supta Tadasana, I a*
- Press 4 corners of the feet into the wall, away from back pelvis
- Create a neutral lumbar, lifting L4 + L5 off the floor
- Bend the left leg, bringing left foot to the floor, *I b*
- Keeping the lumbar curve, bend right leg, bringing it toward the chest, *I c*
- Loop belt inside the right leg, around the back of the heel, *I d*
- Keeping lumbar curve neutral, press front of right thigh away from torso, extending right leg on exhalation, *I e-f*
- Bring the leg no closer than 90° from torso
- Press elbows into floor, lengthening the belt if necessary

ॐ *Once learned well and provided there's no back pain, loop belt before raising leg. Keeping leg straight, lengthen out of back pelvis to lift leg I g-h.*

Sustain

- Draw the elbows toward each other and press them into the floor to lift and open the chest
- Without moving the leg closer to the torso, pull the leg down into the pelvis, making it heavy
- With the pelvis heavy, push the right heel up into the strap, away from back pelvis, *I i*
- Keeping the leg stable, resist the right heel laterally
- Spread the toes, broadening the sole of foot
- Emphasize leg length, not range of motion
- Open the leg gradually
- Without flattening the lumbar spine, draw bottom back ribs toward the floor
- Soften the face and abdomen

Exit

- Hold pose for 8-10 breaths
- Keep the pelvis level and stable
- Bend the right leg into the chest
- Extend both legs to *Supta Tadasana, I a*
- Repeat with the left leg
- After the second side, bend both legs and roll to the right
- Press into the hands and come up from the side to seated

Challenge

1. Lower back strain
2. Tight hamstrings cause legs to bend
3. Leg straightens too easily, or hyperextends
4. Head tilted back, throat tension

Response

1. Bend both legs and press the lumbar spine into the floor to alleviate discomfort.
2. Extend through the right femur, not the hamstring; bring the leg further away from torso and fully extend it. Set up closer to wall, rest heel on wall, *I j*. Practice with the raised leg resting on a door frame, *I k*.
3. Press back pelvis more heavily downward. Practice *I k*, resisting the leg into the door frame. Draw the hamstring into the femur as the femur presses back. Resist the calf into the tibia. Continue to *Explore*.
4. Manually adjust back of the skull away from the shoulders; use a folded blanket under the head sloping forehead toward chest, *I l*.

The hamstrings are often a challenge for yoga practitioners, and can cause some forms of back discomfort. As such, Supta Padangusthasana A is beneficial at all levels of practice. This pose releases the hamstrings and develops leg action for Standing Poses.

Contact Points

Back torso, shoulder blades, elbows, occiput, bottom foot

External Supports

Mat, wall, strap
Blanket, door frame

Essence of Form

Hip flexion, leg extension
Arms and legs in neutral rotation

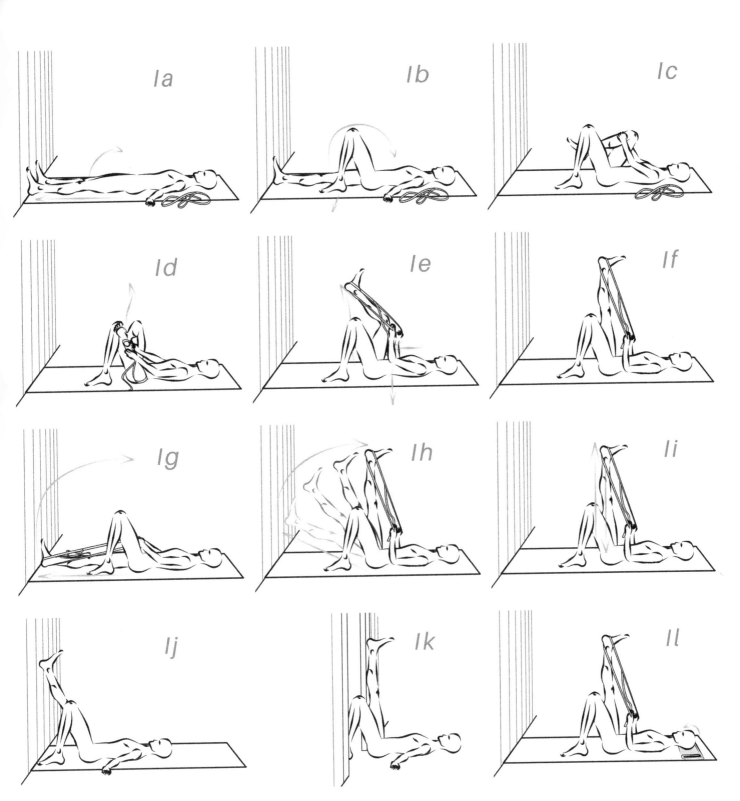

Ia   Ib   Ic

Id   Ie   If

Ig   Ih   Ii

Ij   Ik   Il

Learn + Practice

Once the leg straightens with ease at 90° in Simplify Before deep Forward Bends

Linked Poses

Standing Poses, Forward Bends, Supta Tadasana

Safety Factors

As for Simplify; do not practice Explore until pain and injuries are managed in Simplify

Prepare

- As for *Simplify*, with a folded blanket under the upper thighs in *Supta Tadasana, II a*

Enter

- Push the left heel into the wall, away from the back pelvis and descend left thigh into the blanket
- Without bending left leg, bend the right leg toward the chest, *II b*
- Keeping left leg extension, loop strap as in *Simplify, II c*
- Press right thigh away from torso and extend right leg, *II d*
- Throughout, maintain left heel contact at wall and left thigh contact with blanket
- Once left leg is consistently stable, lift right leg straight, *II e*

Sustain

- Maximize inner leg length from inner groins to big toe mounds
- Without rotating from the knees, roll top inner thighs backward

Sustain

- Gather the front iliums
- Without changing the leg position, resist both heels away from the mid line
- Pushing left foot away from back pelvis, lengthen left groin
- Increase right front groin space by pressing right femur away from the right hip, lifting right hip away from femur
- Exhaling, lengthen the right sitting bone toward the left heel
- Keeping the left leg and foot stable, the lumbar neutral, and without bending at the knee, draw the right leg toward right shoulder, *II f*

Exit

- Inhaling, lengthen both legs
- With left leg stable, bend the right leg on exhalation, lowering foot to the floor
- Extend right leg, *Supta Tadasana*
- Repeat to the second side
- Alternatively, keep leg straight while lowering to the floor
- Bend both legs and roll to the right
- Press into the hands and come up from the side to seated

Challenge

1. Left thigh lifts or left heel moves away from the wall as the right leg extends upward
2. Lower back pain
3. Bottom leg hyperextends while pressing femur into the blanket
4. Lumbar flattens into floor

Response

1. With the left thigh supported, weight the front thigh, *II g*. Resist heel upward and emphasize lengthening back of leg more deeply away from back pelvis.
2. Return to *Simplify*, if pain only occurs when extending the bottom leg along the floor, raise and support the bottom leg, *II h*. Gradually reduce support height.
3. Continue descending upper femur and resist tibia upward, *II i*. Keep back of heel on floor, as calf flesh will often press tibia upward, preventing hyperextension.
4. Open the angle between leg and torso, moving the leg toward wall. Gather front iliums and descend pubis. Descend left femur more heavily.

This variation, with both legs extended, is essential for beginners, while advanced students learn beneficial refinements. Supta Padangusthasana A can alleviate lower back pain by resetting the sacrum.

Contact Points

Bottom foot, bottom femur, back torso, elbows, occiput

External Supports

Wall, mat, strap, blankets
Additional blanket, sandbag, blocks, bolster

Essence of Form

Hip flexion, leg extension
Arms and legs in neutral rotation

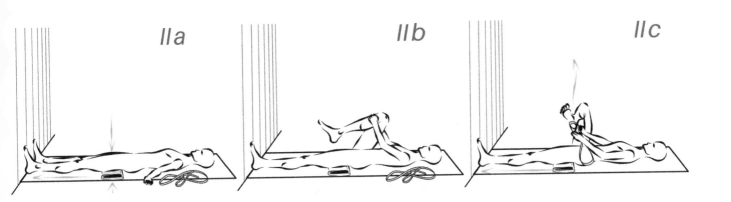

IIa *IIb* *IIc*

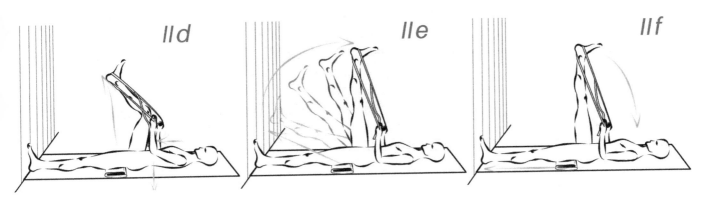

IId *IIe* *IIf*

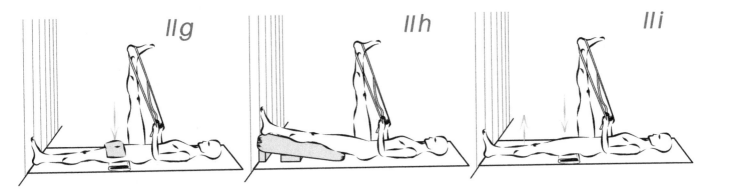

IIg *IIh* *IIi*

Learn + Practice

Once Explore is stable and comfortable, practice after deep Back Bends

Linked Poses

Standing Poses, Forward Bends, Supta Tadasana, Supta Padangusthasana B

Safety Factors

As for Simplify and Explore

Prepare

· Set the mat's short end to wall
· Have a strap within reach

Enter

· Begin by looping strap around right heel as for *Simplify*
· With strap around right heel, extend both legs to *Supta Tadasana, III a*
· Resist heels laterally and gather front iliums
· Keeping right heel contact with wall, bend the left leg and bring foot flat on the floor, *III b*
· Lengthening the right leg away from the back pelvis and pushing heel into strap, raise leg to 90° on exhalation
· Next exhalation, extend left leg and press foot to wall, *III c-d*
· Hold strap with left hand
· Hook right thumb in right inner groin, *III e*
· Manually rotate right thigh flesh externally
· Keeping right thigh flesh in external rotation, internally rotate top of right femur
· Without crossing mid line, draw right leg diagonally toward left shoulder and abduct right upper femur, *III f*

Sustain

· Equalize extension in both legs
· Widen across the back thighs
· Find stretch sensation near the bones rather than near skin at the surface
· With femurs pressing back, draw hamstrings forward
· Differentiate the rotations between right thigh flesh and femur — thigh flesh external, femur internal
· Descend outer right buttock, lengthening right sitting bone toward left heel
· Maximize hip joint space, lifting pelvis away from femur heads as femurs articulate away from pelvis

Exit

· Inhaling, lengthen both legs
· Return right leg to neutral rotation
· Keeping right leg fully extended, lengthen further and bring foot down to floor/wall juncture
· Touch right heel to wall before it reaches the floor
· Repeat to the left
· Rolling to the right, press into the hands and come to seated

Challenge

1. Back pain when raising or lowering the legs straight
2. Raised leg groin binds
3. Pelvis tucks as leg externally rotates

Response

1. Review lower transverse abdominus actions from *Supta Tadasana, Explore*:
· Resist heels laterally, widening greater trochanters, *III g*
· Draw front iliums inward medially, *III h*
· Soften pubis in and up, *III i*
· Engage the lower abdomen no more than 20% of maximum
· Maintain these actions and extend away from the back pelvis when lifting legs
2. Descend femur to back of thigh before lifting. Press hand into thigh before externally rotating leg. Use a second strap from raised leg groin to bottom foot, *see Synthesize*.
3. Broaden sitting bones before externally rotating leg.

ॐ *Once learned well and when there is no back pain, keep left leg extended while raising right leg*

Once the hamstrings release a little and the legs extend with more ease, femur and pelvis articulation can be refined. This variation demonstrates the link between leg action and pelvic alignments.

Contact Points

Bottom foot, bottom femur, back torso, elbows, occiput

External Supports

Mat, wall, strap
Additional strap

Essence of Form

Hip flexion, leg extension; temporary external rotation in raised leg

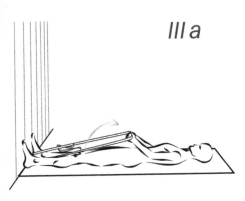
III a

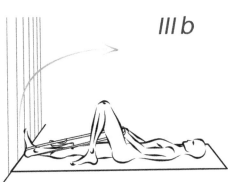
III b

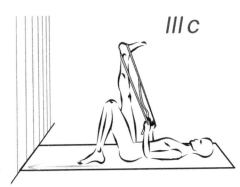
III c

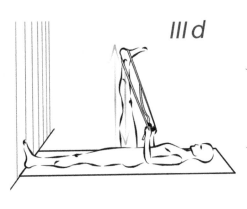
III d

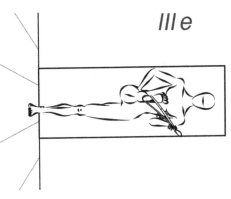
III e

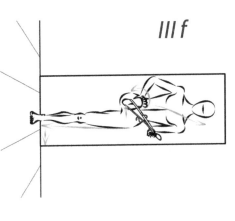
III f

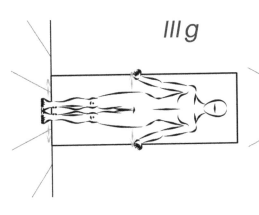
III g

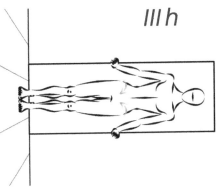
III h

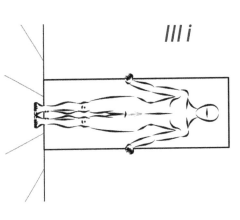
III i

Learn + Practice

*Once legs easily extend to 90°
Before Inversions, Back Bends,
and deep Forward Bends*

Linked Poses

*Back Bends, Inversions, deep
Forward Bends, Supta Tadasana*

Safety Factors

*Same as for Nourish,
High blood pressure,
neck or shoulder injury*

Prepare

- As for *Simplify*, with two straps within reach
- Make a large loop in one strap, at least a leg's length
- Can be practiced without wall, provided leg actions are clear and left leg remains stable

Enter

- Bend left leg and loop strap around left foot, *IV a-c*
- Extend left leg to *Supta Tadasana*, *IV d*
- Bend right leg, bringing it through looped strap, with the across right groin, *IV e*
- Draw right leg toward chest, as for *Simplify*, *IV f*
- With strap connecting left foot and right groin, left leg extension pressurizes right groin, drawing right femur away from pelvis
- If strap is loose, bend left leg slightly, tighten strap, then re-extend left leg
- Continue as for *Simplify* to extend right leg, *IV g-i*
- Bring palms together through strap, loop across inner wrists (thumb side)
- Exhaling, extend arms, *IV j*

Sustain

- Maintain strap tension and establish leg and pelvis actions from *Simplify* to *Nourish*
- Soften right groin, receiving strap pressure into hip crease
- Deepen inner and outer right groin equally as left leg extends
- Soften shoulders away from hands and widen between upper shoulder blades
- Lengthen collarbones laterally
- Keeping arms and legs extended, resist arms and right leg away from each other for 5 breaths, *IV k*
- Without losing extension or neutral lumbar, release resistance and allow right leg to come closer to torso, *IV l*
- Repeat resist/release cycle twice more, do not exceed three repetitions

Exit

- Rest in final position for 5 breaths or more
- Inhale, to lengthen legs, then release to *Supta Tadasana*
- Repeat to the left
- Roll to the right and press into the hands, coming to seated

Challenge

1. Neck and shoulder tension
2. Pain in middle or upper back
3. Hamstring cramp
4. Outer lower leg/ankle fatigue, burning sensation

Response

1. Be careful not to press back of head into floor as the arms resist the strap. Resist by lengthening outer arms away from outer armpits, rather than lengthening from the inner arms, which over-activates the shoulders and trapezius. Roll the outer arms and armpits more clearly toward ceiling.
2. Check strap placement. Strap across wrists affects mid-back and lower ribs; strap between index fingers and thumbs activates upper back and lower trapezius.
3. Resist with less force and do not force each release phase.
4. Extend leg from inner groin to big toe mound rather than shortening outer leg by pulling outer foot down. Deepen hip creases and move femurs more deeply backward.

Developing strength in the hamstrings compliments and stabilizes deeper stretches. This variation establishes a connection between both legs, both femurs, and also strengthens the hamstrings and spinal muscles in preparation for Back Bends and Inversions.

Contact Points

Bottom foot, bottom femur, back torso, elbows, occiput, wrists

External Supports

Mat, wall, 2 straps

Essence of Form

Leg extension, hip flexion, resist/release leg action; arms and legs neutrally rotated

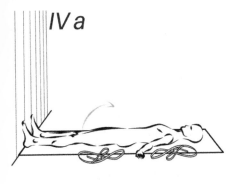
IV a

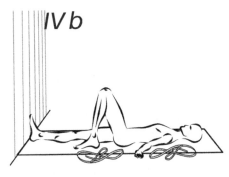
IV b

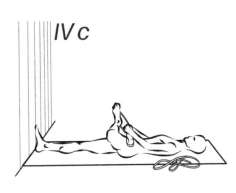
IV c

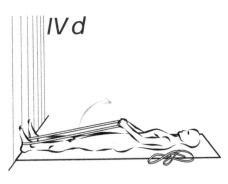
IV d

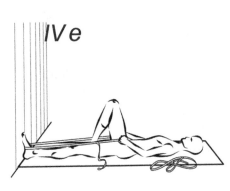
IV e

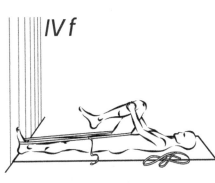
IV f

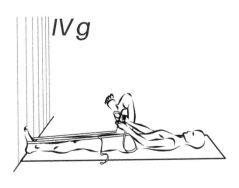
IV g

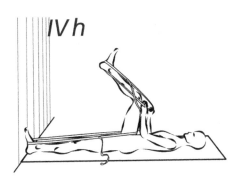
IV h

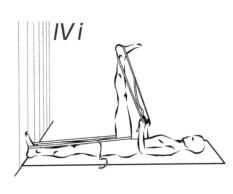
IV i

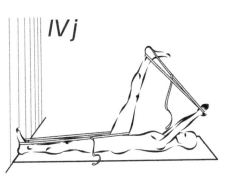
IV j

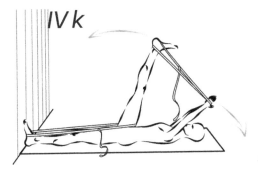
IV k

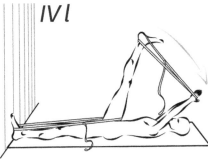
IV l

Learn + Practice

Learn in conjunction with Standing Poses, after Supta Padangusthasana A

Linked Poses

Supta Padangusthasana A, lateral Standing Poses, Baddha Konasana, Upavistha Konasana

Safety Factors

Groin or hamstring injury, SI joint instability

Prepare

- Mat's long edge parallel to and 2.5-3' from wall, have a strap nearby
- Lie on back with right side towards the wall
- Both legs bent, feet hip-width, and neutral lumbar curve, *l a*

Enter

- With abdomen soft, gather front iliums (ASIS)
- Soften pubis inward and resist heels laterally
- Keeping left foot on the floor, bend the right leg and loop belt around heel as in *Supta Padangusthasana A, l b*
- Exhaling, extend right leg to *Supta Padangusthasana A, Simplify, l c*
- Hold strap in the right hand
- Extend left arm at shoulder level
- Turn left palm down and press into the floor, *l d*
- Without rolling the pelvis to the right, and keeping the neutral lumbar, extend right inner leg and take right leg laterally toward wall, *l e*
- Press right foot into wall, instep parallel to floor

Sustain

- Keeping the left thigh neutral, push the left foot into the floor to keep the pelvis level
- Lengthen right sitting bone away from armpit
- Gather right ilium toward the left as right leg lowers to the wall
- Neither internally nor externally rotate the right leg, keeping the instep parallel to the floor
- Release buttocks away from back ribs
- Descend back pelvis symmetrically
- Move L4 + L5 symmetrically in, away from floor
- Soften abdomen, face, throat, and jaw

Exit

- Inhaling, raise the right leg and bring it back to center
- Exhaling, bend and lower the right leg
- Rest with both legs bent, feet hip-width apart and on the floor
- Roll to the right and press to seated
- *Prepare and Enter* with the left side torso to wall, left leg extended
- Once learned well, extend left leg after abducting right leg, *l f*

Challenge

1. Buttocks bind toward shoulder blades, right torso shortens
2. Hips roll rightward and SI joint compression
3. Inner knee strain
4. Head tilts back, throat tension

Response

1. Keep right foot against wall. Pressing into left foot, lift pelvis slightly and tuck right buttock, *l g*. With right buttock moving away from ribcage, lower pelvis symmetrically, *l h,*
2. Move closer to wall and abduct the leg no further than the pelvis can stay level. Support the outer thigh with bolster or block and push from the outer back pelvis to outer foot. Practice *Baddha Konasana.*
3. Release inner femur away from inner thigh toward outer thigh. Resist heel upward to abduct femur head and increase groin space. *See Response 2.*
4. Support head with folded blanket, *l i.*

❧ *See Supta Padangusthasana A for additional Challenges and their Responses*

Supta Padangusthasana B opens the hips laterally and lengthens the adductors. It increases lateral pelvic/abdominal space and prepares for lateral standing poses and hip openers. In this variation, pressing the abducted leg's foot into the wall helps establish that leg's pushing action.

Contact Points

Feet, back pelvis, back ribs, shoulder blades, arms, palm, back of skull

External Supports

*Mat, strap, wall
Blanket, bolster, block*

Essence of Form

Hip flexion, leg extension, lateral abduction; leg rotation neutral, left arm internal, right arm external

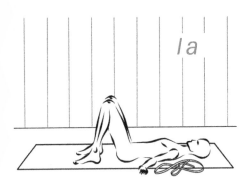

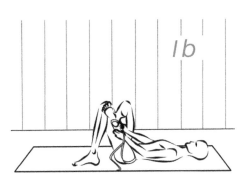

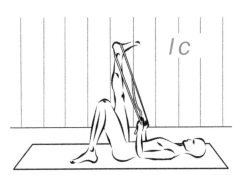

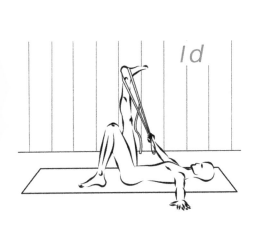

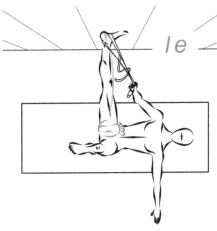

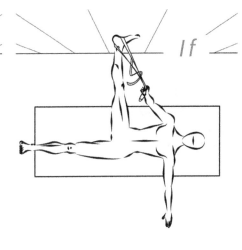

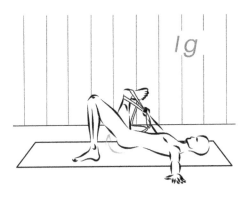

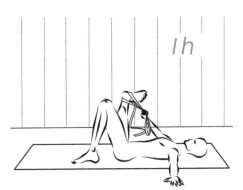

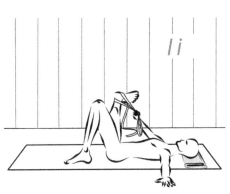

Supta Padangusthasana B
Lying Down Lateral Leg Stretch

Explore

Learn + Practice

After Simplify + Supta Padangusthasana A, Explore

Linked Poses

Lateral Standing Poses, Upavistha Konasana, Janu Sirsasana, open Twists

Safety Factors

Lower back strain, SI joint dysfunction, hamstring or groin injury

Prepare

- Set up mat and 2 blankets as for *Supta Padangusthasana A, Explore, II a*
- Place bolster lengthwise to right of mat, *II b*
- Have strap within reach

Enter

- Lie down in *Supta Tadasana* and follow *Enter* instructions for *Supta Padangusthasana A, Explore, II c*
- Hold the strap with the right hand
- Extend left arm to the side, palm down, *II d*
- Keeping left femur descending, and without shifting pelvis, extend and abduct right leg to the side
- Rest right thigh on bolster, *II e*

Sustain

- Push left heel into wall, away from back pelvis
- Continuously descend left upper femur into blanket
- Descend left inner back thigh more than outer back thigh

Sustain

- Reaching right heel away from back pelvis, lengthen right sitting bone toward wall
- Keep right leg in neutral rotation, with the instep level with floor
- Resist left heel leftward, and the right thigh into bolster
- Soften pubis in and up
- Draw right front ilium toward left front ilium
- Pressing the right femur to back thigh, lengthen the right side torso, freeing the diaphragm
- Descend and broaden bottom back ribs
- Soften unnecessary tension in right arm, rolling right elbow toward wall
- Release abdomen, throat, jaw, and tongue

Exit

- Hold for 10-20 breaths
- Inhaling, raise the right leg and bring it back to center
- Exhaling, lower the right leg
- Extend both legs, then repeat second side
- Roll to the right and press into the hands, coming to seated

Challenge

1. Left thigh lifts or pelvis rolls rightward
2. Right groin or buttock bind toward shoulder
3. Right leg action not clear
4. Lumbar pain
5. Hip or groin pain, right leg internally rotating

Response

1. Ensure left thigh is well supported and apply weight on left thigh. Receiving weight, extend back of left leg more thoroughly.
2. Bend left leg, push foot into floor and lift pelvis. Tuck right buttock, and re-descend back pelvis. Keeping buttock action, extend left leg. Loop a second strap from right groin to left foot, *II f. See also Nourish.*
3. Practice in a corner, both feet to wall, *II g*, or practice *Simplify* with bottom leg extended, *II h.*
4. Raise bottom leg angle with bolster and additional blocks, *II i. See Nourish.*
5. Externally rotate right thigh before abducting. Gradually reduce rotation after abducting.

One of the main challenges in Supta Padangusthasana B is to keep the pelvis level. Descending the bottom leg's femur is a crucial action, and it deepens the lateral space created by the pose, especially in the pelvic area. Practice it to understand poses like Trikonasana well.

Contact Points

Back pelvis, back ribs, shoulder blades, skull, bottom femur, foot, lateral arm

External Supports

Mat, 2 folded blankets, bolster, strap
Additional strap, bolster, 2 blocks

Essence of Form

Hip flexion, leg extension, lateral leg abduction; leg rotation neutral, extended arm internal, strap arm external

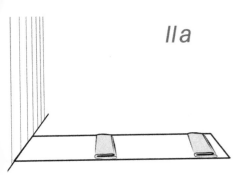

IIa

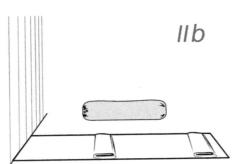

IIb

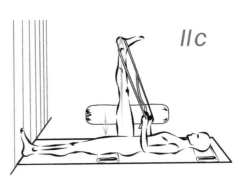

IIc

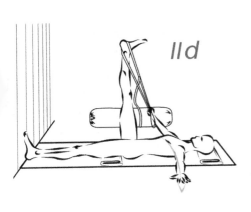

IId

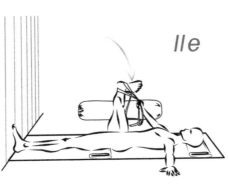

IIe

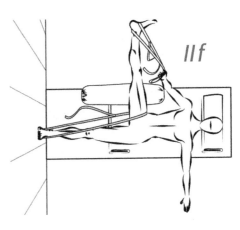

IIf

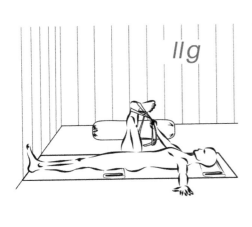

IIg

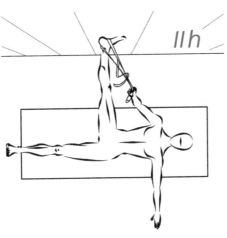

IIh

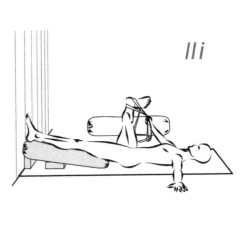

IIi

Learn + Practice

*After Simplify + Nourish,
After Supta Padangusthasana A, Nourish*

Linked Poses

*Lateral Standing Poses,
Parsvakonasana,
Upavistha Konasana, Janu
Sirsasana, open Twists*

Safety Factors

*As for Simplify + Nourish, use
care with hip replacement
and knee injury*

Prepare

· Lie on left side in door frame or
  at outer corner, with the sitting
  bones level with wall *III a*

Enter

· Roll onto back with right leg
  bent and on wall, right sitting
  bone against it and left leg
  bent with foot flat on floor, *III b*
· Extend right leg away
  from back pelvis, *III c*
· Press back of right thigh into wall
· Keeping right sitting bone
  against wall, extend left leg
  to *Supta Tadasana, III d*
· Contact left inner thigh
  against door frame
· Establish leg and pelvis actions
  from *Simplify + Explore*
· Maintain a neutral lumbar
  and level pelvis
· Without losing right sitting
  bone contact, draw right ilium
  leftward and abduct right leg
  to reasonable capacity, *III e*
· Right leg in neutral rotation,
  neither internally nor
  externally rotating
· *Prepare* with support under
  right leg for holds longer
  than one minute, *III f*

Sustain

· Extend left foot away
  from back pelvis
· Press left big toe mound
  away from inner groin and
  descend left inner femur
· Keeping left inner femur
  descending, broaden left inner
  femur away from door frame *III g*
· Release right outer buttock
  away from back ribs,
  lengthening side torso
· Create maximum contact
  with right inner and outer
  back thigh against wall
· Extend through outer right
  leg from outer hip
· Broaden inner groins
  and anterior sacrum
· Soften behind abdominal wall

Exit

· Pressing the left femur downward
  to stabilize pelvis, inhale and
  lift right leg to vertical
· Use right hand to assist lifting
  right leg for holds longer
  than one minute *III h*
· Bend both legs and roll to the left
· *Prepare* for the second side
  and repeat to the left
· Roll to the right and press into
  the hands, coming to seated

Challenge

1. Right knee or lumbar pain
2. Right groin or inner thigh strain
3. SI joint compression
4. Left thigh lifts

Response

1. *Prepare + Enter* further away from
   door frame. Loop strap from
   right groin to left foot as for *Supta
   Padangusthasana A, Synthesize.*
   Bend right leg, sole of foot against
   wall. Use a second strap at back of
   right lower femur and hold strap in
   right hand. Without lifting right foot
   from wall, pull lower femur toward
   torso and extend through left leg,
   creating traction on right hip and
   knee joint, *III i. See Response 2.*
2. Decrease degree of abduction,
   but move inner femur away
   from inner thigh. Support right
   leg and weight inner thigh,
   III j. Resist heel toward mid
   line and lengthen outer thigh
   away from outer back pelvis.
3. Wedge blanket under right
   outer back ilium and roll
   right ilium leftward.
4. Support left thigh and weight top
   of left thigh. Raise left leg angle
   with bolster and blocks, *III k.*

Using a door frame is an excellent way to practice both Supta Padangusthasana A and B. The wall supports the back of the leg, encouraging posterior femur movement. This support also enables longer holds for deeper layers to release.

Contact Points

Back pelvis, bottom thigh, raised leg sitting bone, back torso

External Supports

Door frame or outer corner, chair Wall, 2 straps, 2 blocks, sand bag, blanket, bolster

Essence of Form

Hip flexion, leg extension, lateral leg abduction; arms and legs in neutral rotation

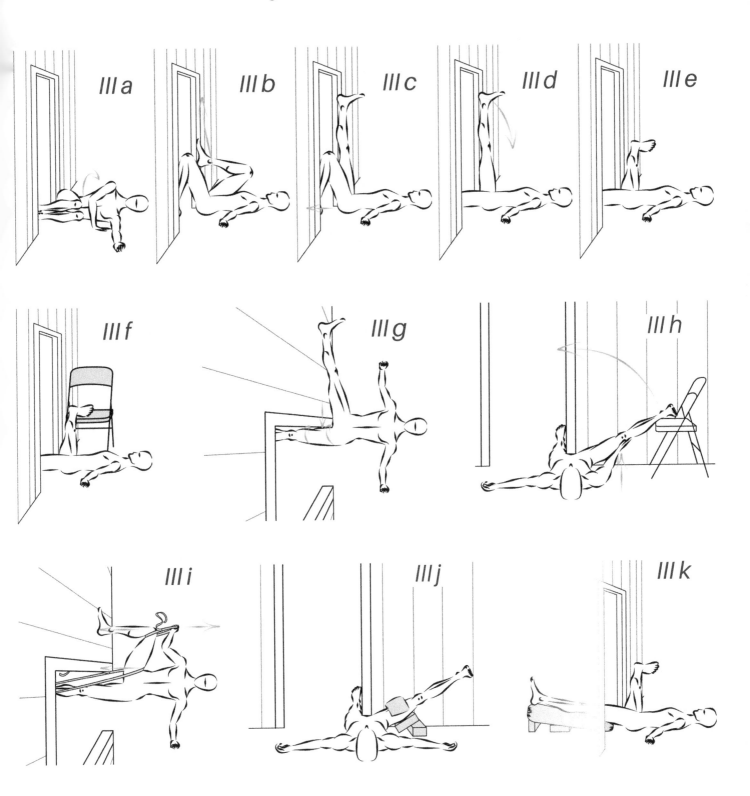

Supta Padangusthasana B
Lying Down Lateral Leg Stretch

Synthesize

Learn + Practice

Learn after Explore + Nourish, used as a lumbar reset after Back Bends. Practice no more than twice a week

Linked Poses

Lateral Standing Poses, Tadasana Urdhva Hastasana, open Twists

Safety Factors

Groin, hamstring, or adductor injury; disc problem, do not practice with hip replacement

Prepare

- With an assistant, away from walls or with a heavy piece of furniture (or other anchor) beyond head
- Set mat away from walls with enough space to extend legs and arms laterally and longitudinally

Enter

- Lie down on mat with legs bent, assistant or anchor beyond head, *IV a*
- Reach arms overhead and interlock fingers behind assistant's ankle or catch anchor
- Assistant steps free leg forward to extend anchor foot backward for traction, *IV b*
- Extend legs to *Supta Tadasana, IV c*
- Descending left thigh, exhale and draw right thigh toward chest, leg bent, *IV d*
- Without lifting left thigh, abduct right leg
- Keeping right thigh close to side body, extend right leg fully then externally rotate, *IV e*
- Keeping external rotation, sweep leg through side plane to *Tadasana*, right heel toward left toes, little toe descending, *IV f*

Sustain

- Maintain full arm extension with traction
- Soften shoulders away from hands
- Descend bottom back ribs away from anchor
- Avoid turning the head and ribcage
- Extend both legs away from back pelvis
- Continually descend left thigh
- Engage lower transverse abdominus 20%
- Keep external rotation as leg sweeps around
- Make leg movement as smooth as possible

Exit

- Bending legs, press feet into floor and lift pelvis to adjust away from anchor to re-create maximum traction
- Alternatively, assistant can step further back for greater traction
- With maximum traction, repeat up to three times with the right leg
- Repeat to the left, up to 3 times
- Bend legs and bring feet to floor
- Release hands and arms
- Roll to the right, pressing into the hands to come to seated

Challenge

1. Grinding and popping noises or sensation in the hip joint
2. Insufficient traction
3. Left hip lifts
4. Groin binding/discomfort

Response

1. Not problematic unless sharply painful. If pain occurs, reduce leg abduction and increase external rotation. Increase traction. *See Response 2.*
2. If practicing with an assistant, assistant lifts heel and steps ball of foot as far back as possible. When partner lowers heel, more traction is created. If practicing alone holding an anchor, bend legs and press feet into floor. Lift pelvis and lengthen away from torso, then keeping length, lower pelvis for more traction.
3. Support under left thigh, pressing thigh against support. If supported, weight can be applied to upper left thigh.
4. Abduct inner femurs. Reach legs more fully away from back pelvis. Completely externally rotate right leg before sweeping leg. Practice *Explore* or *Nourish* immediately before.

Both Supta Padangusthasana A and B are useful for creating a minor spinal adjustment. This is more effective, and safer, when combined with traction. Here, use an assistant to help you create traction for a deep sacro-lumbar adjustment after deep back bends.

Contact Points

Back body, bottom leg, clasped hands

External Supports

Mat, assistant (or other stable anchor)

Essence of Form

Leg extension with abduction; raised leg in deep external rotation, bottom leg neutral, arms neutral

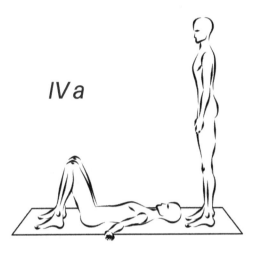

IV a

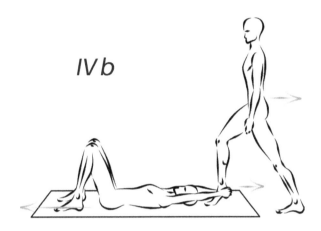

IV b

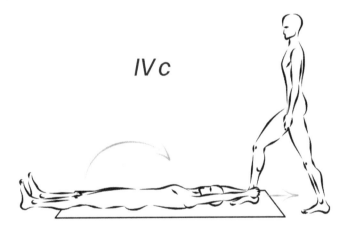

IV c

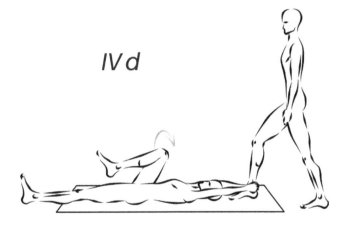

IV d

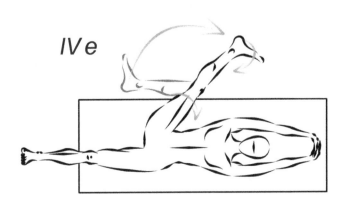

IV e

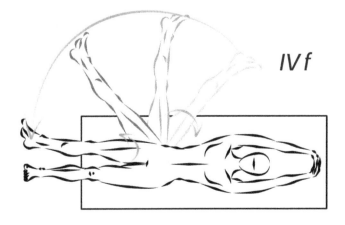

IV f

Ardha Uttanasana
Wall Pushing Downward-Facing Dog Pose

Simplify

Learn + Practice

Before Uttanasana, Inversions, and later stages of Adho Mukha Svanasana

Linked Poses

Standing Poses, Forward Bends, and Inversions

Safety Factors

Hamstring, shoulder, or wrist injury

Prepare

- Place mat's short edge to wall
- Stand facing the wall, an arm's length from it

Enter

- Place hands on wall at shoulder height, with hands shoulder width apart, *l a*
- Have the index fingers parallel to each other, *l b*
- Ensure hands are level
- Spreading fingertips, press hands into the wall
- Push the index finger mounds away from the armpits and fully extend elbows, *l c*
- Without losing index finger mound contact, press pelvis away from wall, walking the feet back, directly below pelvis, *l d-f*
- Set the feet hip-width apart, with the foot mid lines parallel, *l g*
- Descend torso until armpits come into line between wrists and pelvis
- With legs slightly bent, press top femurs backward to straighten legs on exhalation, *l f*
- Once armpits come into line between wrists and groins, practice with hands at chest height, *l h-i*, then at hip height, *l j-k*

Sustain

- Lengthen from back pelvis to big toe mounds
- Pressing 4 points of feet equally into the floor, lift toes and activate arches
- With arch lift, lengthen toes and lightly descend them to the floor on exhale
- Thighs firm, push back pelvis up, away from feet and off femur heads
- Resist heels laterally, widening then deepening inner groins
- Symmetrically lengthen side torso from armpits to pelvis
- Keep head neutral, ears between upper arms

Exit

- Stabilize the hands on the wall
- Pressing into the index finger mounds, exhale and bend the legs
- Look forward between the hands, checking hand height
- If hands are no longer level, adjust and bring them level, then re-stabilize
- Keeping the hands anchored, inhale and step feet forward to standing

Challenge

1. One hand slides down the wall
2. Shoulders lift, neck tension
3. Head hangs below upper arms
4. Legs too close or far away from wall
5. Excessive lumbar lordosis
6. Thoracic kyphosis

Response

1. Push equally from shoulder blades to each hand. Notice any tendency to lean right or left, and minimize that tendency.
2. Pushing hands into the wall, broaden inner shoulder blades and extend them away from the skull.
3. Lift head slightly, lengthening the crown of head toward wall as pelvis extends back.
4. Walk feet slightly forward or back, bringing legs parallel to wall. Ensure both feet are the same distance from the wall.
5. Keeping the belly soft, lift front ribs into the body. Widen sitting bones and descend the tail bone down into that space.
6. Keep hands at shoulder height until kyphosis is corrected. *See Responses 1 + 2.*

The wall pushing variation is appropriate for all levels and is an excellent substitute for Adho Mukha Svanasana. Increasing shoulder mobility and lengthening the hamstrings, it also teaches correct pushing actions applicable throughout the pose's development.

Contact Points

Hands, feet

External Supports

Wall, mat

Essence of Form

Hip flexion; arm, torso, and leg extension; arms and legs in neutral rotation

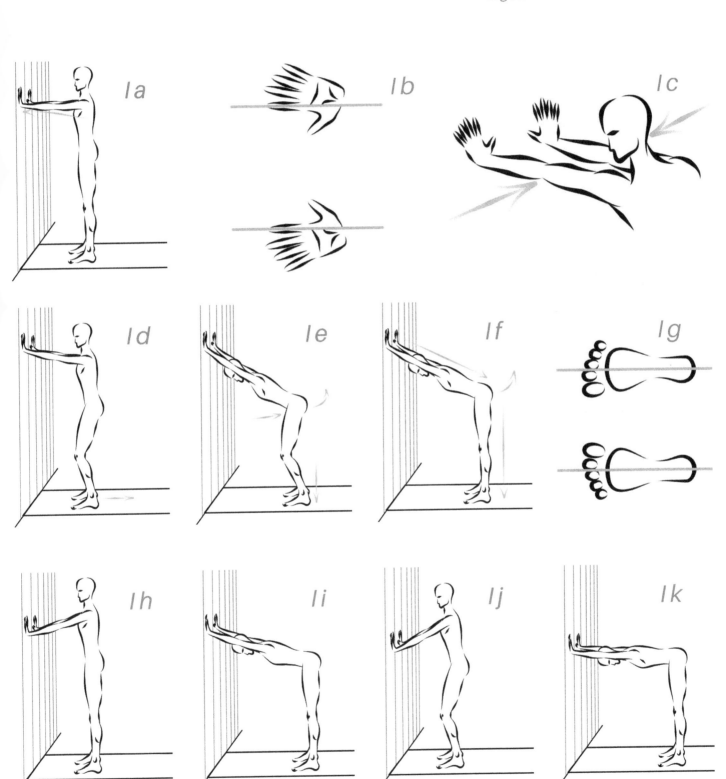

Adho Mukha Svanasana
Chair Pushing Downward-Facing Dog Pose

Explore

Learn + Practice

Once wrists, armpits, and pelvis are level in Simplify, before arm balances and Inversions

Linked Poses

Standing Poses, Forward Bends, and Inversions; All weight-bearing arm poses

Safety Factors

Hamstring or shoulder injury; some lower back injuries
Use care or return to Simplify if unsure or uncomfortable

Prepare

· Place mat's short edge to wall
· Brace a chair against the wall

Enter

· Stand one foot away from the chair
· Exhaling, lean forward and place inner hands on the chair seat, in *Ardha Uttanasana*, *ll a*
· Lift outer hands, bringing palms flush with the chair seat, increasing the pressure through the index fingers and thumbs into the chair seat, *ll b*
· Keeping hand pressure, lengthen the arms fully
· Exhale and bend the legs, stepping the feet away from chair, *ll c-d*
· Press pelvis back until wrists, armpits, and hips are in line, *ll e*
· Extend arms and armpits fully, pressing thighs backward
· Walk feet further away from the chair than the pelvis, legs 90° to the torso
· Bring feet hip-width apart and ensure foot mid lines are parallel
· Anchor heels and without moving pelvis toward wall, press upper thighs back to straighten the legs on exhalation, *ll e-f*

Sustain

· Keep actions from *Simplify*
· Spread and lengthen fingers, to open and broaden the palms
· Continue lifting outer hands away from the floor and chair seat edge
· With arms fully extended, turn inner elbows toward each other
· Broaden between the shoulder blades and descend the outer armpits, *ll g*
· Extend front and back torso equally, bringing volume into the back rib cage
· Balance breath in front and back body
· Press femurs away from hands, extending the side torso
· Resist the heels laterally and widen between the inner upper femurs
· Into that space, extend the pubis backward
· Draw front iliums toward each other

Exit

· Keep both hands stable
· Exhaling, bend the legs and look forward
· Inhaling, walk the feet toward the chair and come to standing

Challenge

1. Weight collapses into shoulders
2. Calves or hamstrings overstretch
3. Shoulder strain or wrist pain
4. Shoulders sway toward floor

Response

1. Use hand pressure to extend thighs and pelvis away from the chair. Move weight more deeply into legs and extend femurs backward, rather than applying pressure through hands by bringing weight forward.
2. Use a tightly rolled mat or slanted board under the heels, *ll h*. Widen stance slightly. Practice *Simplify* and *Supta Padangusthasana A.*
3. Wrap hands around chair sides, pointing thumbs forward on chair seat, *ll i*. If shoulder strain is still excessive, practice *Ardha Uttanasana* with hands on chair seat below shoulders, *ll a*, or return to *Simplify.*
4. Draw front ribs inward and lift mid-thoracic spine between shoulder blades. Lift armpits and emphasize side torso length.

Transitioning from the wall to placing the hands on a chair seat transfers slightly more weight into the hands and arms. This variation deepens the shoulder, torso, and leg extension. It also prepares the circulatory system for partial Inversions.

Contact Points

Hands, feet

External Supports

Chair, wall, mat
Slant board

Essence of Form

Hip flexion, arm, torso, and leg extension; upper arms externally rotated, legs in neutral rotation

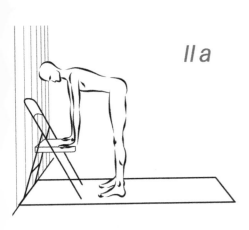
II a

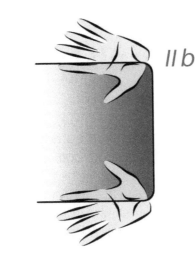
II b

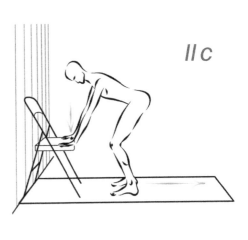
II c

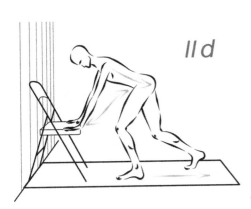
II d

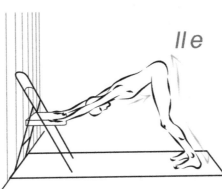
II e

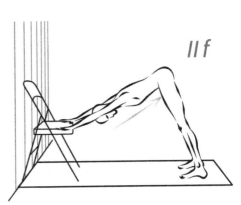
II f

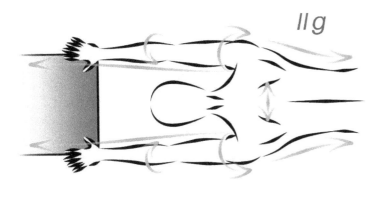
II g

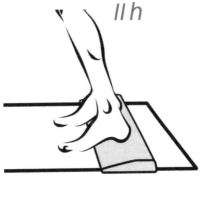
II h

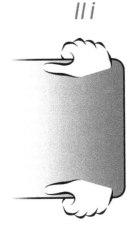
II i

Learn + Practice

*After Simplify + Explore;
before Inversions and
deep Forward Bends*

Linked Poses

*Standing Poses, Forward
Bends, and Inversions;
All weight-bearing arm poses*

Safety Factors

*Hamstring, shoulder, or
wrist injury; hypertension,
migraine, eye pressure*

Prepare

· Set mat's short edge to wall

Enter

· Kneel facing the wall, 2-3' from it
· Place the hands on the floor,
  shoulder-width apart with the
  thumb and index finger tips at
  the wall/floor juncture, *III a*
· Fully extend arms, elbow
  creases facing inward
· Exhaling, lift onto hands and
  knees, toes tucked under
· Walk feet back until knees
  are directly beneath pelvis
· Press hands equally down and
  forward, with greatest pressure
  on the index finger mounds
· From hand pressure, exhale
  and lift knees off the floor, *III b*
· Have equal weight on each foot
· With legs bent and heels raised,
  exhale and press into hands,
  lifting the pelvis toward ceiling, *III c*
· Keeping heels lifted, press upper
  front thighs backward, away from
  hands, and fully extend legs, *III d-e*
· Keeping pelvic height, lengthen
  legs and descend outer heels
  away from outer pelvis, *III f*
· With outer heels heavy, descend
  inner heels also, *III g-h*

Sustain

· Retain actions from
  Simplify + Explore
· Pushing the hands equally
  forward away from both
  shoulder blades, lift the
  pelvis toward the ceiling
· Continually stretch outer
  heels diagonally away from
  big toe mound pressure
· Press femurs backward
  away from hands, reducing
  load on wrists
· Widen and soften between
  shoulder blades
· Extend inner shoulder
  blades toward pelvis
· Keep the head neutral,
  with the ears between
  the upper arm bones
· Extend the occiput away from
  upper shoulder blades
· Soften face and scalp,
  release jaw and tongue

Exit

· Stabilize the hands
· Being careful not to hit the
  head on the wall, exhale and
  lower knees to the floor
· Rest in *Uttana Balasana* for a
  few breaths before repeating
· Repeat 3-5 times, 5-15
  breaths each

Challenge

1. Hamstring restriction causes
   rounding of the lower back
2. Shoulder restriction causes
   upper back to round
3. Excessive sitting bone lift,
   straining the upper hamstrings
4. Shoulder laxity and
   lumbar collapse

Response

1. Take feet mat width, bend legs
   deeply to move L4 + L5 inward,
   tilting pelvis anteriorly, *III i*.
   Keeping pelvic tilt and wider
   stance, press upper femurs
   back and re-straighten legs.
2. Lengthen from sternum to
   pubis, extending front body
   and descend upper back.
3. Push sacrum directly backward
   and descend tail bone,
   extending lower spine.
4. Inhaling, draw inner armpits
   inward, and roll outer armpits
   downward. Lengthen from
   bottom back ribs to back pelvis.

ॐ *For Responses 1 + 2, place
hands on blocks, III j, go
back to Simplify + Explore.
For Responses 3 + 4, de-
emphasize stretch sensations.*

To maintain the forward pushing action through the hands, the wall provides useful feedback when transitioning to the more classic form of Adho Mukha Svanasana. For many practitioners, this will be the first Inversion, bringing the head and heart below the pelvis.

Contact Points

Feet, hands, tips of thumb and forefinger

External Supports

Mat, wall
Blocks

Essence of Form

Hip flexion; arm, torso, and leg extension; arms in external rotation, legs in neutral rotation

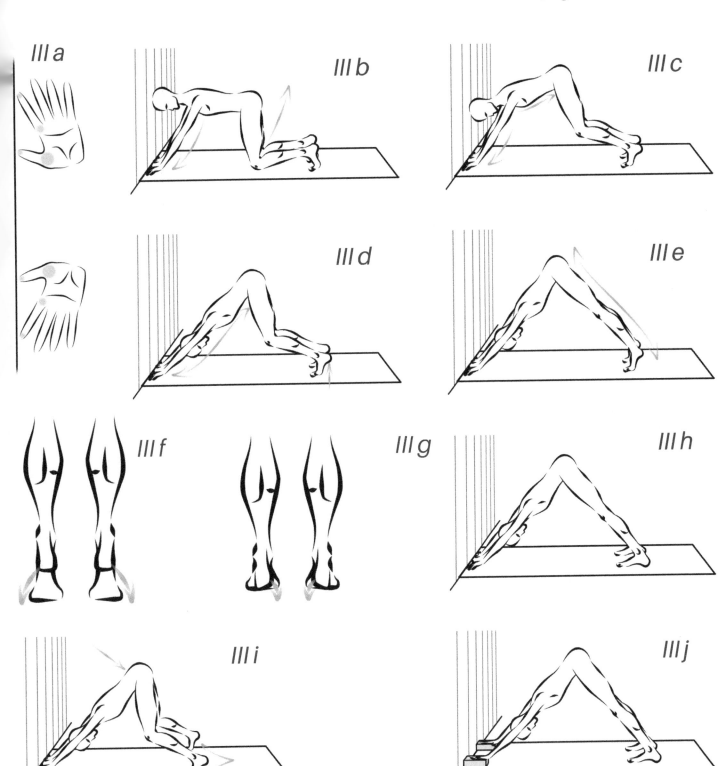

III a

III b

III c

III d

III e

III f

III g

III h

III i

III j

Adho Mukha Svanasana
Downward-Facing Dog Pose

Synthesize

Learn + Practice

*After Simplify + Explore;
before Inversions and
full Surya Namaskara*

Linked Poses

*Standing Poses, Forward
Bends, and Inversions;
All weight-bearing arm poses*

Safety Factors

Same as Nourish

Prepare

- Place mat's short edge to wall
- Set a block near mat, within reach

Enter

- Kneel on mat with
  back to wall, *IV a*
- Place a block between
  the upper thighs
- Walk hands forward and lie
  face-down on mat, *IV b*
- Bring the heels to the wall, balls
  of feet in wall/floor juncture, *IV c*
- Place hands under the
  armpits, index fingers parallel
  to each other, *IV d*
- Pressing hands into the
  floor, exhale to lift onto
  hands and knees
- Next exhalation, deepen index
  finger mound pressure
- Without losing index finger
  mound pressure, exhale and
  lift knees off the floor, *IV e*
- Keeping legs bent, extend
  pelvis up and back, *IV f-g*
- Squeeze block symmetrically
  and press the block backward
  to straighten the legs, *IV h-j*
- With pelvis lifted, press the heels
  symmetrically into the wall

Sustain

- Build on actions from *Simplify,
  Explore, + Nourish*
- Internally rotate from the tops of
  thighs and lift the block backward
- Widen the sitting bones
- Keep the knees and
  ankles neutral
- Draw lower shoulder blades
  toward spine and widen
  upper shoulder blades
- Lengthen torso's shorter side
- Without lifting big toe mounds, lift
  inner ankles toward outer ankles
- Lift and deepen inner groins
- Soften and release tension
  in the space between
  sacrum and pubis

Exit

- Keep the hands stable
- Exhaling, bend legs
  and look forward
- Step or jump feet to *Uttanasana*
- Thighs firm, descend back
  pelvis and inhale press
  torso up to *Tadasana*
- Repeat without the wall, *IV k*
- In *IV k*, keep leg length and
  symmetrically descend outer
  heels, then inner heels

Challenge

1. Hyperextended elbows
2. Elbows don't straighten
3. Weight collapses into
   one arm/shoulder
4. Wrist compression

Response

1. Belt elbows and press outward,
   IV l. Avoid externally rotated
   hand position as in *Nourish*.
2. Keep externally rotated
   hand position from *Nourish*,
   extend from bottom
   shoulder blades to hands.
3. On alternate practice days,
   support with mat remnant
   beneath heel of hand on
   collapsed side. Lift collapsed
   armpit until weight comes
   more equally into the
   opposite hand and arm.
4. Extend fingertips much more
   fully away from back of wrists.
   Keeping palms broad, lift
   palm centers away from floor.
   Lift groove between heel of
   thumb and outer heel of hand.
   Draw undersides of forearms
   upward and distribute weight
   forward through all bones
   of each hand, not resting
   solely into the heel of hand.

As a preliminary Inversion, Adho Mukha Svanasana prepares the circulatory system for deeper Inversions while teaching necessary physical actions in the arms, torso, and legs. In this variation, both a block and the wall are used to emphasize the leg actions.

Contact Points

Feet, hands, inner thighs

External Supports

Wall, mat, block
Strap

Essence of Form

Hip flexion, arm, torso, and leg extension; upper arms externally rotated, legs slightly internally rotated

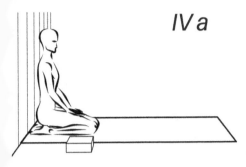
IV a

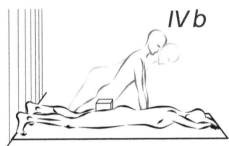
IV b

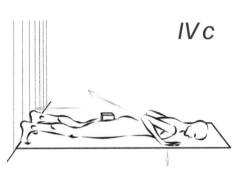
IV c

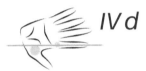
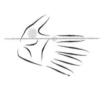
IV d

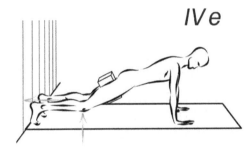
IV e

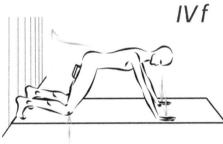
IV f

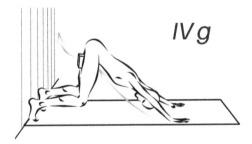
IV g

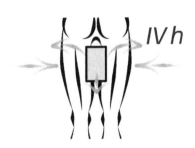
IV h

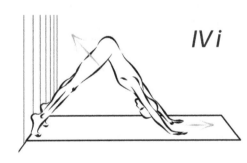
IV i

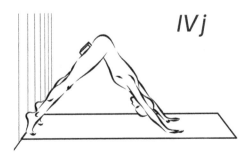
IV j

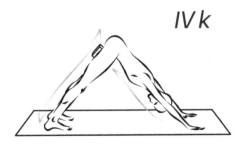
IV k

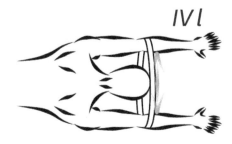
IV l

Uttitha Hasta Padasana
Parallel Wide Stance Pose

Learn + Practice

Learn early, within the first few classes; practice before and with Standing Poses

Linked Poses

Tadasana, Prasarita Padottanasana, Parsva Hasta Padasana, lateral Standing Poses Use a narrower stance

Safety Factors

for ankle or groin injury and hip replacement

Prepare

· Set the mat away from walls

Enter

· Stand in *Tadasana*, with the heels at mat's long edge, *I a*
· Inhaling, raise hands to collarbones with the middle fingers touching and elbows lifted to the sides at shoulder level, *I b*
· Gather front iliums and resist heels laterally
· Pushing feet away from back pelvis, soften pubis in and up
· Exhaling, bend the legs slightly, *I c*
· Inhaling, step right foot 1.5-2' to the right, away from the mid line, then step left foot the same amount to the left
· Coordinate extending arms to the sides at shoulder level as the feet step apart, *I d-g*
· Separate the feet until the ankles are aligned under the wrists, *I h*
· Ensure the back of both heels remain on the mat's long edge, neither heel forward
· Keep foot mid lines parallel throughout with the kneecaps facing directly forward

Sustain

· Symmetrically push feet away from the back pelvis
· Firm the thighs, lifting the kneecaps
· Continue gathering the front iliums and resisting the heels laterally
· Lift and spread the toes, activating arches
· Without tucking pelvis, descend the tail bone heavily
· Lift both torso sides equally
· Extend arms from bottom shoulder blades through elbows to fingertips
· Soften trapezius and widen chest and upper back equally

Exit

· Exhaling, bend the legs slightly
· Inhaling, step right foot back to the mid line, then step left foot in, coming to *Tadasana*
· Alternatively, heel-toe feet inward symmetrically
· Bring hands to collarbones as feet step in
· Fully extend legs and rest arms to sides
· Repeat *Enter* and *Exit* up to 10 times to increase hip joint mobility, alternating leading leg with each repetition

Challenge

1. Difficulty stepping feet apart
2. Feet and legs turn out
3. Inner arches collapse
4. Outer ankle strain

Response

ॐ *Adductor restriction contributes to Challenges 1 + 2. Practice Baddha Konasana to release.*

1. Reduce stance width. Gradually widen stance as capacity increases. Do not bend legs to increase stance width. Instead, press upper femurs away from each other without stepping feet further apart.
2. Emphasize moving the heels out, not the toes. Roll the inner thighs back and press heels out.
3. Without lifting big toe mounds, pressurize outer feet. Roll inner arches toward outer ankles. Without widening stance, press heels and upper femurs laterally.
4. Reduce stance width slightly. Keep inner ankles lifted and draw outer ankles inward. Increase big toe mound pressure.

This pose increases hip and ankle mobility and is the foundation of several Standing Poses, usually learned before other Standing Poses, after Tadasana. Hasta, meaning hand, and Pada, meaning foot, here refer to having the feet the hand-width when the arms extended to the sides.

Contact Points

Feet

External Supports

Mat

Essence of Form

Leg abduction
Arms and legs neutral

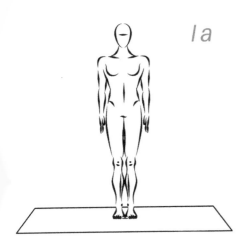

I a

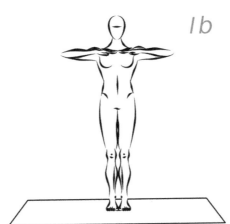

I b

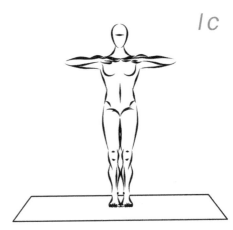

I c

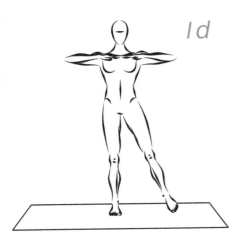

I d

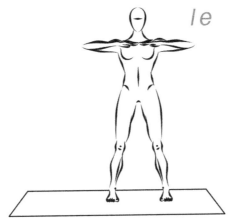

I e

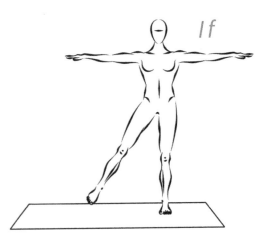

I f

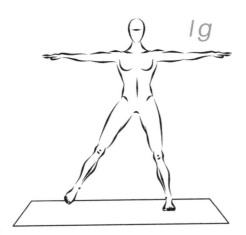

I g

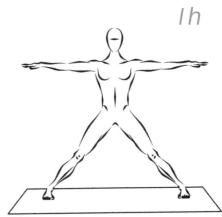

I h

Uttitha Hasta Padasana
Parallel Wide Stance Pose

Once Simplify is smooth, before jumping in Surya Namaskara and more complex transitions

Linked Poses

Tadasana, Prasarita Padottanasana, Parsva Hasta Padasana, lateral Standing Poses

Safety Factors

Do not jump with major joint or spinal injuries, or if pregnant

Prepare

- Set the mat away from walls

Enter

- Stand in *Tadasana*, with the heels at mat's long edge
- Bring hands to collarbones, elbows bent, *II a*
- Exhaling, bend the legs, *II b*
- While inhaling, jump feet apart
- Extend arms while jumping, *II c-e*
- Bend the legs on landing, backs of heels flush with mat's long edge, *II f*
- Adjust foot position if necessary
- Pushing the feet away from back pelvis, extend the legs, *II g*

Sustain

- Gather front iliums and resist heels laterally
- Lift front iliums up and away from upper front femurs
- Descend tail bone and slide it gently forward
- Soften pubis inward and upward
- Without poking bottom front ribs, maximize side torso length from hips to armpits

Sustain

- Softening front ribs inward, extend arms from center of chest through arms to fingertips
- Externally rotate arms from deep in shoulder joint, turning palms upward, *II h*
- Release trapezium as arms rotate, drawing bottom shoulder blades forward
- Maximize arm span from fingertip to fingertip
- Keeping upper arms externally rotated, turn palms back downward, *II i*

Exit

- Exhaling, bend the legs slightly
- While inhaling, jump the feet back together
- Coordinate bringing the hands to the collarbones while jumping
- Cushion landing by bending legs
- Land with heels flush with mat's edge
- Extend legs fully in *Tadasana*
- Exhaling release arms to side torso
- Repeat up to 10 times until jumping movements are smooth and symmetrical

Challenge

1. Joint impact on landing
2. Feet come forward or back, or land asymmetrically
3. Inner arches collapse
4. Knees collapse in and feet turn out

Response

1. Inhale while jumping. Don't jump as high and land with bent legs to soften impact. If impact is still too great, do not jump. Instead, step feet apart as for *Simplify*.
2. Observe asymmetry and refine landings with each repetition. Ensure correct foot alignment does not result in pelvic twist.
3. Lift the toes and pressurize outer feet.
4. Lead outward movement with heels. Broaden upper femurs while jumping. Think less of separating feet, more of separating thighs. Reduce stance width until landing is better aligned, walking feet apart after landing. Gradually increase jump width as landing alignment improves.

Once hip and ankle mobility is established by stepping the feet apart, Uttitha Hasta Padasana can be entered into by jumping. Doing so is more symmetrical, develops strength in the legs, builds spinal resilience, and further increases hip mobility. Use care if impact is a risk.

Contact Points

Feet

External Supports

Mat

Essence of Form

Jumping while abducting legs; arms and legs in neutral rotation

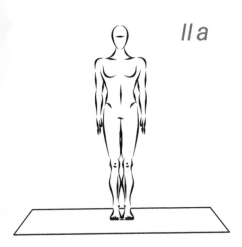

II a

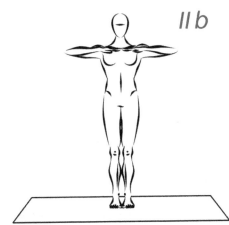

II b

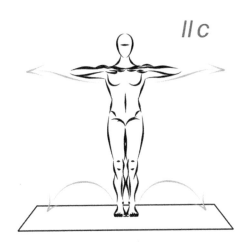

II c

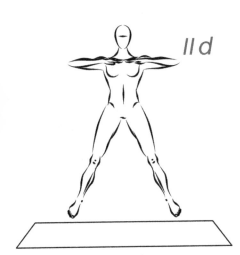

II d

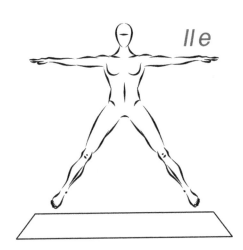

II e

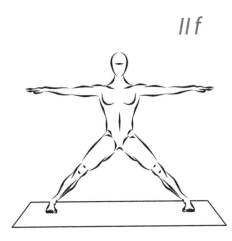

II f

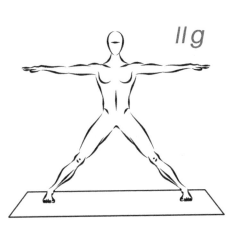

II g

II h

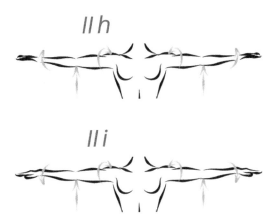

II i

Parsva Hasta Padasana
Lateral Wide Stance Pose

Learn + Practice

Learn before lateral Standing Poses; after Uttitha Hasta Padasana, Simplify

Linked Poses

Lateral Standing Poses, Trikonasana, Parsvakonasana, Virabhadrasana B

Safety Factors

Groin injury, use care with knee injuries

Prepare

- Set mat's short end to wall

Enter

- Stand in *Tadasana*, left side toward wall, an arm's length from it
- Extend left arm at shoulder level and press left hand into wall, *III a*
- Step left foot's outer edge to wall, *III b*
- Pressing into left outer heel, step right foot out to *Uttitha Hasta Padasana*, ankles below wrists, *III c-d*
- Push outer heels equally away from back pelvis
- Gather front iliums and soften pubis inward and upward
- With the left thigh firm, press left outer heel into the wall and turn left foot in 15°-30°
- Firm right thigh and lift kneecap
- Draw right ilium up, off of right femur and roll it slightly leftward
- Without shifting abdomen to the right, inhale and externally rotate right thigh 90° pivoting on right heel, *III e*
- Hips horizontally level, roll the left hip slightly forward
- Both heels along one line perpendicular to wall

Sustain

- Continue pressing feet away from back pelvis
- Lift toes to establish arches
- Keeping pelvis level, descend right buttock and deepen external rotation from top of right thigh
- Lift both sides of the torso equally

Exit

- Keeping pelvis level, stabilize left heel
- Exhaling, turn right leg in
- Push into outer right heel and left hand
- Bend legs and step left foot to mat's center, then step right foot to *Tadasana*
- Alternatively, heel-toe the feet inward
- Keep pelvis as level as possible
- Stand in *Tadasana*, resting arms to the sides
- Repeat to the left, reversing left/right instructions
- Rotate each leg up to 10 times each side to increase hip joint mobility
- Keep arm extension during leg rotation repetitions to develop endurance

Challenge

1. Inner knee or outer ankle strain
2. Pelvis drops on the right side
3. Torso turns as the right leg turns out
4. SI joint compression or instability
5. Ankle compression

Response

1. Turn left foot in, 30°-45°. Lift heel up wall, with the outer edge of foot to wall. Wedge a slant board under left heel and/or outer foot and abduct left femur.
2. Keep navel shifting to the left as right leg turns out. Soften internal abdominal organs and shift them to the left as well, *III f*. Tuck right buttock more strongly and increase vertical space between right femur and front ilium.
3. Push more firmly through left arm to hand. Resist left side rib cage backward as leg turns. *See Response 2.*
4. Without dropping right hip, allow left hip to roll forward.
5. Stretch the front and back of each foot away from ankles. *See Response 1, or Responses in Synthesize.*

From Uttitha Hasta Padasana, Parsva Hasta Padasana is the foundation of lateral Standing Poses. It differentiates leg and torso actions while developing external thigh rotation and hip mobility. Practicing it with the wall helps clarify the back leg's actions, and keeps the torso upright.

Contact Points

Feet, outer heel, hand

External Supports

Wall, mat

Essence of Form

Leg abduction, leg/hip articulation; legs externally rotated, arms neutral

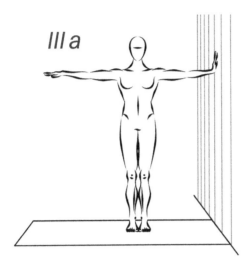

III a

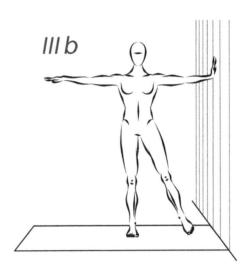

III b

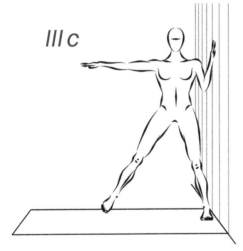

III c

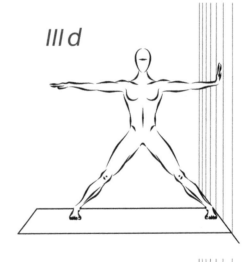

III d

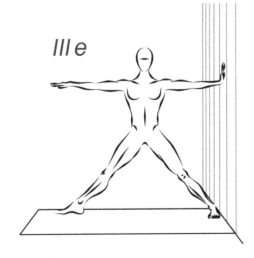

III e

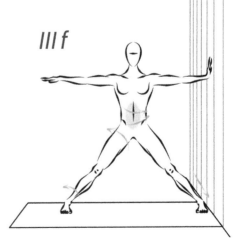

III f

Parsva Hasta Padasana
Lateral Wide Stance Pose

Synthesize

Learn + Practice

Once leg and pelvis actions are clear in Nourish, before lateral Standing Poses

Linked Poses

Lateral Standing Poses, Upavistha Konasana, Janu Sirsasana

Safety Factors

Groin injury, use care with knee injuries

Prepare

- Set mat away from wall

Enter

- Stand in *Tadasana* at mat's center
- Step or jump to *Uttitha Hasta Padasana, IV a*
- Follow instructions for *Nourish*, except:
- With left wrist neutral and palm horizontal, extend left arm as if pushing into wall to keep torso from turning as right leg rotates, *IV b*
- When turning right leg out, lift right heel and turn from ball of foot 45°, then lift ball of foot and turn from heel for remaining 45° to align right heel and left foot arch
- Soften right buttock while externally rotating leg; firm the lower buttock once leg is rotated to stabilize pelvis
- Rotate from as high in the right thigh as possible, at head of femur
- Vertically stack throat, respiratory, and pelvic floor diaphragms, keeping them level from side-to-side and front-to-back

Sustain

- Deepen left outer heel pressure and lift inner left arch and femur, *IV c*
- Externally rotate both legs while gathering front iliums, *IV d*
- Lift the right ilium up and away from the upper right femur
- Without rolling pelvis back, draw right front ilium to the left
- Laterally resist inner right femur toward outer right thigh
- Soften upper buttocks, firm lower buttocks
- Keeping upper buttocks soft, descend back pelvis and draw right sitting bone forward
- Without hardening buttocks or groins, activate quadriceps
- Release shoulders and extend both arms away from inner shoulder blades, *IV e*

Exit

- Increase left outer heel pressure
- Exhaling, turn the right leg in to *Uttitha Hasta Padasana*, and repeat, turning to the left
- Return to *Uttitha Hasta Padasana*, then inhale and step or jump to *Tadasana*, as for *Simplify* or *Explore*
- Release the arms and rest

Challenge

1. Right big toe mound lifts, straining knee ligaments as weight shifts to the outer foot
2. Right knee misalignment or hyperextension
3. Side body shortens from hips to armpits, shallow breath
4. Right groin binds as thighs firm

Response

1. Without internally rotating, push diagonally from right greater trochanter to right big toe mound, *IV f*. Keeping external rotation, lift right outer ankle and draw it inward.
2. Keep kneecaps lifted and in line with center of ankles. Increase external rotation from top thighs. Without bending the legs, widen backs of the knees and resist calves toward tibias. To learn this, wedge a block diagonally behind front calf, *IV g*.
3. Raise arms to *Urdhva Hastasana*. Lengthen side body from hips to armpits. Maintaining length, descend arms back to shoulder level.
4. Lighten right heel pressure to release groin. Alternatively, raise ball of foot on block, *IV h*.

Once the back heel action in Parsva Hasta Padasana is clear using the wall, transfer that activity without tactile feedback. If reasonable, jump to Uttitha Hasta Padasana, then turn the feet. With practice and repetition the movement progressively becomes smoother.

Contact Points

Feet
Back of calf in IV g
Ball of foot in IV h

External Supports

Mat
Block

Essence of Form

Leg abduction, leg/hip articulation; legs externally rotated, arms neutral

IV a
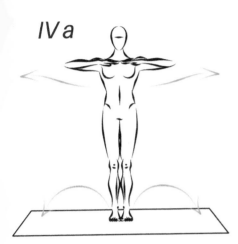

IV b
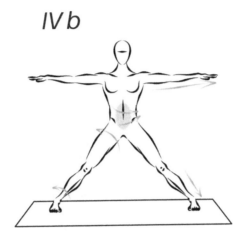

IV c
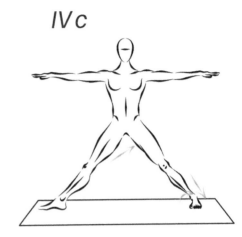

IV d
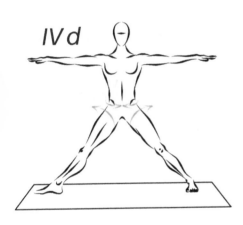

IV e
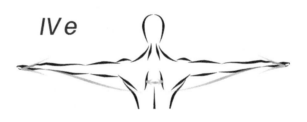

IV f
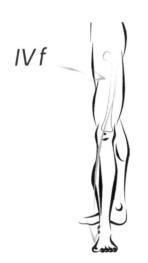

IV g
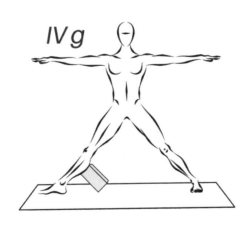

IV h
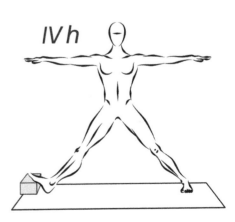

Prasarita Padottanasana A
Standing Wide-Legged Forward Bend

Simplify

Learn + Practice

Learn before deep Forward Bends and full Inversions

Linked Poses

Lateral Standing Poses, Upavistha Konasana, Uttanasana, and Sirsasana

Safety Factors

Groin, hamstring, or adductor injury; disc problem

Prepare

- Set the mat away from walls
- Place blocks on their ends at mat's long edge

Enter

- Stand in *Tadasana*, heels flush with opposite mat edge, *I a*
- Inhaling, step or jump to *Uttitha Hasta Padasana*, aligning heels on mat edge, *I b*
- Place hands on hips
- Press 4 corners of the feet away from back pelvis, into the floor
- Lift front iliums away from upper femurs, vertically aligning pubis and iliums
- Resist the heels laterally
- Gather the front iliums, engaging lower transverse abdominus no more than 20%
- Soften the pubis inward and draw the back of the pubis up
- Lift iliums up and over femur heads, rolling them diagonally toward opposite inner thighs
- Press weight into outer edges of feet and move L4 + L5 inward while folding pelvis up and over femurs, *I c*
- Place hands directly under shoulders on blocks, arms straight, *I d*

Sustain

- Once folded, redistribute weight symmetrically into all four corners of each foot, pushing them away from back pelvis
- Firming the thighs, press the upper femurs back and resist upper tibias forward
- Resisting heels laterally, draw lower inner femurs medially
- Broaden across back pelvis
- Continually lengthen the spine from coccyx to crown
- Without lifting heels, transfer weight forward into balls of feet
- Keeping hands pressing into blocks, lift torso away from floor
- Extend chest away from pubis
- Draw the chin slightly inward and extend occiput away from back ribs to lengthen back neck

Exit

- Press firmly into big toe mounds
- Inhaling, further lengthen spine
- Exhaling, place hands on hips
- With thighs firm, descend back pelvis lift the torso on inhalation
- Heel-toe the feet back to *Tadasana*
- Repeat, reducing block height, until the hands are flat on the floor with straight arms, *I e-g*

Challenge

1. Back rounds and chest collapses
2. Back inner knee pain
3. Ankle discomfort
4. Buttocks shift backward behind heels, *I i*

Response

1. Raise hands onto a chair instead of using blocks, *I h*. Widen between upper back femurs. Maintain *Enter* instructions while *Sustaining* the pose.
2. Without turning feet out and keeping big toe mound pressure, increase outer foot pressure and resist inner upper femurs laterally. Ensure inner knees are not pressing backward, rotate from the top thigh instead of knee joints.
3. Without changing foot pressure or leg rotation, draw the outer ankles inward. Slightly narrow stance and increase big toe mound pressure.
4. Walk hands forward on fingertips, shifting the weight into balls of feet. Keeping weight forward, walk hands under shoulders, *I j-k*.

This pose tones and lengthens the inner thighs, increases hip and ankle mobility, and releases the outer hamstrings. For some practitioners, the wider stance aids in tilting the pelvis over the femur heads, creating lumbar space.

Contact Points

Feet, hands

External Supports

Mat, 2 blocks
Chair

Essence of Form

Hip flexion, leg extension with abduction; legs slightly internally rotated, arms neutral

I a

I b

I c

I d

I e

I f

I g

I h

I i

I j

I k

Prasarita Padottanasana A
Standing Wide-Legged Forward Bend

Explore

Learn + Practice

Once hands reach floor in *Simplify*, before deep Forward Bends and Inversions

Linked Poses

Lateral Standing Poses, Upavistha Konasana, Uttanasana, and Sirsasana

Safety Factors

As for *Simplify*; hip replacement, meniscal tear, ankle injury

Prepare

· As for *Simplify*

Enter

· Follow the instructions for *Simplify, Enter*
· Place hands on floor or blocks
· Keep the arms fully extended and chest lifted
· Press the outer heels down and draw the outer ankles in
· Resisting the upper tibias back and without losing neutral spinal curves, exhale and bend the legs deeply, *II a*

Sustain

· All actions from *Simplify*
· Lift and widen inner back femurs
· Continue resisting the upper tibias backward as the legs bend
· Tuck pelvis if lumbar curve is excessively concave; untuck pelvis if lumbar is flattened or rounding, *II b*

Sustain

· Observe asymmetry in pelvic movement
· On side that folds less, move that ilium toward opposite inner thigh
· Soften and deepen both inner groins
· Equalize the inner groin spaces by widening the narrower side
· Lengthen pubis upward and backward while extending the chest forward, *II c*
· With the legs bent, tilt the pelvis more deeply and move the front iliums between the upper inner femurs, *II d*
· Keeping the iliums between the upper femurs, press upper femurs backward
· Widening upper femurs, hug lower femurs in
· Exhaling, press upper femurs backward to re-straighten the legs, *II e*

Exit

· As for *Simplify*, once legs are straight and firm
· Once in *Tadasana*, observe groin spaces and lower abdominal breath

Challenge

1. Pelvis tucks
2. Outer knee pain when legs are bent
3. Chest collapse
4. Outer buttock restriction

Response

1. Increase internal thigh rotation and establish deeper leg and pelvis actions in *Sustain*. Wrap a strap across and under the back iliums, around outer groins, over inner groins, between the legs and across the back thighs. Folding forward, pull strap ends laterally then forward, *II f-h* (also applicable to *Uttanasana*).
2. The pelvis is likely tucking or legs are externally rotating. Internally rotate from the top inner femurs and untuck the pelvis, lifting the sitting bones. *See Response 1.*
3. Use height under the hands. Resist hands toward the legs and away from each other. Externally rotate the upper arms. Extend from pubis to sternum. Practice *Simplify* more before moving to *Explore*.
4. Turn toes inward and deepen internal rotation at the upper femurs. *See Response 1.*

Bending the legs usually deepens the groins and increases the experience of folding the pelvis over the femurs. Doing so in a wide stance also creates lateral space in the hip joints. Use care, as this can be near end-range joint movement.

Contact Points

Feet, hands

External Supports

Mat, 2 blocks (if hands do not reach floor with neutral spine)
Strap

Essence of Form

Leg abduction, hip and knee flexion, arms and legs neutrally rotated

II a
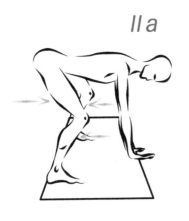

II b
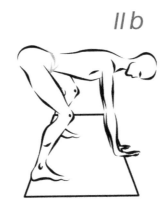

II c
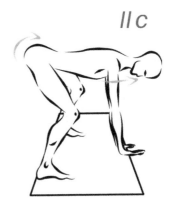

II d
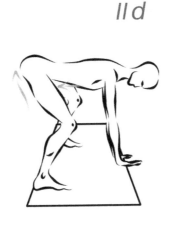

II e
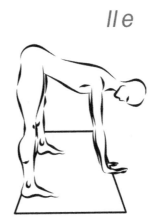

II f
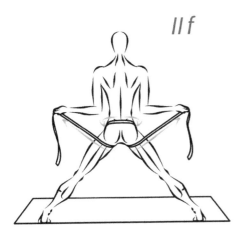

II g
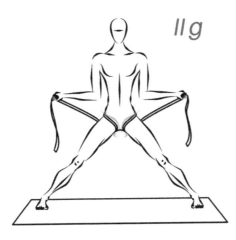

II h
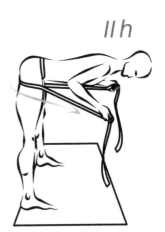

Learn + Practice

Once hands easily reach
the floor in *Simplify*,
alternative to Sirsasana

Linked Poses

Uttanasana, Sirsasana, Upavistha
Konasana, Chaturanga
Dandasana,
all bent-arm arm balances

Safety Factors

As for *Simplify + Explore*; be
cautious of leg hyperextension,
low blood pressure, neck injury

Prepare

- As for *Simplify*
- If head does not reach
  the floor, use a bolster
  perpendicular to mat
- In *III d*, set up with buttocks on
  the wall, heels slightly forward

Enter

- Follow instructions for
  Simplify, pressing more
  weight into the outer feet
- Without losing lumbar
  curve, place hands to floor
  directly under shoulders
- Inhaling, lengthen from
  pubis to sternum
- Exhaling, walk the hands between
  the feet, bending at the elbows
- Keep the hands and elbows
  shoulder-width apart, index
  fingers parallel to each other
- Forearms perpendicular to floor
- With a long spine, exhale
  and release the head to
  the bolster or floor, *III a-b*
- Transfer weight of pelvis
  forward as torso descends
- Do not strain to lower
  the torso and head
- Do not tilt or turn the head once
  it contacts the floor or support

Sustain

- Continue the leg actions
  from *Sustain* in *Simplify*
- Press index finger mounds
  down and lengthen fingers
  away from palms
- Inhaling, lengthen inner elbows
  away from inner armpits
- Exhaling, roll the outer
  elbows inward, *III c*
- Broaden across the collarbones
- Widen the upper shoulder
  blades and draw the lower
  shoulder blades inward
- Press crown into bolster or
  floor and lengthen spine
  from head to tail bone
- Lift inner groins away from
  skull, increasing torso length

Exit

- Increase big toe mound pressure
- Pressing into index finger
  mounds, inhale and extend
  arms, lifting torso
- Keeping the spine long
  and lifted, place hands
  on hips on exhalation
- With big toe mounds heavy,
  descend back pelvis and inhale
  to *Uttitha Hasta Padasana*
- Step or jump to *Tadasana*

Challenge

1. Leg hyperextension
2. Weight shifts backward
3. Elbows collapse outward
4. Blood pressure drops
   when *Exiting*
5. Eye strain and high
   blood pressure

Response

1. Without bending the legs,
   resist the tibia heads forward
   as the upper femurs press
   back. Move outer groins back
   and shift weight forward.
   See also Response 2.
2. Keeping pressure through
   balls of feet, lift the kneecaps.
   Practice with buttocks against
   wall, progressively moving
   heels closer to the wall, *III d*, until
   back thighs are against wall.
3. Turn hands outward. Strap
   elbows and draw outer
   elbows away from strap, *III e*.
4. Exhale (not inhale) to lift the torso
   in *Exit*, then rest forehead on the
   wall to balance blood pressure.
5. Rest the head and elbows on
   a chair, *III f*, to reduce inversion.
   Soften the jaw, lips, throat,
   tongue, and back of neck.

Prasarita Padottanasana's wide stance enables some practitioners to fully invert the torso, resulting in an important preparation and alternative to Inverted Poses. Helpful arm actions are also learned in this variation before significant weight is applied in later poses.

Contact Points

Feet, hands, crown

External Supports

Mat
Bolster, wall, strap, chair

Essence of Form

Hip, elbow, and wrist flexion, leg extension with abduction; arms externally rotated

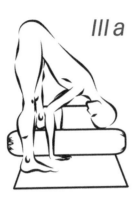

III a

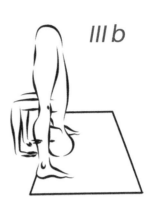

III b

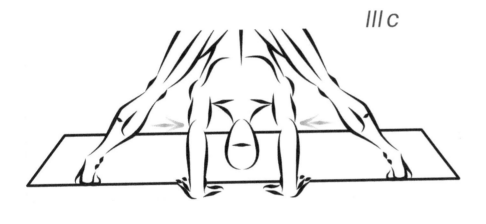

III c

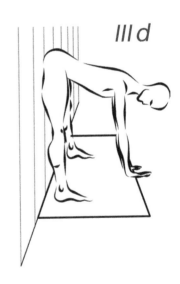

III d

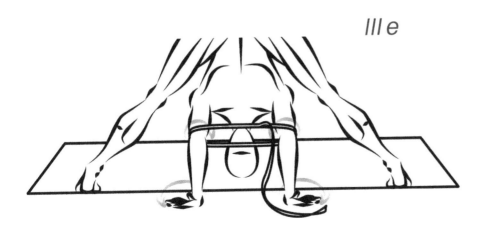

III e

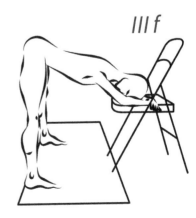

III f

Prasarita Padottanasana A
Standing Wide-Legged Forward Bend

Synthesize

Learn + Practice

Refinements can be learned at any stage

Linked Poses

All Forward Bends and poses with abductions and deep hip flexion

Safety Factors

As for Simplify, Explore, + Nourish; greater neck risk if head is touching floor

Prepare

- As for *Simplify*, use necessary props

Enter

- Enter the pose as for *Simplify* or *Nourish*

Sustain

- Transferring minimal weight into hands, lift heels off the floor, raising pelvis, *IV a*
- Keeping the pelvis lifted, descend outer heels, then inner heels, *IV b*
- Repeat, but initiate heel lift by lifting groins first
- Holding groin height, descend heels away from back pelvis
- Practice with arms straight first, lower hands and bend elbows only when necessary
- Keeping new leg length, deepen internal rotation at upper inner femurs
- With inner femurs moving

Sustain

- back, move outer femurs back to neutralize rotation
- Widen outer hamstrings away from inner hamstrings, *IV c*
- Rotate the big toe mounds internally and broaden the pelvic floor
- Soften the space between pubis and tail bone, and release both halves of that space equally
- With the lower pelvic space soft, release the tail bone into it
- Gently draw both halves of the lower pelvic area inward
- Soften pelvic floor and interior pelvic space
- Lengthen from hips to armpits

Exit

- Increase big toe mound pressure
- Keeping front iliums toward each other, think of drawing back iliums together as well at 5% engagement
- From this stability, place hands on hips
- Firm the thighs and lift kneecaps
- Descending the back pelvis, inhale and raise torso
- Return to *Tadasana* as for *Simplify* or *Nourish*

Challenge

1. Upper hamstring strain near insertion
2. Thoracic spine rounds
3. Ankle strain, despite previous *Responses*

Response

1. Further widen outer hamstrings away from inner hamstrings and resist hamstrings forward as femurs move back. Broaden sitting bones, but slightly tuck pelvis, drawing front iliums away from upper femurs.
2. Practice back to wall with bolster:
   - Stand facing the wall in *Uttitha Hasta Padasana*, 1.5'-2' from wall
   - Hold bolster behind upper back, *IV d*
   - Without twisting, bend the legs and fold forward
   - Walk toward the wall, leaning into the bolster, *IV e*
   - Resting toward the wall, straighten the legs, lifting pelvis, *IV f*
   - Continue with to *Sustain*
3. Broaden inner calves inward, away from outer calves, *IV g*. Squeeze mid-outer tibias toward each other, *IV h*.

bducting the legs can bring awareness to the pelvic floor. The wide stance is often more
table when refining groin and hamstring actions, making these actions more accessible. Once
earned, these refinements are applicable to nearly all poses, particularly deep Forward Bends.

Contact Points

Feet, hands
Back (IV d-f)

External Supports

Mat, (hand and head
support can be used)
Wall, bolster

Essence of Form

Hip flexion, leg extension with
abduction, heel lift + groin
depth; arms externally rotated

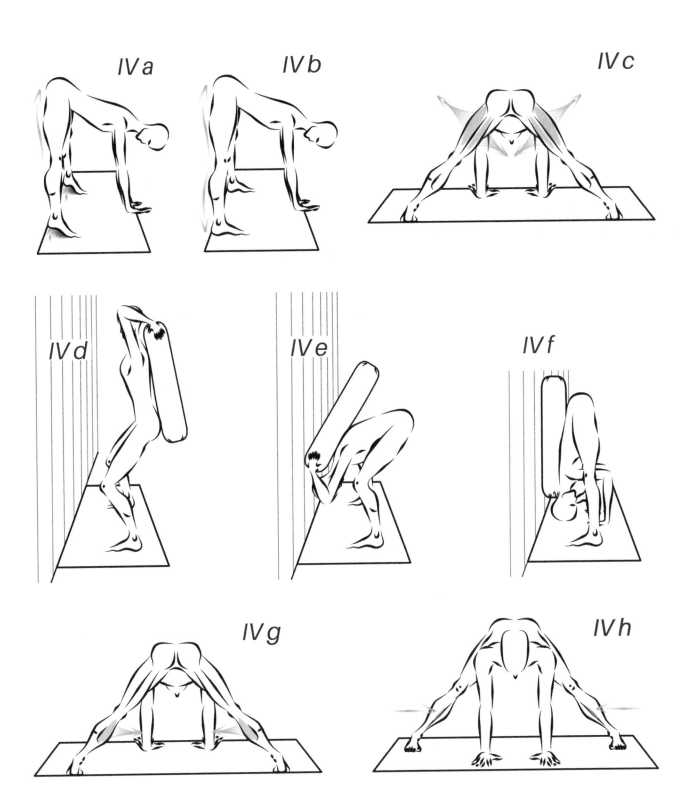

IV a

IV b

IV c

IV d

IV e

IV f

IV g

IV h

Learn + Practice

Once leg action is learned
in Tadasana, before
deep Forward Bends

Linked Poses

All Forward Bends, Adho Mukha
Svanasana, and Sirsasana

Safety Factors

Hamstring injury, disc problems,
low blood pressure

Prepare

- Place mat's short edge
  against the wall
- Set chair 1.5-2' away from
  wall, seat facing the wall
- Place bolster across chair seat
- Alternatively, set bolster
  lengthwise, through chair back

Enter

- Stand in *Tadasana*, with
  the heels to wall, *I a*
- Visually note foot
  distance from wall
- Resting buttocks on wall, step
  heels one foot length from wall
- Feet hip-width apart,
  mid lines parallel
- Place hands on hips, *I b*
- Press 4 corners of feet
  away from back pelvis
- Without hyperextending
  legs, firm the thighs and
  lift kneecaps upward
- Pushing through big toe
  mounds, resist heels outward
- Inhaling, lift pelvis up
  and over firm thighs
- Exhaling, press pelvis into wall
  and slide buttocks upward, *I c*
- Rest forehead and elbows
  on bolster, elbows clasped
  with opposite hands, *I d*

Sustain

- Spreading toes, equalize
  downward pressure through
  each foot, and all 4 corners of feet
- Press pelvis upward,
  widening sitting bones as
  feet press downward
- Press both sitting bones
  equally backward into wall
- Roll front iliums toward each other
- Soften pubis inward, lifting
  back of pubis upward
- Laterally release spinal muscles
- Lengthen torso away from wall
- Ensure forehead skin slides
  toward nose, not scalp, and
  extend occiput away from neck

Exit

- Exhaling, press hands into
  bolster or chair seat
- Inhaling, extend arms
  to lift torso, *I e*
- For short holds of one minute or
  less, firm thighs, descend back
  pelvis, inhale to standing, *I f*
- In longer holds, bend legs
  and press hands into front
  thighs, using arms to assist
  standing up on inhalation, *I g*
- Place forehead against wall to
  equalize blood pressure, *I h*

Challenge

1. Pelvic movement restricted by
   tight hamstrings, lumbar strain
2. Hyperextension at the knee
3. Soft thighs, knee instability
4. Legs externally rotate
   as pelvis folds
5. Inner arch collapse

Response

1. Place blocks under bolster
   until head is supported, *I i*.
   Practice over a table with whole
   torso supported, *I j*. Revisit
   *Supta Padangusthasana,
   Simplify + Explore*.
2. Without bending the legs, resist
   tibia heads forward, lift kneecaps
   using the Vastus Medialis, or
   lower inner quadricep muscles.
3. Increase big toe mound
   pressure, consciously lift
   kneecaps to firm thighs. Bend
   the legs very slightly and push
   the floor away to straighten legs.
4. Turn feet and legs inward,
   squeeze block between thighs
   and slide it backwards.
5. Keeping big toe mound
   pressure, lift and roll inner
   arches toward outer ankles, *I k*.
   Strap big toes together, spread
   toes away from strap, *I l*.

Supported Uttanasana allows the spine and torso to release slowly. Resting the buttocks on the wall helps encourage the pelvis tilt forward as the hamstrings lengthen. This semi-Restorative variation can be placed early in sequences or near the end as it is usually calming.

Contact Points

Feet, sitting bones, forehead, hands

External Supports

Mat, wall, chair, bolster
Table, strap; blocks may be used to elevate bolster

Essence of Form

Hip flexion, leg extension; legs slightly internally rotated, arms passively internal

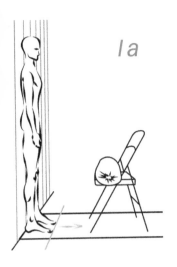 Ia

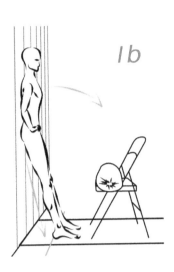 Ib

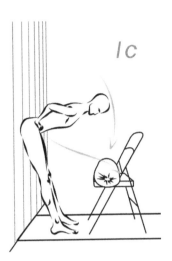 Ic

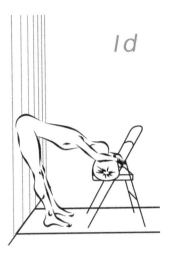 Id

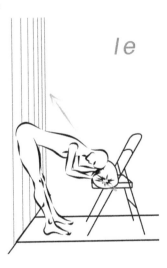 Ie

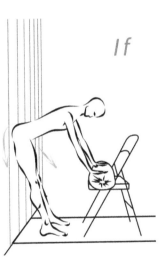 If

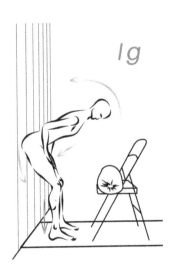 Ig

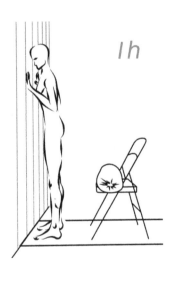 Ih

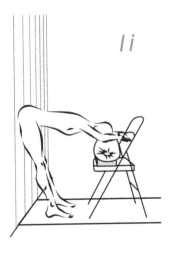 Ii

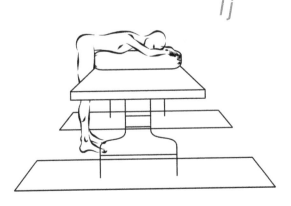 Ij

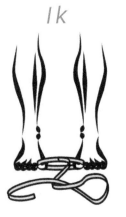 Ik

 Il

Standing Forward Bend — *Simplify*

Learn + Practice

After Simplify, when pelvis can fold over femurs with firm legs

Linked Poses

All Forward Bends, Adho Mukha Svanasana, and Sirsasana

Safety Factors

As for Simplify

Prepare

- Set 2 blocks on end, shoulder-width apart
- Arrange additional blocks between first two for head support, adjusting if necessary after *Entering*

Enter

- Stand behind blocks in *Tadasana*, with the feet hip-width apart
- Inhaling, raise arms to *Urdhva Hastasana* to lengthen torso
- Keeping torso length, exhale and place hands on hips, *II a*
- Resist heels and greater trochanters laterally
- Inhaling, gather front iliums and lift them upward
- Lifting kneecaps, roll iliums up and over thighs, toward each other on exhalation
- Move pelvis backward minimally while folding, with weight centered over ankles
- Without dropping chest, place hands on blocks, arms fully extended, *II b-c*
- Inhale, lengthen from pubis to sternum
- Keeping length, bend elbows and lower head to central blocks, *II d-e*

Sustain

- As for *Simplify*, but keep pelvis over ankles
- Sharpen big toe mound pressure
- Lift inner arches and roll them toward outer ankles
- Without pushing knees back, maintain lifted kneecaps
- Keeping legs straight, resist tibia heads forward
- Internally rotate from top thighs
- Continually lengthen from pubis to sternum, sternum to pubis
- Pressing hands into blocks, resist them toward feet to lengthen side torso
- Keep head in line with spine
- In , *II d-e*, roll outer elbows inward and lengthen them away from armpits
- Extend occiput away from shoulder blades and lift pelvis away from head pressure

Exit

- Firm the thighs
- Inhale, push hands into blocks to straighten arms and lift chest, *II b-c*
- Exhale, place hands on hips
- Resisting heels laterally, descend back pelvis and inhale to standing

Challenge

1. Weight sinks back into heels
2. Leg hyperextension
3. Overstretch sensation in hamstrings or back of knees
4. Blood pressure drops on standing

Response

ॐ *Responses 1 + 2 are related:*

1. Without lifting heels, transfer weight forward into balls of feet. Increase big toe mound pressure and lift quadriceps.
2. Do not compensate for weight transference by jamming knees backward; resist tibia heads forward as upper femurs press back. Ensure knees are not internally rotating more than upper femurs and keep inner arches lifting.
3. Reduce intensity by 10% and broaden laterally where overstretch is felt. Resist flesh toward bone, bone toward flesh. Keeping pelvis lifted, release tail bone downward.
4. *Exit* with an exhalation instead of inhalation. Rest forehead on a wall or drag forehead skin down with heel of hand after standing.

In Uttanasana, the head is below the heart, which both rests and invigorates the brain increasing circulation. Supporting the hands and bending the elbows can lower heart rate, and supporting the head helps regulate blood pressure changes.

Contact Points

Feet, hands, crown of head

External Supports

Mat, 4-6 blocks
Strap

Essence of Form

Hip flexion, leg extension, elbow flexion; legs slightly internally rotated, arms slightly external

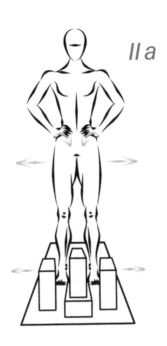

II a

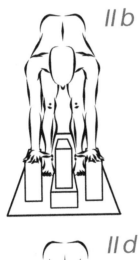

II b

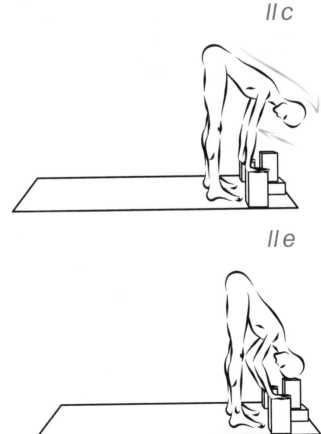

II c

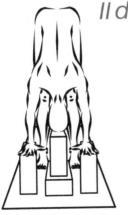

II d

II e

Learn + Practice

Once pelvis folds with relative ease in *Simplify* or *Explore*, near the end of practice

Linked Poses

All Forward Bends,
Adho Mukha Svanasana,
Sirsasana and Inversions

Safety Factors

As for *Simplify*; ensure pressure is on groins, not abdomen

Prepare

- Set mat's short end to wall
- Lean folded chair against wall, seat facing outward, *III a*

Enter

- Stand facing the wall in *Tadasana*, 2-3' from it
- Tilt the chair and place the chair legs in the wall/floor juncture
- Step forward or backward bringing the chair to the groins, at the level of the pubis, *III b*
- Stabilizing the legs, press chair back into upper femurs while lifting pelvis up, *III c*
- Exhaling, fold the pelvis up and over the chair (and femurs)
- Walk the hands down the chair legs, descending the torso to reasonable capacity, *III d*

Sustain

- Lean into chair, pressing the femurs back and lifting groins
- With groins lifted, reach heels away from back pelvis
- Continually softening groins, receive chair pressure

Sustain

- Lift front iliums away from femurs, gradually lengthening torso over chair
- Resist heels laterally and gather front iliums
- Release spinal muscles laterally
- To deepen the pose: shift weight forward and lift heels, tipping chair closer to wall, *III e*
- Chair angle lifts groins and pelvis more fully
- With heels lifted, and keeping groin height, walk feet closer to wall, under pelvis, *III f*
- Reaching away from new pelvic height, descend outer heels, then inner heels, *III g*

Exit

- Walk hands up chair legs and press chair back into femurs
- Shift weight backward and bend legs symmetrically, *III h*
- Without twisting or hitting head on wall, press chair into femurs and descend back pelvis
- Inhaling, lift torso as back pelvis descends, *III i*
- Set chair against wall and step forward, resting forehead on wall to equalize blood pressure, *III j*
- Once blood pressure is equalized, step away from wall

Challenge

1. Chair is too low, not reaching hip creases
2. Chair is too high
3. Chair too close to wall, causing twist in *Enter* and *Exit*
4. Chair unfolds when *Entering* or *Sustaining*
5. Chair pressure is too hard, irritating groins

Response

1. Set blocks against wall and stand chair legs on blocks, *III k*.
2. Step away from wall, tipping the chair further.
3. Set blocks against wall as in *Response 1*, but use blocks as spacer between chair and wall, *III l*.
4. Hold chair legs together to keep chair folded, or tie a strap around closed chair legs.
5. Pad chair back with a folded mat or blanked. Ensure the chair back is in the hip creases, between femurs and iliums. Recede the pubis and soften the groins.

🕉 *Responses 1 + 3 can be combined, using 4 or more blocks to raise chair and increase space from wall*

Supporting the pelvis over a chair in Uttanasana both deepens the fold at the groins and maintains space between the femurs and front iliums. Learn before deep Forward Bends to help incorporate that action. Moving the femurs back facilitates a feeling of calm stability.

Contact Points

Feet, groins, hands, possibly forehead

External Supports

Mat, wall, chair
2-4 blocks, strap, blanket

Essence of Form

Hip flexion, leg extension; arms passively externally rotated, legs slightly internal

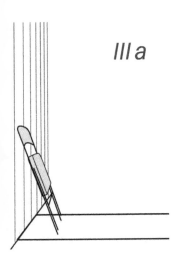

III a

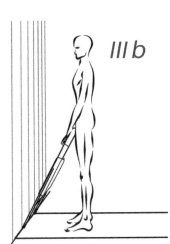

III b

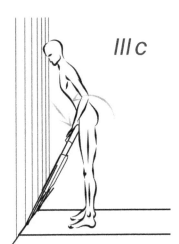

III c

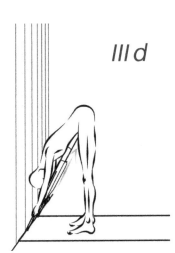

III d

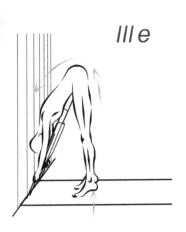

III e

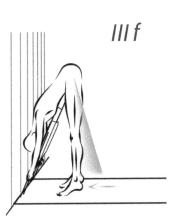

III f

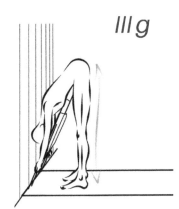

III g

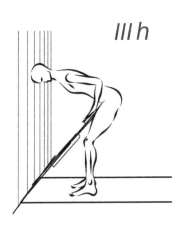

III h

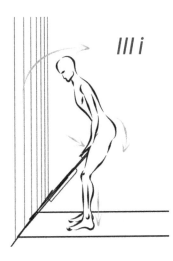

III i

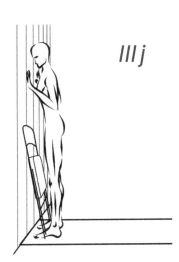

III j

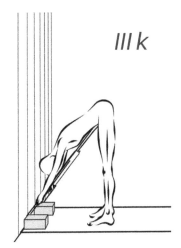

III k

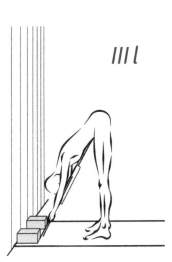

III l

Uttanasana
Standing Forward Bend

Synthesize

Learn + Practice

Once pelvis folds with relative ease in Explore, near the end of practice

Linked Poses

All Forward Bends, Adho Mukha Svanasana, Sirsasana and Inversions

Safety Factors

As for Simplify; be sure not to work beyond capacity or to force fold

Prepare

- Stand in *Tadasana*, big toes together, heels slightly apart

Enter

- Firming the thighs, inhale and raise arms, *IV a*
- Engage preparatory actions from *Simplify, Explore, + Nourish*
- Moving pelvis minimally backward, lift pelvis up and over femurs, folding forward
- Bring hands to floor, *IV b*
- Inhaling, lengthen from pubis to sternum, lifting to fingertips if necessary, *IV c*
- Keeping torso length, exhale and fold torso toward thighs
- Walk hands beside, then behind feet if reasonable, *IV d*

Sustain

- As for *Explore*
- Lift and separate all 10 toes to activate arches
- Keeping arches active, lengthen toes outward and lightly lower them to floor

Sustain

- Using lift action from arches, press back pelvis toward ceiling, away from feet
- Feel directional leg length: one lengthens down, the other upward, *IV e*
- Equalize both directions in each leg, *IV f*
- Lengthen shorter feeling leg
- Widen across back of thighs
- Press upper femurs back and lift front iliums, maximizing that space
- Extend side torso, increase spaces between each rib, between ribs and pelvis
- Distribute stretch sensation through entire posterior chain from feet to forehead

Exit

- Inhale to lift torso and look forward, coming to fingertips
- Exhale bring hands to hips, or if uninjured, sweep arms to sides
- Pushing into big toe mounds, descend back pelvis
- Firming thighs and using buttocks and hamstrings to lift, inhale to raise torso
- Release hands to sides and rest in *Tadasana*

Challenge

1. Pelvic space narrows
2. Overstretch in lumbar spine
3. Neck tension (also applicable to *Explore*)

Response

1. Broaden stance. Resist heels and femurs laterally to widen groins. Without narrowing groin space, narrow stance as capacity permits. Internally rotate thighs and feet deeply, beyond neutral rotation.
2. Reduce intensity 10%. Without compressing sacrum, minimally gather posterior iliums. Lift front iliums away from front femurs. *Also see Response 1.*
3. Soften scalp and face, release occiput away from back ribs. Widen upper shoulder blades, narrow lower shoulder blades. Lengthen from armpits to inner elbows, releasing trapezius. Rest shoulders on 2 chairs (with foam blocks if height is needed), *IV g.*

※ *Refer to Prasarita Padottanasana for additional Challenges, Responses, and ways to work*

Standing Forward Bends generally facilitate a deeper fold in the pelvis than when seated. Practicing Uttanasana without props balances release and stability, and can reduce insomnia, fatigue, and depression when done regularly.

Contact Points

Feet, hands
Shoulders (IV g)

External Supports

Mat
2 chairs, 2 foam blocks

Essence of Form

Hip flexion, leg extension;
arms slightly externally
rotated, legs slightly internal

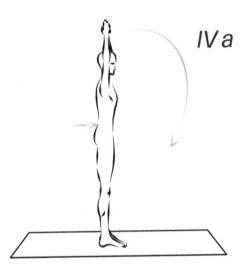

IV a

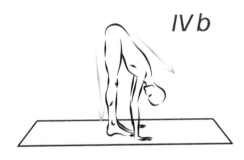

IV b

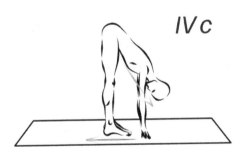

IV c

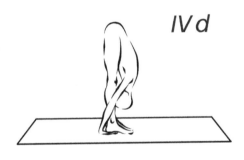

IV d

IV e

IV f

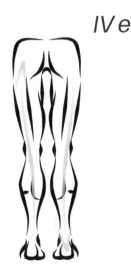

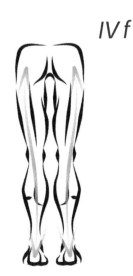

IV g

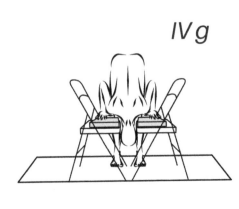

Simplify

Learn + Practice

Learn early, once Tadasana is stable and before bent-leg Standing Poses

Linked Poses

All bent-leg Standing Poses; particularly Virabhadrasana A

Safety Factors

Use care with knee injury; do not raise arms if hypertense

Prepare

- Set mat's short end to wall

Enter

- Stand with back to wall
- Walk feet forward, 18-24", until legs are 45° to wall and floor, *I a*
- Have the feet hip-width apart, foot mid lines parallel
- Rest back pelvis and back ribs on wall
- With the lumbar spine neutral, bring hands to hips
- Spreading toes, anchor 4 corners of feet
- Gather front iliums and resist heels laterally
- Soften pubis in and up
- Exhaling, bend both legs 90°, sliding pelvis down wall until femurs are parallel to floor and tibias are vertical, *I b*
- Keeping back ribs against wall, extend arms forward, *I c*
- Without losing back rib contact, raise arms to *Urdhva Hastasana, I d*

༄ *For a deeper arm/shoulder opening, place hands on wall beside head before descending pelvis and press hands to wall as legs bend, I e-f*

Sustain

- Maintain *Enter* actions
- Without collapsing knees inward, increase big toe mound pressure
- Equalize inner and outer heel pressure
- Keeping thighs parallel, circularly roll inner ankles toward outer ankles, *I g*
- Extend back femurs away from back pelvis
- Lift front pelvis up as femurs descend
- Resist tibia heads backward toward wall/pelvis, *I h*
- Balance back pelvis against wall
- Minimally gather posterior iliums

Exit

- Stabilize pelvis and big toe mounds
- Firm both thighs
- Pushing feet away from back pelvis, inhale and straighten legs, sliding pelvis up wall
- Extend legs until kneecaps are fully lifted
- Bring hands to hips (if raised overhead)
- Walk feet back toward wall
- Rest, and repeat up to 10 times

Challenge

1. Tibias not vertical
2. Pelvis slides below knee level
3. Knees fall inward or splay outward
4. Knee pain
5. Lumbar strain

Response

1. Do not adjust while in the pose. *Exit* and move the feet forward or back, then re-*Enter*.
2. Feet too far from wall, see *Response 1*. Press feet forward while drawing tibia heads back
3. For inward collapse, strap lower thighs and resist outward. For splaying knees, squeeze a block between knees.
4. Ensure femurs are horizontal. Draw heels backward to engage hamstrings, *I i*. Strengthen quadriceps with seated leg raises and leg extensions, *I j-k. See Responses 2 + 3*.
5. Strap big toes and resist laterally, *I l*. Decrease leg bend, but always keep tibias vertical. Flatten lumbar against wall, increase neutral curve over time. *See prior Responses.*

Utkatasana builds strength in the legs, particularly the thighs and hamstrings. Practicing with a wall teaches the legs to bend at 90° with the femurs parallel to the floor and the tibias vertical, which is an important relationship in bent-leg Standing Poses.

Contact Points
Feet, back pelvis, back torso

External Supports
Mat, wall
Chair, block, strap

Essence of Form
Hip and knee flexion; arms and legs in neutral rotation

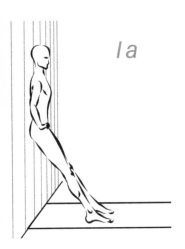
I a

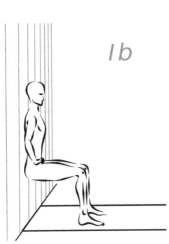
I b

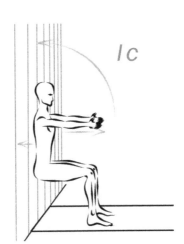
I c

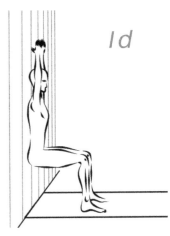
I d

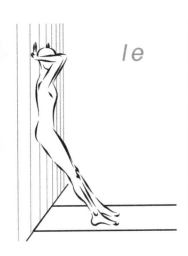
I e

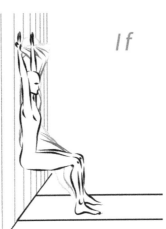
I f

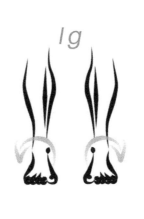
I g

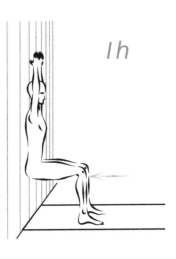
I h

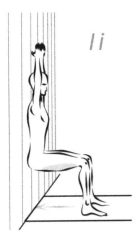
I i

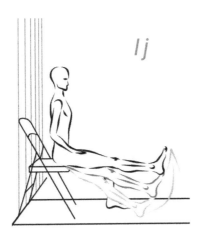
I j

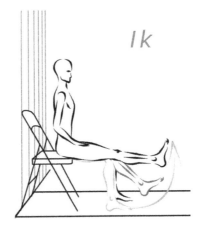
I k

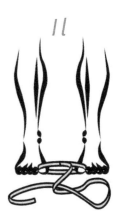
I l

Utkatasana
Fierce/Chair Pose

Learn + Practice

As soon as Simplify is stable, before practicing jumping transitions

Linked Poses

All bent-leg Standing Poses; jumping movements and transitions

Safety Factors

Use care with knee injury; keep hands on hips if hypertense

Prepare

- Place a chair on the mat
- Set a block near the chair

Enter

- Sit at chair's edge, feet hip-width apart and parallel, legs bent 90°
- Place block between lower femurs, *II a*
- Extend arms to *Urdhva Hastasana, II b*
- Gather the front iliums
- Squeezing the block, resist heels laterally and widen greater trochanters
- Without collapsing arches, increase big toe mound pressure and stabilize feet
- Pushing feet away from back pelvis, shift weight slightly forward and stand straight up on inhalation, *II c-g*
- Fully extend legs and arms in *Tadasana Urdhva Hastasana, II h*
- Keeping arm and torso lift, fold legs and pelvis to sit back on chair on exhalation
- Repeat standing and sitting 5-10 times

🕉 *Once stable, do not sit on chair — lower to 1" from chair and press back up to standing*

Sustain

- Maintain equal pressure through 4 corners of each foot
- Keep thigh and pelvis actions throughout
- Minimize lateral wobble and shift at ankles, knees, and pelvis
- Push evenly through both feet and legs
- Limit and reduce forward torso pitch with each repetition
- Use arm extension to assist lift when standing and control descent when sitting back down
- Resist tibias forward when standing up, backward when sitting down
- Without externally rotating legs, tone lower buttocks and release upper buttocks
- Each repetition, gradually reduce weight into chair until sitting bones barely touch chair

Exit

- On last repetition, remain standing in *Tadasana*
- Lower arms and remove block
- Once movement is smooth, steady, and symmetrical, practice without block, keeping leg integrity and actions

Challenge

1. Not enough force generated to stand
2. Torso shifts too far forward
3. Pelvis too far from chair when sitting

Response

1. Instead of raising arms, press hands into front thighs, *II i*. Push thighs downward and resist torso upward during both sitting and standing phases. Squeeze block to activate thighs and generate lift. Raise chair seat height with foam blocks or folded blankets until standing and sitting are easy, *II j-k*. Gradually reduce height as mobility increases.
2. *Prepare* facing the wall. Attempt to not touch the wall on both sitting and standing, *II l*. Set-up closer and closer to the wall as torso shift decreases. Descend back pelvis while sitting rather than pushing sitting bones backward in anterior tilt. *See also Nourish*.
3. Sit further back in the chair. Raise seat height as in *Response 1*.

Moving in and out of Utkatasana increases mobility in the hips, knees and ankles while further strengthening the thighs. It also exercises the diaphragm, balancing upper and lower torso breath while developing overall breath capacity.

Contact Points

Feet, sitting bones, inner knees

External Supports

Mat, wall, chair, block
Foam blocks or folded blanket

Essence of Form

Leg extension from flexion, flexion from extension; Arms and legs neutral

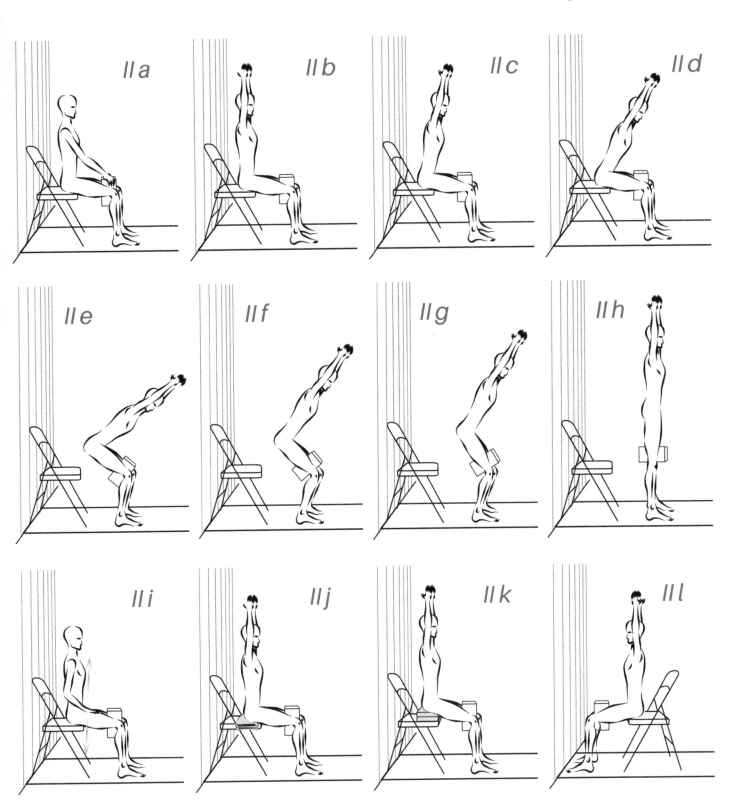

Utkatasana
Fierce/Chair Pose

Learn + Practice

When Explore movement is smooth and the torso pitches forward minimally

Linked Poses

Bent-leg Standing Poses, Virabhadrasana A, Back Bending poses

Safety Factors

Use care with knee and some back injuries; do not raise the arms if hypertense

Prepare

- Practice in a door frame

Enter

- Holding a 2-4' stick, stand in a door frame in *Tadasana*
- Bring feet hip-width apart, foot mid lines parallel, *III a*
- Raise stick overhead, hands shoulder-width apart, palms facing forward, *III b*
- For deeper armpit/chest opening, externally rotate arms, turning palms to face backward, *III c*
- Increasing big toe mound pressure, resist lower femurs inward
- Resist heels laterally and gather front iliums, softening pubis inward
- Bending the legs, descend pelvis
- Bring tibia heads back as femurs lengthen forward, *III d*
- Without collapsing knees, descend until femurs are parallel to floor, *III e*
- Keep arms and torso as vertical as possible
- Move closer to door frame over time, with door frame between lower thighs *III f*

Sustain

- Maintain leg and pelvis actions
- Keep heels firmly anchored
- Lift inner arches
- Lengthen femurs away from back pelvis
- Soften between pubis and tail bone, then move them toward each other
- Without tucking, descend back pelvis
- Lift back ribs away from back pelvis, *III g*
- Draw front ribs inward, lift sternum, *III h*
- Keep arms as vertical as possible
- Make descending and ascending actions smoother with each repetition

Exit

- Anchor outer heels and big toe mounds
- Inhaling, extend legs away from back pelvis to straighten
- Resist tibia heads forward and femurs back when extending legs
- Repeat 5-10 times, moving closer to door frame edge as possible
- When finished, lower arms

Challenge

1. Arms do not straighten in *Tadasana*
2. Heels lift on full descent
3. Lumbar and/or thoracic pain, shoulder restriction

Response

1. Press stick up into top of door frame while bending the legs until the arms straighten. Keep pushing stick up, attempting to maintain contact with top of door frame as legs bend.
2. Descend until just before heels lift. Practice calf stretches *III i-j*. Elevate the heels on a wedge or board, *III k* on alternate practice days.
3. Slightly tuck pelvis. Widen sitting bones and move tail bone forward. Minimally gather back iliums. Lift back ribs away from back pelvis and widen grip on stick to bring arms vertical. Descend only to point immediately before pain. Hang from top of door, with a mat over door for grip, blocks under feet to create traction on shoulders and spine, *III l*.

The torso often pitches forward in Utkatasana to counterbalance bending at the hips and knees. Practicing in a door frame helps teach keeping the torso more vertical as the legs bend, the knees on either side of the door frame. This variation challenges and strengthens the spinal muscles.

Contact Points

Feet, hands (holding stick)

External Supports

Door frame, stick
Wall, slanted board,
door, blocks, mat

Essence of Form

Knee and hip flexion with arm
and torso extension; arms
externally rotated, legs neutral

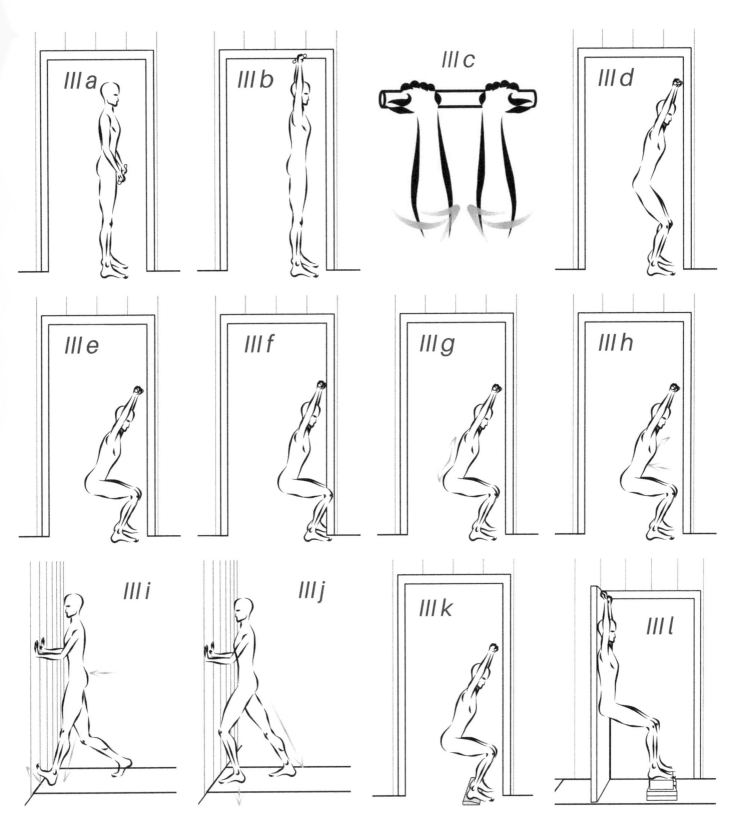

Learn + Practice

Once challenges are addressed in *Simplify, Explore, + Nourish*

Linked Poses

Virasana, Malasana, Pashasana, Bakasana

Safety Factors

Do not raise arms if hypertense; do not tolerate knee pain

Prepare

- With or without mat, away from wall

Enter

- Stand in *Tadasana*
- Inhaling, raise arms to *Urdhva Hastasana, IV a*
- Resist lower femurs medially; heels laterally
- Gather front iliums, soften pubis in and up
- Resisting tibia heads backward, lengthen femurs away from back pelvis
- Exhale and fold legs and pelvis until femurs are parallel to floor, *IV b*

Sustain

- Continue *Sustain* actions from *Simplify, Explore, + Nourish*
- Lift inner ankles and draw outer ankles inward, *IV c*
- Keeping tibia heads drawing back, pull heels back as well, activating hamstrings
- Widen calves and hamstrings

Sustain

- Lengthen inner and outer femurs equally
- Deepen front and inner groins
- Broaden across back pelvis
- Tone lower buttocks
- Release upper buttock flesh down and outward, away from lumbar, *IV d*
- Descend upper femurs, *IV e*
- Lift pelvis away from femurs
- Soften lower sternum inward and lift upper sternum
- Deepen armpits and roll outer armpits forward, *IV f*
- Lengthen inner shoulder blades down, and widen upper shoulder blades, *IV g*
- Roll trapezium downward while extending undersides of arms, *IV h*
- Extend back of skull away from mid-shoulder blades

Exit

- With big toe mounds and tail bone heavy, push into floor and inhale to extend legs to *Tadasana*
- Resist tibia heads forward and femurs back while extending legs
- Exhaling, lower arms and rest

Challenge

1. Buttocks and front ribs protrude, *IV i*
2. Groins bind
3. Arches collapse
4. Thigh fatigue

Response

1. Shift pelvis forward and torso back. Descend back pelvis and draw sitting bones toward back knees, *IV j*. Increase heel pressure.
2. Press more firmly into balls of feet and decrease heel pressure.
3. Resist big toes toward each other. Without collapsing knees inward, ensure heels are further apart than big toes. Keeping big toe mound pressure, increase outer heel pressure and roll inner ankles toward outer ankles.
4. Not usually problematic unless accompanied by knee pain. *See Responses in Simplify, Explore, + Nourish*. Build endurance for longer holds progressively and practice long holds and repetitions on alternate practice days. Engage inner quadriceps, especially when *Exiting*.

Freestanding Utkatasana strengthens the lower leg muscles. As the arms extend upward and the pelvis descends, the diaphragm tones and lifts. This also tones the pelvic floor and develops resilience in the deep postural muscles.

Contact Points

Feet

External Supports

Mat

Essence of Form

Hip and knee flexion, arm extension; Arms and legs in neutral rotation

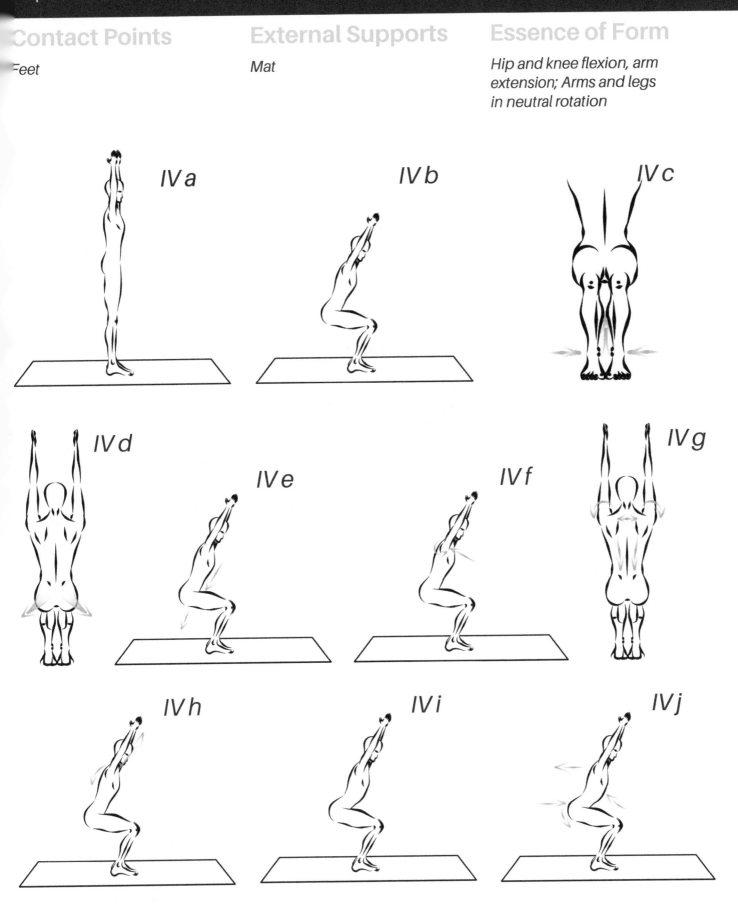

Simplify

Learn + Practice

Learn before bent-leg Standing Poses and practice before Back Bends

Linked Poses

Virabhadrasana A, Supta Virasana, all Back Bends

Safety Factors

Knee, groin, or quadricep injury

Prepare

- Place mat's short end to wall
- Set blocks on end on either side of mat, around mid-mat

Enter

- Kneel with back to wall, sitting on heels, toes close to wall, *I a*
- Lean forward and place hands on blocks
- Inhaling, lift pelvis off heels, *I b*
- Do not stand on knees for long
- Exhaling, step right foot forward between or beyond blocks, *I c*
- Bring right tibia vertical, stepping further forward if necessary
- Walk hands and blocks forward to each side of right foot
- Keep right knee directly on top of right ankle
- Flex left foot and press ball of foot into floor
- Lift left knee slightly off floor and bring left heel to wall, ball of foot at wall/floor juncture, *I d*
- Maintain left heel pressure and rest left knee on floor with minimal weight

ॐ *Once stable and groin and quadricep length develops, fully extend left leg, pushing back through heel into wall*

Sustain

- Pressing back through left heel, draw left ilium forward
- Keeping left knee contact with floor, lift left upper femur, *I e*
- Increasing right big toe mound pressure, draw right outer hip back and down, *I f*
- Soften and deepen right groin
- Keeping tibia vertical, lengthen right femur from groin to inner lower thigh
- Descend right inner thigh as left inner thigh ascends
- Lift right armpit away from right groin and equalize length along both sides of torso, *I g*
- Pressing hands down into blocks, lift chest away from hands, *I h*

Exit

- Increase left heel pressure
- Lift left knee slightly from floor
- Pressurize hands into blocks
- Step right leg back on exhalation
- Bring both knees to floor and sit back on heels in *Vajrasana*
- Rest for a few breaths, and repeat on the second side
- If continuing to other Back Bends, do not fold forward in *Uttana Balasana*

Challenge

1. Front tibia is not vertical, *I i*
2. Knee pain from floor pressure
3. Groin binds, obstructing step forward and closing front body
4. Lower back discomfort

Response

1. Step right foot forward, but avoid inching front foot forward or back, which destabilizes the knee. Instead, press hands into blocks and lift foot completely off the floor. With foot lifted, step forward or back to verticalize tibia, *I j*. Resist head of right tibia backward.
2. Place folded blanket across mat to pad under knees in *Prepare*, *I k*. Press left heel more deeply into wall to reduce weight on left knee and increase front foot and hand pressure.
3. Increase space between leg and torso, using a chair instead of blocks, *I l*. See also *Response 1 in Explore and Response 4 in Nourish.*
4. Without increasing knee pressure, move pelvis slightly backward, *I m*. Lengthen left femur away from back pelvis. Roll left ilium forward.

Lunges strengthen the legs, tone the buttocks, and lengthen the groins and quadriceps. Practicing lunges with the back leg bent lengthens the quadriceps; extending the leg has a deeper effect on the groins. They are an excellent preparation for Standing Poses and Back Bends.

Contact Points

Feet, hands, back knee

External Supports

Mat, wall, 2 blocks
Blanket, chair

Essence of Form

Front leg and hip flexion back leg flexion, hip extension; arms and legs in neutral rotation

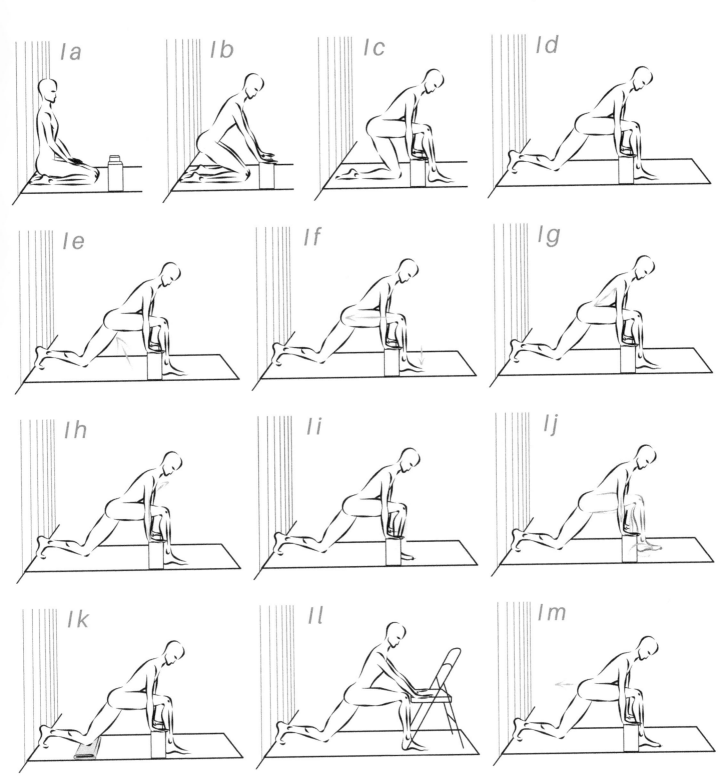

Learn + Practice

Once back leg fully extends in *Simplify*, before *Virabhadrasana A*

Linked Poses

Virabhadrasana A, all asymmetrical Standing Poses, Back Bends

Safety Factors

Knee, groin, or quadricep injury

Prepare

· Note front foot's distance from wall in *Simplify*
· Place blocks this distance from wall

Enter

· Stand in *Tadasana* between blocks
· With thighs firm, lift pelvis and fold to *Uttanasana*, hands to blocks, *II a-b*
· Anchor right big toe mound
· Keeping left leg straight, bend right leg and step left foot back toward wall, *II c*
· Bring left heel to wall, bending right leg to 90° with right tibia vertical, *II d*

Sustain

· Fully extend left leg, pressing left heel away from back pelvis into wall
· Draw left ilium forward away from heel
· Without lifting pelvis, ascend left femur, *II e*

Sustain

· Keeping left leg in neutral rotation, firm left buttock
· Keep right knee tracking straight forward and without collapsing right knee inward, increase big toe mound pressure
· Lift and spread toes, lengthening them forward as they lower
· Descend right femur, *II f*
· Extend right sitting bone backward, toward wall, *II g*
· Bring pelvis level relative to floor and wall
· Resist heels laterally
· Release tail bone symmetrically
· Equalize side body length
· Pressing into hands, lift and widen chest
· Keep head neutral, lengthening the back of the neck, *II h*

Exit

· Press hands to blocks
· Increase right big toe mound pressure
· Keeping left leg straight, inhale and step left foot forward to *Uttanasana*, *II i*
· Repeat, stepping right leg back
· After the second side, from *Uttanasana* firm the thighs and descend the back pelvis, inhaling to *Tadasana*

Challenge

1. Front leg groin binds
2. Back thigh and groin sag
3. Back leg knee pain

Response

1. Lift front heel 1" from floor. Release groin and upper femur, *II j*. Keeping groin released, descend heel to floor. Once learned, reduce heel pressure without losing floor contact. Partially straighten right leg, reduce heel pressure, and return to 90° fold.
2. Support back leg thigh with blocks, *II k*. Lift thigh away from this contact. Dig ball of foot into floor and lift femur. Push through the back leg heel and emphasize length in back of thigh rather than seeking stretch sensation in the front of the thigh.
3. Change pressure through back heel, either increasing or decreasing, balance inner and outer heel pressure. Often caused by tight quads — return to *Simplify* or practice quadricep stretches, *II l*.

Lunges also teach the front leg groin to soften and deepen — an essential action for Standing Poses and Forward Bends. Stepping backward from Uttanasana is often more accessible than stepping forward from Adho Mukha Svanasana, and emphasizes depth in the front groin.

Contact Points

Hands, Feet

External Supports

Mat, wall, 2 blocks
Additional blocks

Essence of Form

Back leg and hip extension, front leg and hip flexion; arms and legs neutrally rotated

II a

II b

II c

II d

II e

II f

II g

II h

II i

II j

II k

II l

Anjaneyasana
Lunge Pose

Nourish

Learn + Practice

Once Explore transitions are smooth, in conjunction with hip openers

Linked Poses

Parsvakonasana, Marichyasana A, Pincha Mayurasana, Eka Pada Koundinyasana

Safety Factors

Groin or quad pull, knee injury, some lower back injuries — do not practice if pain is caused

Prepare

- Mat's short end to wall
- Blocks on each side of mat's far end

Enter

- Lie on the belly, heels to wall, hands under shoulders, *III a*
- Anchor both heels against wall
- Exhaling lift to all fours position, *III b*
- Keeping heels to wall, press into hands and exhale to lift thighs up and back into *Adho Mukha Svanasana, III c*
- Keep left heel pressing into wall
- Step right foot forward between hands, bending right leg 90°, *III d*
- Once right leg is stable, move blocks under hands and press into them, *III e*

🕉 *If capacity allows, continue to deepen by stepping right foot to outer side of right hand, with the right shoulder inside the right lower leg, III f*

- Descend right buttock to reasonable capacity
- If capacity allows, keep left femur lifted and descend torso, lowering forearms to blocks or floor, *III g-h*

Sustain

- Resist heels laterally, broadening upper femurs away from pubis
- Hug lower right thigh inward; in *III f-h*, squeeze right outer arm with leg
- Without lifting right heel, reduce pressure to release groin
- Keeping ankle lift descend inner right groin, then descend outer groin
- Descend right femur and ascend left femur in equal opposition
- Draw inner and outer right groin equally back
- Roll outer left hip forward away from heel
- Lengthen from outer hips to armpits
- Lengthen from pubis to sternum

Exit

- Extend arms and press hands into floor
- Increasing hand pressure, exhale and step right leg back to *Adho Mukha Svanasana, III c*
- Repeat to the second side
- Step or jump forward to *Uttanasana*, or lower knees and rest in *Uttana Balasana*

Challenge

1. Lumbar rounds, causing strain
2. Left thigh and left side of pelvis drop
3. Chest collapses
4. Right inner groin narrows

Response

1. Use adequate support under elbows or keep arms extended, do not lower to elbows. Initiate forward bend from pelvis by softening and deepening groins, not from the waist or chest. Bring right ilium inside right femur. Minimally draw back iliums toward each other.
2. Dig left ball of foot down to elevate thigh. Stretch back of the muscle rather than the surface, *III i*. Descend right buttock. Rest left knee lightly on floor, lifting groin and femur.
3. Resist hands (or elbows) back and engage triceps to extend sternum forward.
4. Lift pelvis and pass a strap around right inner thigh, both ends to the right. Hold ends with right hand and pull femur downward and laterally. Maintain this pull direction and bend leg, descending pelvis, *III k-l.*

Once the groins start to lengthen and deepen, step into the lunge from Adho Mukha Svanasana. Further increase this depth by descending the torso inside the forward leg, which also encourages length through the back of the extended leg groin.

Contact Points

Feet, hands, elbows, forearms

External Supports

Wall, mat, 2 blocks
Strap

Essence of Form

Back leg and hip extension, front leg and hip flexion with abduction; arms and legs neutrally rotated

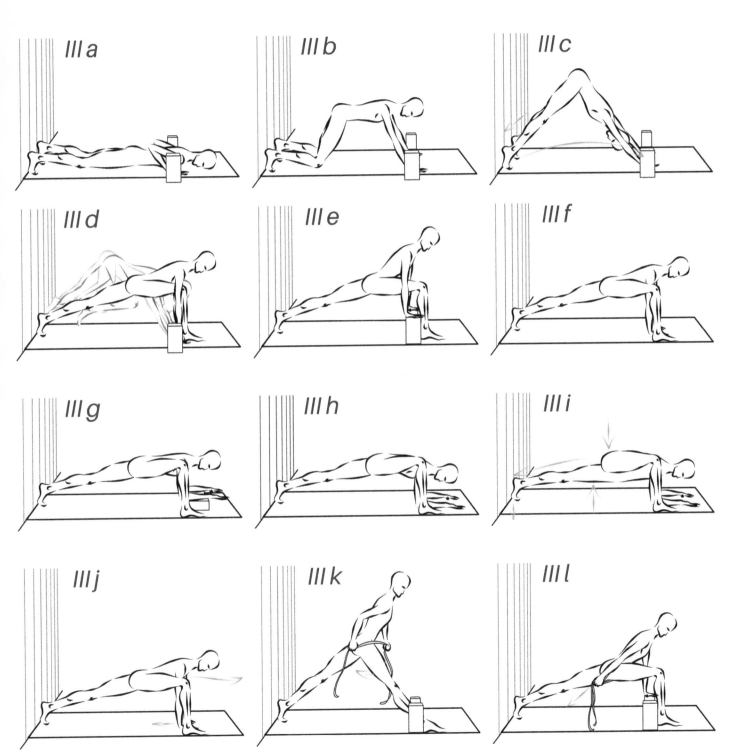

III a

III b

III c

III d

III e

III f

III g

III h

III i

III j

III k

III l

Learn + Practice

After Explore, before deep Back Bends

Linked Poses

Virabhadrasana A, Virabhadrasana C, Viparita Dandasana

Safety Factors

As for Simplify, Explore, + Nourish; for hypertension bring hands to hips

Prepare

· Same *Preparation* as for *Nourish*, with or without blocks

Enter

· Follow *Enter* instructions from *Nourish* up to *III d*
· Resist right tibia head backward, *IV a*
· Stabilize right big toe mound and left heel
· Without lifting pelvis or torso, extend arms forward, palms facing each other, *IV b*
· Extend from left heel to fingertips, *IV c*
· Draw front iliums toward each other and lift iliums away from top femurs
· Keeping right leg bent to 90°, bring pelvis toward vertical, torso upright, arms raised, *IV d*
· Alternatively, from *Tadasana*, stabilize right big toe mound and step left foot back, heel to wall, *IV e*
· Extend both legs and neutralize pelvis
· Inhaling, raise arms overhead, *IV f*
· Pushing through left heel, keep torso lifted and fold right leg to 90°, *IV g*

Sustain

· Engage leg and pelvis actions from *Simplify, Explore, + Nourish*
· Pressing into right big toe mound, roll inner arch circularly to outer ankle
· Without collapsing right knee inward, draw right outer ankle in
· Resist right tibia head backward while lengthening right femur forward
· Keeping pelvis height, recede left groin
· Glide sacrum forward away from left heel
· Lift back ribs away from back pelvis, *IV h*
· Extend arms fully from side ribs to fingertips

Exit

· Stabilize right big toe mound
· Lifting chest, lead with the sacrum and step left leg directly forward to *Tadasana*, *IV i-k*
· Exhaling, release arms to sides, *IV l*
· Repeat to the second side
· Alternately, perform repetitions moving between *IV f* and *IV g* before stepping forward to *Tadasana*

Challenge

1. Lumbar compression
2. Arm lift raises blood pressure
3. Foot drags, pelvis lags, and other problems with stepping forward

Response

1. Lean torso forward slightly. Descend back pelvis and ascend front pelvis to bring torso upright. *See Enter, IV b-c.* Use arm extension to lengthen lumbar and descend pelvis away from torso. Review leg and pelvis actions in *Simplify, Explore, + Nourish*. Increase groin length in *Simplify, Explore, + Nourish* before bringing torso upright.
2. Hands to hips. Do not raise arms overhead.
3. Lead with the sacrum. Maintain big toe mound pressure. Keep maximum back leg length before and while stepping. Keep the chest lifted. Step up rather than forward, *IV j*. Shorten holds before stepping forward, gradually increase hold over time.

Active length helps maintain structural integrity as poses become more challenging. Stepping forward to Tadasana from Anjaneyasana trains the groin muscles, particularly the psoas, to remain long when activated. Progressively increase time spent in lunge before stepping.

Contact Points

Feet, hands

External Supports

Mat, wall, blocks (optional)

Essence of Form

Back leg and hip extension, front leg and hip flexion, arm and torso extension; arms and legs neutrally rotated

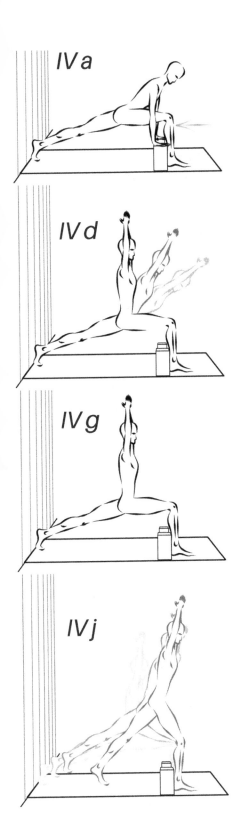

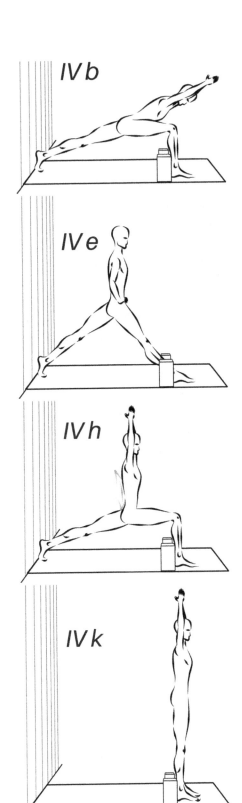

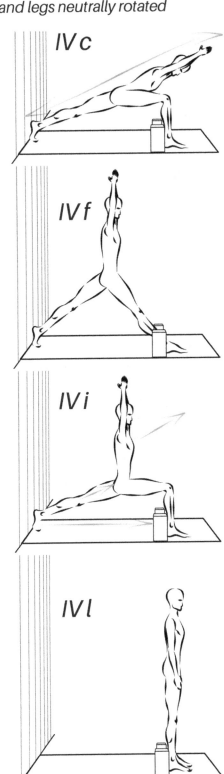

Virabhadrasana A
First Warrior Pose

Simplify

Learn + Practice

Once Anjaneyasana
(lunge) is stable, before
Back Bending poses

Linked Poses

Anjaneyasana, Parsvottanasana,
Virabhadrasana C

Safety Factors

Knee or groin injury, SI
joint dysfunction; do not
raise arms if hypertense

Prepare

· Mat's short end to wall
· Place blocks on mat at each
  long edge, one and a half
  leg lengths from wall

Enter

· Stand between blocks facing
  away from wall in *Tadasana*
· Step left leg back, heel to wall,
  folding right leg and bringing
  hands to blocks, *I a-b*
· Pressing hands into blocks, draw
  ball of foot away from wall
· Without collapsing right knee
  medially and minimally moving
  left hip backward, externally
  rotate left leg 15-45°
· If capacity allows, without
  torquing knee, bring
  left heel to floor
· Push left outer heel deeply
  into wall and draw left hip
  forward, extending left leg
· Without lifting pelvis, increase
  right big toe mound pressure
· Keeping left outer heel
  pressure, extend arms
  forward on inhalation, *I c*
· Maintain left outer heel
  pressure and descend
  back pelvis on exhalation,
  lifting torso to vertical, *I d*

Sustain

· Differentiate external rotation
  of left femur and forward
  action in left hip, *I e*
· Extend left hip forward, away
  from left outer heel pressure, *I f*
· Using left outer heel pressure,
  lift left femur upward
· Soften pubis in and up
· Increase right big toe mound
  pressure and draw right outer
  hip crease back and down
· Keeping right leg bent, resist
  right tibia head backward, *I g*
· Soften right groin and
  descend right femur
· Descend back pelvis;
  ascend back ribs
· Wrap outer armpits forward
  and extend arms from bottom
  back ribs, softening trapezium

Exit

· Exhaling, lower hands to blocks
· Return left leg to neutral rotation,
  lifting left heel up wall
· Pressing into right big toe
  mound, step left leg forward, *I h*
· Alternately, straighten right
  leg and turn leg and torso to
  Uttitha Hasta Padasana, then
  heel-toe feet to *Tadasana*
· Repeat, stepping right
  leg back in *Enter*

Challenge

1. High blood pressure
2. Right knee extends
   beyond right ankle
3. Right groin binds
4. Lower back pain
5. Left knee strain

Response

1. Bring hands to hips or
   extend elbows to sides,
   forearms vertical, *I i.*
2. Pressing hands into blocks,
   lift right foot off floor and step
   foot forward. Do not move
   foot while bearing weight.
3. Before extending and raising
   arms, lighten right heel pressure
   to release groin, *I j.* Keeping
   groin released and femur
   descending, re-stabilize foot
   before raising arms and torso.
4. Extend torso forward before
   coming upright, creating lumbar
   length. Retain length and lift
   torso. Keeping previous leg
   and pelvis actions, engage
   multifidus by minimally
   gathering back iliums.
5. Rotate at hip joint from the
   uppermost part of the thigh,
   not the knee. Allow the pelvis
   to turn slightly leftward, *I k-l.*

The First Warrior Pose builds on the groin opening from Anjaneyasana, and develops further hip articulation. Although the only major difference between Virabhadrasana A and Anjaneyasana is the back leg's rotation, which deepens and complicates the pose significantly.

Contact Points

Feet, hands (transitional)

External Supports

Wall, 2 blocks

Essence of Form

Front leg flexion, back leg extension, torso extension; front leg in neutral rotation, arms and back leg external

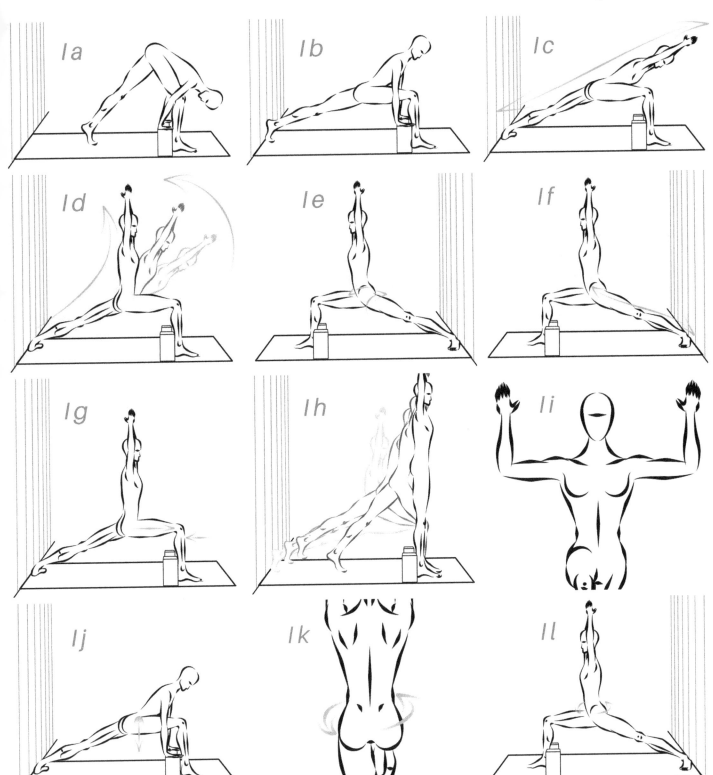

Learn + Practice

After Anjaneyasana, once lumbar discomfort is diminished in Simplify

Linked Poses

Anjaneyasana, Urdhva Mukha Svanasana, Marichyasana C

Safety Factors

Use care with lower back injury, SI joint dysfunction, knee or groin injury

Prepare

· Set mat's short end to wall

Enter

· Stand facing the wall and place hands on wall at waist height, elbows bent, *II a*
· Step right foot forward, 1" from wall and step left foot generously backward, *II b-c*
· Externally rotate left thigh 45-60°, *II d*
· Keeping leg rotation, lower left heel, *II e*
· Ensure center of left thigh, head of left tibia, and left foot's mid line face the same direction
· Push left outer heel away from back pelvis
· Keeping left outer heel pressure, press both hands into the wall and fold right leg to 90° on exhalation, *II f-g*
· If right knee moves beyond ankle before thigh descends fully, straighten right leg and step left foot further back
· Lower hands if above shoulder level

❀ *Left leg can be kept in neutral rotation, II h*

Sustain

· Extend femurs away from pelvis while lifting pelvis up off femur heads
· Press left pelvis away from left outer heel
· Lift left inner arch and inner left femur, *II i*
· Differentiate external thigh rotation from forward ilium action
· Stabilize right big toe mound
· Resist right tibia head backward
· Soften right groin and descend right femur
· Level pelvis but do not force pelvis to "square" to wall
· Use arm extension to retain upright torso
· Pressing hands to wall, resist downward to lift chest, *II j*

Exit

· Stabilize right big toe mound
· Pressing into left outer heel, lift left inner femur to straighten right leg
· Extend right leg until right kneecap lifts, engaging right quadricep
· Neutralize left leg rotation
· Pressing into hands, step right foot back
· Repeat, stepping left foot forward

Challenge

1. Right knee extends beyond ankle, tibia action unclear
2. Pelvis and torso fold forward, elbows bend
3. Lumbar pain

Response

1. *Enter* with ball of right foot in wall/floor juncture, toes up. Holding a block in the right hand, fold the leg and wedge the block between wall and tibia head. Lengthen right femur forward to hold block. Without dropping block, draw tibia head away from block pressure, *II k.*
2. Due to lumbar stiffness and/or groin tightness. *Enter* further from wall and lean torso forward. Descend back pelvis to bring torso more vertical. Practice with left leg in neutral rotation, *II h*, as for *Anjaneyasana*. Externally rotate leg only once groin lengthens and lumbar region is more limber.
3. Lengthen both torso sides equally while carrying left side torso up and forward, right ribcage receding slightly in a subtle twist. *See also Solution 2, and* Simplify, *Solution 2.*

Virabhadrasana A also introduces Back Bending actions, mild Twisting, and stabilizes the pelvis and lower back. Pressing the hands into a wall helps establish the line of extension from the back heel to the same-side armpit as the front leg folds.

Contact Points

Feet, hands
Head of tibia

External Supports

Wall, mat
Block

Essence of Form

Front leg flexion, back leg extension, torso extension; front leg in neutral rotation, arms and back leg external

II a

II b

II c

II d

II e

II f

II g

II h

II i

II j

II k

Learn + Practice

*After Anjaneyasana,
Once Simplify is stable*

Linked Poses

*Anjaneyasana, Urdhva Mukha
Svanasana, Marichyasana C*

Safety Factors

*Use care with knee, groin,
and lower back injury*

Prepare

- Set a chair slightly less than a leg's length from wall, seat facing wall

Enter

- Stand between wall and chair, *III a*
- Step right leg through chair back, sitting right thigh and buttock on chair seat, *III b*
- Keep right thigh perpendicular to wall, foot mid line neutral
- Ensure right tibia is vertical
- Extend left leg, first with heel to wall and the leg in neutral rotation, *III c*
- Extend left leg from back pelvis to heel
- Gather front iliums and resist heels laterally
- Once neutral rotation is not problematic, keep left ilium rolling forward and externally rotate top of left thigh
- Bring outer left heel to wall/floor juncture, edge of foot 15-30° from wall *III d*
- Press hands into chair back, with elbows bent and held close to side torso, *III e*

☸ *Left leg can also be kept in neutral rotation, III f*

Sustain

- Resist heels laterally, broadening upper femurs away from pubis
- Soften pubis inward and upward
- Keeping left heel pressure into wall, roll left ilium forward and draw sacrum inward
- Press hands downward and hug elbows inward, lifting chest
- Lift back ribs away from back pelvis
- Descend inner shoulder blades and broaden between bottom shoulder blades
- Draw bottom shoulder blades forward and toward each other
- Roll outer back armpits forward
- Descend trapezium and lengthen inner elbows down

Exit

- Lift left heel and bring leg to neutral rotation, *III f,* then bend the leg
- Push hands into chair seat and lift pelvis, sliding right leg out of chair
- Use hand pressure to reduce weight on legs during transitions
- Avoid unnecessary torque
- Repeat to the second side

Challenge

1. Right heel does not reach floor
2. Right buttock does not descend into chair seat
3. Stepping through chair back is difficult
4. Left knee pain

Response

1. Use mat remnants, wood boards, or foam blocks under right heel. Use only as much height as necessary.
2. Build up chair seat height with blankets or foam blocks. Gradually reduce height over time.
3. Tilt chair back toward floor before stepping in and while stepping out. Use chair with backrest removed, *III g.*
4. In neutral rotation, support tibia head with bolster and blocks. Resist tibia head into that support, *III h.* Equalize inner and outer heel pressure. When externally rotating, ensure rotation is at thigh, not knee or ankle. Reduce rotation and lift heel, bringing foot's outer edge to wall, *III i.* Lift inner femur and increase outer heel pressure.

With the support of a chair, the depth of the front leg groin can be explored as the back groin is challenged. This supported form provides stability, but is also more intense than it may at first appear. Build up longer holds gradually.

Contact Points

Feet, thigh, sitting bone, hands

External Supports

Mat, chair, wall
Bolster, blocks, blankets, mat remnants

Essence of Form

Front leg flexion, back leg extension, torso extension; front leg in neutral rotation, arms and back leg external

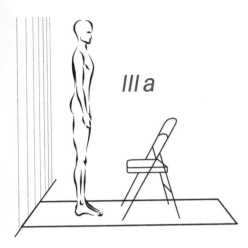

III a

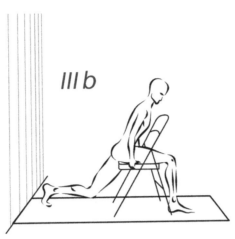

III b

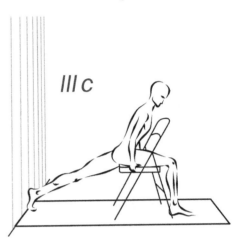

III c

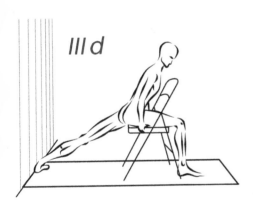

III d

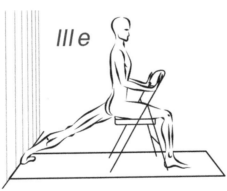

III e

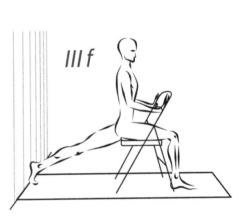

III f

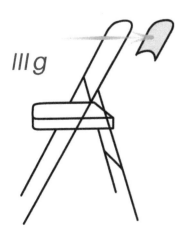

III g

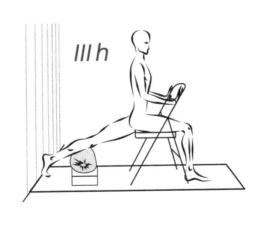

III h

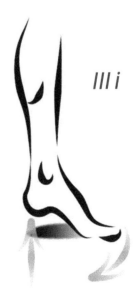

III i

Synthesize

Learn + Practice

After Nourish, before deep Back Bends, especially those with arms overhead

Linked Poses

Salabhasana, Viparita Dandasana, Urdhva Dhanurasana

Safety Factors

As for Simplify, Explore, + Nourish

Prepare

- Can be done with left outer heel against wall or without wall support
- Take a long strap or tie two straps together: the loop should be 4.5-6'

Enter

- Step left foot in one end of looped strap
- Turn left leg and foot out 45-60° from mid line, anchoring strap with outer foot, *IV a*
- Step right foot forward, lunge distance, leg extended and kneecap lifted, *IV b*
- Holding strap in left hand, bring strap over left shoulder with elbow forward, *IV c*
- Bring right arm to same position, hooking thumbs in strap behind head, *IV d*
- Draw elbows toward each other, lifting chest
- Exhaling, push into left heel and fold right leg 90°, extending arms to keep strap taut, *IV e*
- Coordinate arm extension with folding right leg as one movement
- Resist right tibia back as leg folds, *IV f*

Sustain

- Leg and pelvis actions from *Simplify, Explore, + Nourish*
- Soften space between pubis and sacrum
- Glide sacrum forward
- Without tucking pelvis, heavily descend tail bone
- Resisting strap with left foot and hands, lift chest and ribcage away from pelvis
- Broaden back ribs and draw thoracic spine deeply inward
- Lengthen top and bottom sternum away from each other
- Maximize side torso length

Exit

- Stabilize right big toe mound
- Pressing into outer left heel, inhale to straighten right leg
- Exhaling, release arms from strap
- With both legs straight, turn right leg and pelvis leftward to *Uttitha Hasta Padasana*
- Heel-toe the feet to *Tadasana* and *Prepare + Enter* the second side
- Repeat, shortening strap to increase back bend if capacity allows

Challenge

1. Chest and ribcage collapse
2. Torso rotation incomplete
3. Neck compression

Response

1. Back Bend is too deep. Lengthen strap. Maximize negative space between strap and back body, bowing away from strap, *IV g*. Emphasize upward extension more than backward extension by resisting arms and torso up into strap. Lift chest more deeply before folding right leg.
2. Soften right groin and descend right femur. Lift right ilium off femur head. Lengthen left side torso, lifting left side ribs away from left heel to rotate torso forward, *IV h*. Maintain left thigh rotation as torso lifts.
3. Draw chin downward. Lift posterior sternum and move throacic spine deeply inward. Extend occiput away from thoracic spine. Keeping length, lift skull up and back, initiating from mid-thoracic spine.

One of Virabhadrasana A's most important roles is as a preparation for Back Bends. In this variation, the strap's resistance helps teach the lengthening action of Back Bends, as well as establishing a kinetic connection from the back foot through the entire body's arc to the hands.

Contact Points

Feet, hands

External Supports

Mat, 2 straps

Essence of Form

As for Simplify, Explore, + Nourish; groin, torso, neck, and arm extension

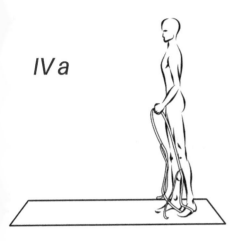

IVa

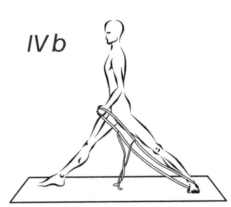

IVb

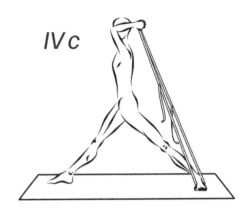

IVc

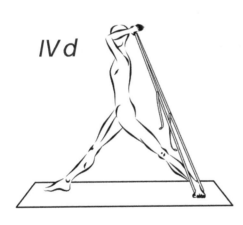

IVd

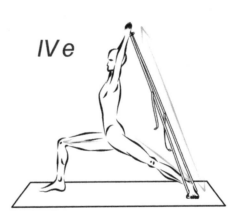

IVe

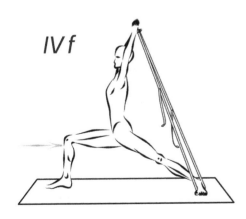

IVf

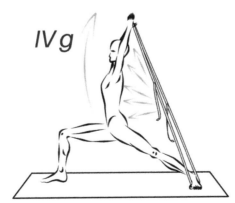

IVg

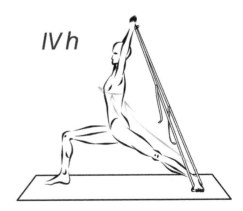

IVh

Learn + Practice

*After basic hip opening
and in conjunction with
lateral Standing Poses*

Linked Poses

*Parsvakonasana, Vrksasana,
Virabhadrasana A, Janu
Sirsasana, Baddha Konasana*

Safety Factors

*Lower back and knee injuries,
SI joint pain, hip replacement,
3rd trimester of pregnancy*

Prepare

- Place mat's short edge
  against wall

Enter

- From *Tadasana*, come to *Uttitha Hasta Padasana* with the left outer heel against the wall, *I a*
- Externally rotate right leg to *Parsva Hasta Padasana*, heel-to-heel alignment, *I b*
- With right arm extended, exhale and place the left hand in left hip crease, *I c*
- Push all 4 corners of feet away from the back pelvis
- Gather front iliums and resist heels laterally, *I d*
- Align the pubis and front iliums vertically, with the left hip slightly forward
- Keeping pelvis level, tuck right buttock
- Lifting right ilium, deepen left heel pressure
- Pressing left hip crease inward, *I e*, fold right leg 90°, femur parallel to floor, *I f*
- Do not move right tibia beyond vertical
- Keep spine as vertical as possible, resisting left side rib cage back as right leg folds

Sustain

- Push equally from back pelvis to both feet
- Pressing into outer left heel, lift left inner arch
- Ascend left femur as right femur descends
- Lengthen right inner thigh more fully than outer thigh and descend right buttock
- Resist torso toward wall
- Lift torso sides equally from hips to armpits

Exit

- Increasing outer left heel pressure, inhale to straighten right leg
- Firm right thigh, fully engaging inner quadricep, kneecap lifted
- Repeat *Enter + Exit* 5-10 times to increase hip mobility
- Keep right arm extended during repetitions, increasing endurance
- After last repetition, straighten right leg and turn leg inward to *Uttitha Hasta Padasana*
- Step feet to *Tadasana* at mat's center
- Set up and *Enter* with the right heel to wall and repeat left

Challenge

1. Strain on left inner knee
2. Pelvis drops on the right side
3. Right buttock untucks
4. Legs internally rotate

Response

1. Turn left foot in, up to 30°. Bring left outer foot against wall, lifting heel 1-2" up wall, *I g*.
2. Lift right ilium as leg bends. Emphasize descending right femur instead of pelvis to bend leg. Keep navel shifting to the left as right leg externally rotates. Soften internal abdominal organs and shift them to the left as well, *I h*. See also *Nourish*.
3. Strongly tuck right buttock before folding the leg. Deepen external rotation from the top of both thighs. *See Response 4. See also Nourish.*
4. Loop a strap around each upper thigh, buckles at inner back thighs. Wrap ends snugly 2-3 times, from inner, over front, and around outer back thighs. Hold and lift straps while *Entering*, pulling thighs into external rotation, *I i-j*.

Virabhadrasana B develops strength in legs, opens the hips, builds endurance, and increases physical and mental stability. Its primary action is moving the extended leg's hip inward, which is often an unfamiliar action. Pressing the hand into the hip crease encourages this movement.

Contact Points
Feet
Hand (on hip)

External Supports
Mat, wall
2 straps

Essence of Form
Leg abduction, knee and hip flexion, groin and leg extension; legs externally rotated, arms neutral

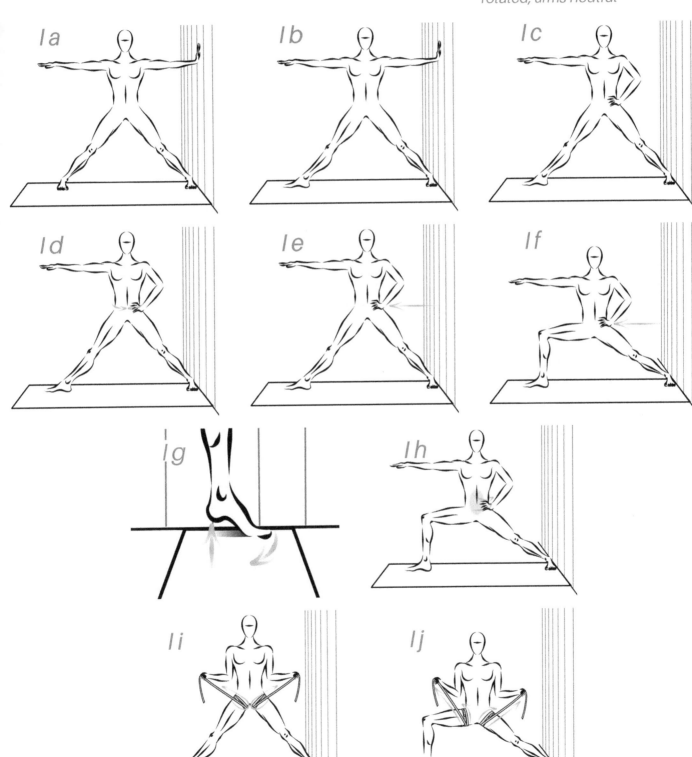

Virabhadrasana B
Second Warrior Pose

Explore

Learn + Practice

After or in conjunction with Simplify and lateral Standing Poses, after Baddha Konasana

Linked Poses

Parsvakonasana, Vrksasana, Trikonasana, Ardha Chandrasana

Safety Factors

As for Simplify; groin injury

Prepare

· As for *Simplify*

Enter

· Come to *Parsva Hasta Padasana* as for *Simplify*
· Bring the left hand to wall at about waist height, elbow slightly bent and pointing downward, *II a*
· Resisting heels laterally, gather front iliums, and soften pubis in and up
· Consciously externally rotate both thighs
· Descend tail bone heavily
· Ensure pelvis is level, with pubis and iliums vertically aligned
· Resisting right tibia backward, move left hip crease into body and away from wall
· Deepen pressure through left outer heel and left hand
· Exhale and bend right leg, descending pelvis until right femur is parallel to floor, *II b*
· Extend left arm, keeping right hand in contact with wall
· Keep right tibia vertical, perpendicular to floor
· Without turning torso and keeping gaze level, turn head to look over right hand, *II c*

Sustain

· Press outer left heel both down into floor and back into wall, *II d*
· Gathering front iliums, roll upper left thigh outward, *II e*
· Strongly tuck right buttock, lifting front iliums
· Without untucking pelvis, abduct right inner thigh
· Lift both sides of the torso equally
· Keep left torso opening laterally
· Pushing left hand into wall, press torso away from wall, extending left arm more fully
· Draw left side torso backward as hand presses into wall
· Extend right arm completely, reaching right hand away from left hand
· Roll trapezium downward as arms extend

Exit

· Firm the legs and descend left outer heel
· Without increasing right heel pressure, inhale and straighten right leg
· Turn right leg in and heel-toe feet together
· Turn to face the other direction and repeat to the left

Challenge

1. Back leg bends
2. Right knee goes past right ankle, *II f*
3. Torso shifts excessively leftward
4. Torso leans forward and/or pelvis untucks excessively

Response

1. Extend to the outer left heel away from the back pelvis, pushing the wall away to extend the leg fully. *See also Sustain actions in Nourish.*
2. Stance is too short. Do not move right foot after bending the leg. Instead, *Exit* and widen the stance by stepping the right foot further away from the wall in *Uttitha Hasta Padasana*. Lift left femur toward wall as right leg bends.
3. The torso will shift leftward in this variation. Depending on body proportions, this may be excessive. If so, press a block into the wall with left hand while *Entering* to keep torso vertical, *II g*.
4. Practice with back against wall, back heel in corner if possible, *II h*.

Symbolically, Virabhadrasana B represents standing firm between opposing courses of action. Often, the torso leans toward the bent leg, which shifts that equanimity into action rather than resting in the present. Pressing the back hand into the wall counters this tendency.

Contact Points

Feet, hand

External Supports

Mat, wall
Block

Essence of Form

Leg abduction, knee and hip flexion, groin and leg extension; legs externally rotated, arms neutral

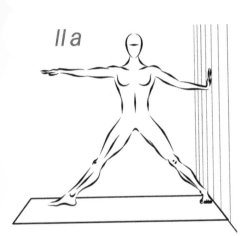

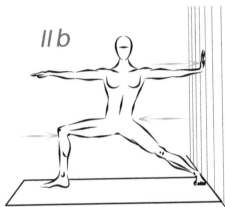

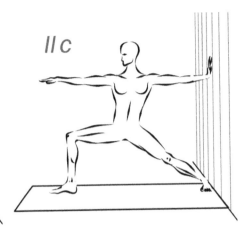

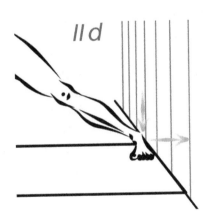

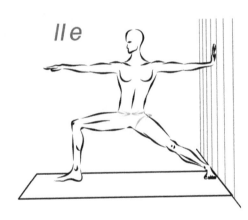

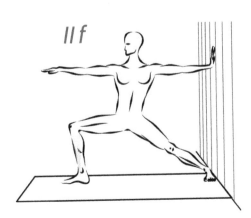

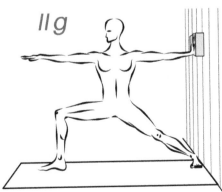

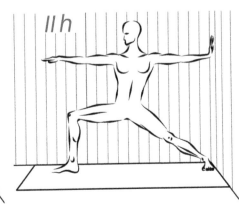

Virabhadrasana B
Second Warrior Pose

Nourish

Learn + Practice

Once Simplify + Explore are clear, before deep hip openers

Linked Poses

Lateral Standing Poses, Baddha Konasana, Vamadevasana

Safety Factors

As for Simplify + Explore; particularly SI joint pain and hip or groin injury

Prepare

· Set mat away from walls

Enter

· Step or jump to *Uttitha Hasta Padasana* and externally rotate right leg to *Parsva Hasta Padasana*, the right heel aligned with the left heel
· Keep leg and pelvis actions from *Simplify + Explore*
· Deepen right big toe mound pressure
· With pelvis level, draw outer right buttock diagonally away from right big toe mound, *III a*
· Without lifting right heel, decrease pressure to release right groin
· Keeping right groin released, increase external rotation from top of right femur, *III b*
· Lift right ilium and descend back pelvis
· Resisting right tibia head inward and without losing right outer buttock action, deepen left hip crease and fold right leg 90°
· Ensure torso is vertical and reach equally through both arms

Sustain

· Stabilize left outer heel
· Without losing left outer heel pressure, bend left leg slightly
· With left leg slightly bent, tuck right buttock strongly, *III c*
· Keep buttock descending and press left upper femur toward back of left thigh
· Without hyperextending left leg, continue pressing left femur backward and extend heel away from back pelvis to re-straighten left leg
· Lift left inner femur away from pubis, widening inner groin
· Soften right groin, descending femur
· Without changing right leg position, draw right calf and tibia toward each other

Exit

· Firm the legs, and press heavily into the left outer heel
· Without increasing right heel pressure, increase right big toe mound pressure
· Lifting from left inner femur, inhale and straighten right leg fully
· *Enter* and repeat to the left

Challenge

1. Sacroiliac joint pain
2. Right groin binds
3. Left femur action is unclear
4. Right knee collapses inward, *III e*

Response

1. Turn left foot in and move left ilium forward until pain dissipates. Once pain is consistently managed, externally rotate left leg over time, *III d*.
2. Increase pressure through ball of right foot. Without destabilizing knee joint, lift right heel 1" from floor and externally rotate right thigh, releasing groin. Reduce heel lift as groin softens.
3. + 4. Practice with back to wall, feet 3-6" from it. Wedge blocks between wall and outer right thigh and back of left thigh. Maintain outer right thigh contact and press left femur back.

ॐ *Assisted: partner sits in front with feet pressing into mid-upper thighs, rolling thighs upward, III f (do not assist without blocks)*

A deep groin and hip opening, Virabhadrasana B can reveal a variety of postural compensations. By bending the back leg, some freedom is created in the groin, which makes descending the folded leg's buttock more accessible. From there, the extended leg's groin can lengthen.

Contact Points

Feet

External Supports

Mat
Wall, 2 blocks, assistant

Essence of Form

Leg abduction, knee and hip flexion, groin and leg extension; legs externally rotated, arms neutral

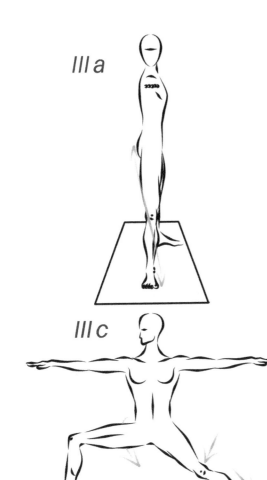

III a

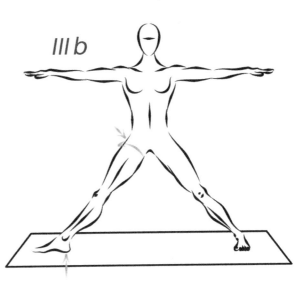

III b

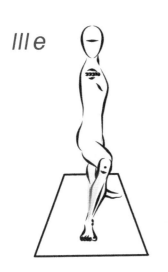

III c

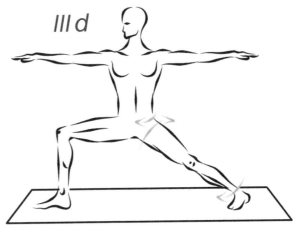

III d

III e

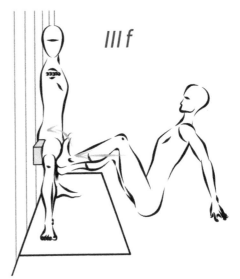

III f

Learn + Practice

Once Simplify + Explore are clear, once thighs reach floor in Baddha Konasana

Linked Poses

Baddha Konasana, Upavistha Konasana, Parivritta Janu Sirsasana

Safety Factors

As for Simplify, Explore + Nourish; do not raise arms if hypertense

Prepare

· Set mat away from walls

Enter

· Step or jump to *Uttitha Hasta Padasana* and externally rotate right turn leg out to *Parsva Hasta Padasana*, arms extended to the sides
· Align right heel with left arch if thighs reach floor in *Baddha Konasana, IV a-b*
· Keep *Enter* actions from *Simplify, Explore, + Nourish*
· Without protruding front ribs, lift arms to *Urdhva Hastasana, IV c*
· Extend up from pelvis, through armpits, to fingertips, lengthening torso sides
· Reaching arms upward, descend pelvis away from upward reach, folding right leg to 90° on exhalation as in *Simplify, Explore, + Nourish*
· Keeping torso length, lengthen arms out and down to shoulder height
· Resist left arm and torso back to keep upper torso parallel to mat's long edge
· Without turning torso or tilting head, turn head to look beyond right fingertips

Sustain

· Vertically stack pelvic, respiratory, and throat diaphragms
· Soften pelvic floor and release tail bone directly forward
· Without pushing lower ribs forward, lift chest from the back body
· Broaden torso from armpit to armpit
· Descend inner shoulder blades
· Lengthen collarbones away from sternum and continue extension through arms to fingertips

Exit

· Practice longer holds on alternate practice days, from 1-6 minutes
· Maintain torso lift and position
· Pressing into outer left heel, lift left inner femur to straighten legs
· Turn right foot 15-30° in and left leg out 90°, coming to *Parsva Hasta Padasana* to the left, left heel aligned with right arch
· *Enter* and *Sustain* to the left then return to *Uttitha Hasta Padasana* and step or jump to *Tadasana*

Challenge

1. Torso length is lost after folding leg
2. Neck strain when turning the head
3. Shoulder strain

Response

1. Repeat arm lift actions from *Enter, IV d*. Increase torso lift as arms descend to shoulder level, *IV e*. If exhaling to lower arms, inhale as arms lower instead.
2. Without tilting the head back, keep gaze level while turning the head. Broaden between shoulder blades and initiate head turn from upper thoracics rather than upper cervicals. *See also Response 3.*
3. Initiate arm lift from bottom shoulder blades, not shoulders or trapezius by lengthening before lifting. Inhaling, externally rotate arms, turning palms and inner elbows upward. Roll front shoulder flesh over the top toward back shoulders. Exhaling, keep maximum upper arm rotation with inner elbows lifted and turn palms down to face floor, *IV f-g*

Extending the arms bilaterally broadens the chest and increases breath capacity, which may develop cardiac resilience. This same arm extension can also cause discomfort across the neck and shoulders. Refining the arm actions helps ensure Virabhadrasana B's benefits are enjoyed.

Contact Points

Feet

External Supports

Mat

Essence of Form

As for Simplify, Explore, + Nourish; overhead arm extension, external upper arm rotation

IV a

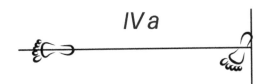

IV b

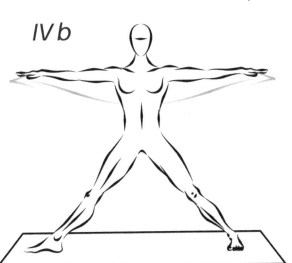

IV c

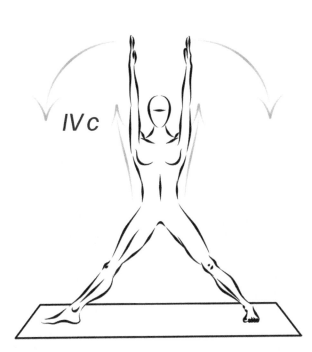

IV d

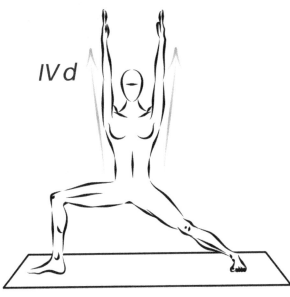

IV e

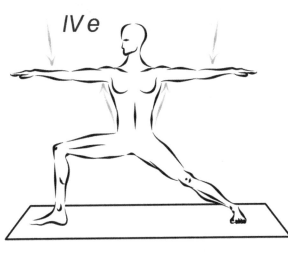

IV f

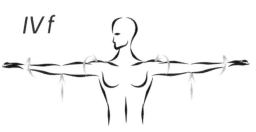

IV g

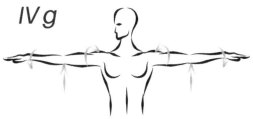

Uttitha Trikonasana
Extended Triangle Pose

Simplify

Learn + Practice

Learn early, after Tadasana, Parsva Hasta Padasana, and Baddha Konasana

Linked Poses

Supta Padangusthasana A + B, Janu Sirsasana, Ardha Chandrasana

Safety Factors

Groin, hamstring, or knee injury, hip replacements, SI joint discomfort

Prepare

- Mat's short end to wall

Enter

- Come to *Parsva Hasta Padasana* with left outer heel to wall,
- Press outer left heel away from back pelvis and into wall/floor juncture
- Heavily descend right big toe mound
- Bring hands to hip creases, *I a*
- Press right thumb into outer buttock, moving it away from right foot, *I b*
- Deepening the right hand into hip crease, lift right ilium away from right hand, *I c*
- Keeping right torso lift and length, fold pelvis and torso laterally over right leg
- Lift left ilium with left hand as right hip crease deepens, *I d*
- Continuously deepen right big toe mound pressure at each stage
- Increase external rotation while folding pelvis over right thigh
- Allow left ilium to roll forward as torso folds laterally
- Keep left rib cage opening toward the ceiling

Sustain

- Push both feet away from back pelvis with the thighs firm and kneecaps lifted
- Descending outer left heel, lift left inner arch
- Without opening left hip backward, externally rotate left thigh, *I e*
- Keeping right big toe mound pressure, draw outer ankle inward
- Ensure center of right foot, ankle, tibia head, knee, and thigh face the same direction
- Equally lengthen inner and outer right thigh, drawing right buttock inward
- Maximize length from right hip to armpit, *I f*

Exit

- Gather front iliums
- Pressing into left outer heel, inhale and descend left ilium and lift right ilium, lifting torso to *Parsva Hasta Padasana*
- Turn right leg inward to *Uttitha Hasta Padasana*
- Step or jump to *Tadasana*
- Turn to face the mat's other long edge and repeat to the second side

Challenge

1. Right leg hyperextends
2. Inner knee pain
3. Right waist shortens
4. Buttocks protrude and torso falls forward

Response

1. Resist right tibia head forward, *I g.* Deepen external rotation at top of right femur, as hyperextension is often related to internal rotation. Wedge a block behind the right calf, *I h.*
2. Ensure upper femurs are fully externally rotated. Without untucking pelvis, resist right greater trochanter to outer right thigh. If necessary, roll left ilium toward the floor and turn left foot in slightly.
3. Set up off the mat with a chair to the right, past the foot. Resting right hand on the chair, slide it away from the torso while folding over the leg, *I j-i.*
4. Deepen external rotation in right leg. Do not force left hip to stack atop right hip, which throws pelvis backward and torso forward. *See also Explore and Synthesize.*

Trikonasana lengthens the groins and hamstrings, increases hip mobility, aids digestion, and can alleviate back pain. Pressing the back heel against the wall emphasizes the back leg's action and strengthens the outer hamstring in the back leg.

Contact Points

Feet, hands (on hips, chair in I i-j), calf in I h

External Supports

Mat, wall
Block, chair

Essence of Form

Leg abduction, lateral hip flexion, groin extension; external leg rotation

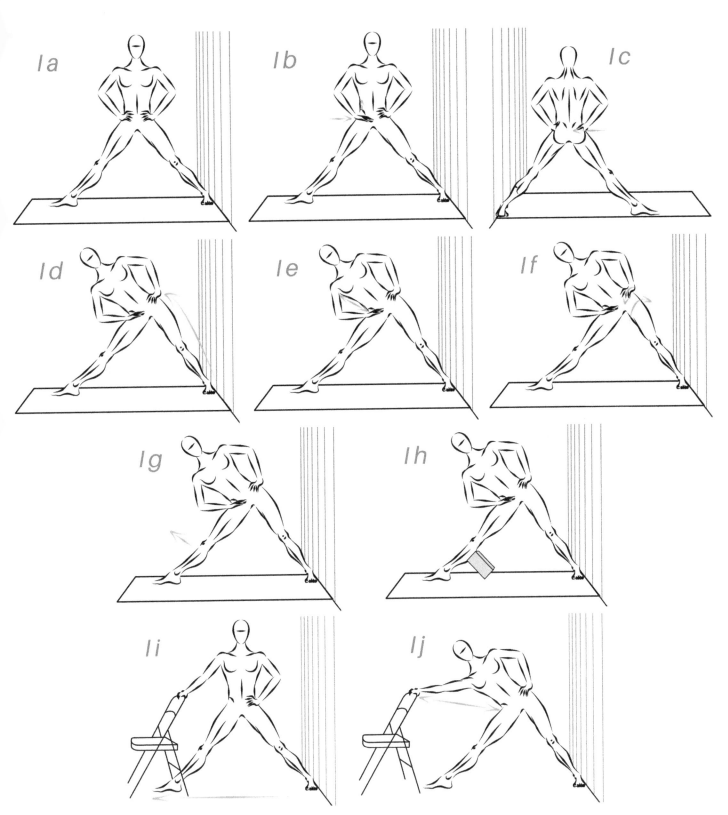

Learn + Practice

After Parsva Hasta Padasana and Baddha Konasana; well before Inversions

Linked Poses

As for Simplify; Parsvakonasana, Parivritta Janu Sirsasana, Sirsasana

Safety Factors

As for Simplify; do not raise top arm or turn head if there is neck discomfort or hypertension

Prepare

· Set blocks against wall, Uttitha Hasta Padasana distance, II a

Enter

· Stand in Tadasana with back to wall, heels 4-8" from it
· Come to Parsva Hasta Padasana, II b
· Blocks will be between heels and wall
· Lifting right ilium up and over hip crease, fold torso laterally over right leg
· Without losing torso length or dropping right shoulder, lower right hand to block, directly under shoulder, II c
· Bring both shoulders against wall, with navel, sternum, throat, and nose in one line
· Keeping left hip forward, externally rotate left leg
· Extending through right arm to right hand on block, turn eye of right elbow outward
· Extend left arm forward, then open upward, stacking joints vertically from right wrist, elbow, shoulders, left elbow, to wrist II d
· Lengthen crown and turn head upward II e-f

Sustain

· Maintain actions from Simplify
· Resist right heel laterally and lift inner left femur
· Lift left ilium away from left outer foot, II g
· Move left buttock away from wall as leg rotates
· Use right hand pressure to widen across shoulder blades and reach left hand maximally upward, II h
· Rest shoulder blades equally into the wall
· Descend left ribcage and extend right ribs away from hip crease, II i
· Extend spine from tail to crown, II j
· Turn head from mid-thoracic spine

Exit

· Increase outer left heel pressure and gather front iliums
· With legs firm, inhale and lift torso to Parsva Hasta Padasana
· Turn legs for left side and repeat left
· When finished, return to Uttitha Hasta Padasana and step to Tadasana

Challenge

1. Inner foot lifts as right buttock tucks
2. Right groin binds
3. Limited twisting capacity, neck strain
4. Lumbar/SI pain while Exiting

Response

1. Push diagonally from right greater trochanter to base of right big toe. Keep right inner heel heavy and draw outer ankle inward.
2. Lighten heel pressure before Entering. Reduce heel pressure again while in the pose to release groin. If this increases binding, wedge a block under ball of right foot, II k.
3. Prepare and Enter facing wall, 12-18" away from it. Place hands on wall, elbows bent. Press into left hand to turn left torso away from wall, drag right hand toward pelvis to lengthen right torso, II l. See also Response 1 in Synthesize.
4. Descend left ilium and ascend right ilium when Coming out. Minimally gather back iliums while gathering front iliums. Firm buttocks during Exit.

This iconic pose teaches fundamental actions of Standing Poses, Back Bends, Forward Bends, and Twists. It also strengthens the neck and spine in preparation for Inversions. Resting the back body against the wall minimizes forward flexion at the hips and reduces strain.

Contact Points

Feet, hands, shoulder blades

External Supports

Wall, 2 blocks
3 blocks for II k

Essence of Form

Leg abduction, lateral hip flexion, groin extension; external leg rotation

II a
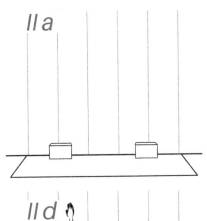

II b
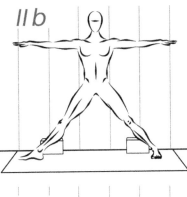

II c
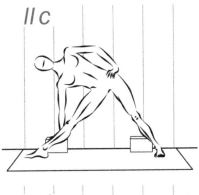

II d
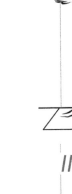

II e
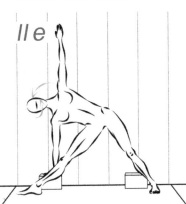

II f
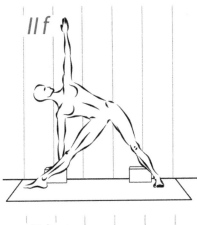

II g

II h
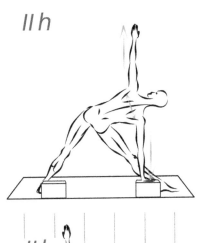

II i
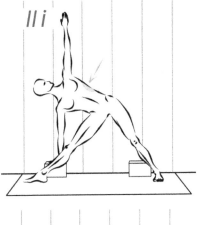

II j
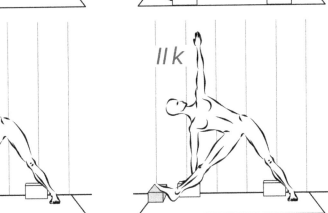

II k

II l
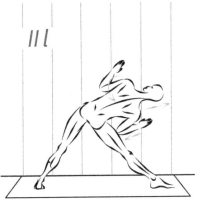

Uttitha Trikonasana
Extended Triangle Pose

Nourish

Learn + Practice

*After Simplify; used as
a therapeutic pose and
to minimize effort*

Linked Poses

*Supta Padangusthasana
A + B, Janu Sirsasana,
Ardha Chandrasana*

Safety Factors

*As for Simplify + Explore,
but much lower risk*

Prepare

- Set up a table 2-3.5′ from wall with mats under table legs, third mat between to stand on, *III a*
- Stack folded blankets on table to support torso and head while in the pose, *III b*
- Set blocks for feet to raise hip creases to table height if needed

Enter

- Stand facing the table, *III c*
- Press hands into table, reducing leg effort
- Step left foot back, outer heel to wall/floor juncture, outer foot 15-30° from wall, *III d*
- Step right foot forward, underneath table, bringing right hip crease to table edge, *III e*
- Ensure right ilium is above table height— stand on blocks if necessary
- Exhaling, lift and fold torso laterally across table and rest torso on blankets
- Extend right arm, supporting head and lengthening side torso, *III f*
- Press left hand into table, in front of chest

Sustain

- Leg and pelvis actions from *Simplify*
- Without sinking pelvis, extend legs and feet away from back pelvis
- Rest right side torso into table, lengthening from hip to armpit
- Pressing into left hand, roll left side torso away from table
- Soften the chest and abdomen
- Use table support to reduce effort
- Decreasing effort, gradually deepen twist

Exit

- Exhaling, turn torso to face table
- Bring both hands to the table, under the armpit/chest
- Pressing into both hands, inhale and raise torso to upright
- Still pressing into hands to take weight off of feet and legs, step right foot back from under the table
- Step left foot forward
- Inhale and come to *Tadasana* or rest in *Ardha Uttanasana* over the table for a few breaths
- Repeat to the left

Challenge

1. Right shoulder strain
2. Right side shortens, spine curves, or torso does not reach table
3. Lower back pain

Response

1. Rest arm in front of torso instead of extending overhead. Support the head so that its axis is in line with the spine
2. Ensure the table is at or below hip level before folding — stand on blocks if necessary. If using more than one layer of blocks, sandwich a mat between each block layer to prevent sliding. Raise blankets with foam blocks, and/or use additional blankets to fill gaps between torso and table. Support head adequately.
3. *See Solution 2*, as incorrect set-up can cause pain. Reduce twist by rolling torso toward table and adding blankets under chest. Place bolster on a mat behind torso and lean into it. *See also Synthesize.*

Contact Points

Feet, side torso, outer arm and armpit, hand, side of head

External Supports

3 mats, table, blankets, wall Blocks, extra mats, blankets, and bolsters may also be used

Essence of Form

Leg abduction, lateral hip flexion, groin extension; external leg rotation

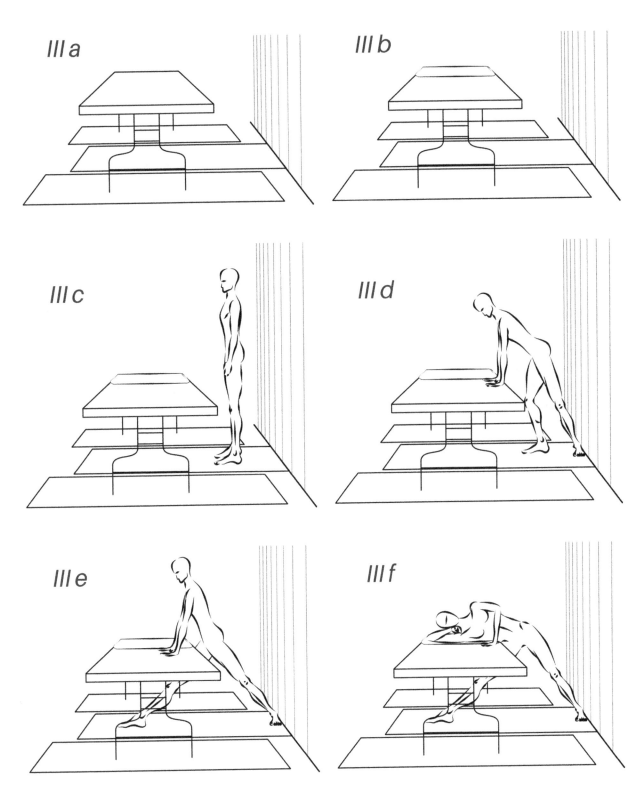

IIIa
IIIb
IIIc
IIId
IIIe
IIIf

Uttitha Trikonasana
Extended Triangle Pose

Synthesize

Learn + Practice

After Simplify + Explore; before learning Twists and Inversions

Linked Poses

Parsvakonasana, Ardha Chandrasana, Baddha Konasana, Upavistha Konasana

Safety Factors

As for Simplify + Explore. Use care with shoulder, elbow, or wrist injury.

Prepare

· Set mat away from wall
· Place blocks at each end of mat's long edge

Enter

· Stand in *Tadasana*, a block's width from mat's long edge
· Step or jump to *Uttitha Hasta Padasana*, arms extended, *IV a*
· Lifting right ilium, continue to *Parsva Hasta Padasana*, externally rotating right leg
· Gather front iliums and resist heels laterally
· Soften pubis in and up
· With left outer heel heavy, and pressurizing the right big toe mound, lift right ilium up and over right hip crease to fold torso laterally over right leg
· Without losing torso length, bring right hand to block, turning arm outward
· Extend left arm vertically
· Facing forward, tilt head slightly to the right
· Turning from the thoracic spine, turn head to the left and gaze up at left hand
· Drawing right buttock in and forward, take head slightly back

Sustain

· Pressing into outer left heel, lift inner left femur, *IV b*
· Keeping outer left heel pressure, bend left leg
· With left leg bent, tuck right buttock, *IV c*
· Maintain tucked right buttock, pressing left femur backward to re-straighten leg
· Lift left front ilium as left femur moves back to lengthen groin
· Without losing external rotation in right leg, draw right ilium forward and toward left ilium
· Extend right outer buttock away from right armpit, lengthening back side body
· Continuously extend both sides of torso evenly from hips to armpits

Exit

· As for *Explore*, and then continue to the left side
· When finished, step or jump from *Uttitha Hasta Padasana* to *Tadasana*

ॐ *Once stable, Enter aligning right heel to left arch if thighs reach floor in Baddha Konasana*

Challenge

1. Neck strain
2. Shoulder/wrist compression
3. Left arm falls behind torso

Response

1. Deepen back leg's external rotation. Without turning torso, turn head to neutral or down to look at floor. Externally rotate right arm, turning hand so that fingertips point back toward left heel, *IV d*. Use a stick or external corner at mid-shoulder blades, *IV e*. Pressing left hand into corner or stick, extend thoracic spine and release trapezium, *IV f*. Support head on chair or high stool with folded blanket on top, *IV g. See also Solution 3.*
2. Increase left outer heel pressure. Pushing right hand down, lift torso away from right wrist, extending through right arm, back, chest, and left arm to left fingertips, *IV h*.
3. Bring left arm in front of chest line, *IV i*. Pressing into right hand, rotate ribcage until chest faces forward. Practice with back to wall, as in *Explore*, bring left shoulder blade to wall before raising left arm.

Trikonasana is the foundation of intermediate and advanced poses, incorporating the entire body in actions that are prevalent in nearly every yoga pose. In this variation, continue activating the back leg and rest the upper torso backward as in the earlier stages.

Contact Points

Feet, Hand
Mid-shoulder blades in
IV e-f, side of head in IV g

External Supports

Mat, 2 blocks
Stick, outer corner, chair

Essence of Form

Leg abduction, lateral hip flexion, groin extension; external leg rotation

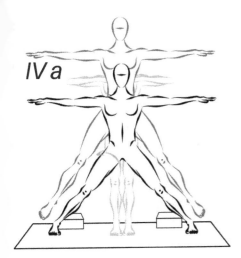

IV a

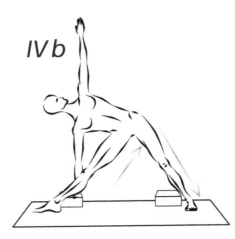

IV b

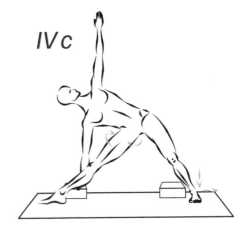

IV c

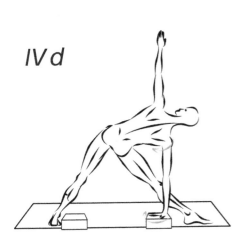

IV d

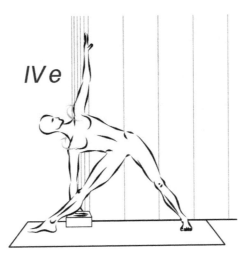

IV e

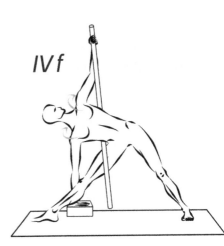

IV f

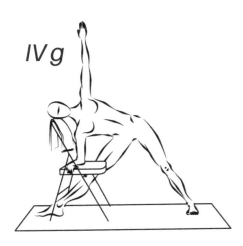

IV g

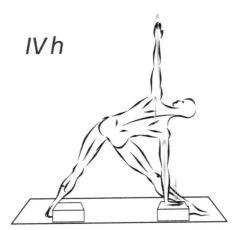

IV h

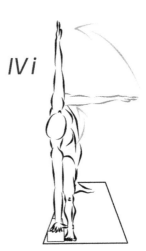

IV i

Extended Triangle Pose — Synthesize

Uttitha Parsvakonasana
Extended Side-Angle Pose

Simplify

Learn + Practice

After Virabhadrasana B
+ Anjaneyasana; before
deep hip openers

Linked Poses

Trikonasana, Virabhadrasana
B, Supta Padangusthasana
B, Marichyasana A

Safety Factors

Hip replacement, groin injury;
use care with knee or ankle injur-

Prepare

· Set mat's short end to wall

Enter

· Step to *Uttitha Hasta Padasana*,
  with left outer heel pressing into
  the wall, heel-to-heel alignment,
  arms raised to sides, *I a*
· Keeping arms extended,
  externally rotate right thigh to
  Parsva Hasta Padasana, I b
· Exhaling, fold right leg 90° and
  descend to *Virabhadrasana B, I c*
· Push outer left heel away
  from back pelvis into wall,
  lifting inner arch and femur
· Keeping right femur descending,
  lift right ilium off femur head, *I d*
· Exhale, deepen right hip
  crease, reaching right arm
  and torso over right thigh, *I e*
· Place right upper outer
  forearm on right thigh,
  rolling thigh outward, *I f*
· Inhaling, sweep left arm forward
  and extend left arm, lengthening
  from left heel to fingertips, *I h-g*

Sustain

· Tucking right buttock,
  increase external rotation and
  roll right ilium forward, *I i*
· Without internally rotating right
  thigh, resist right heel laterally
· Soften pubis in and up
· Lengthen inner right thigh
  away from pubis
· Extend right outer buttock
  toward left heel
· Pressing left femur backward, lift
  left ilium toward left armpit, *I j*
· Lengthen from right
  hip to armpit, *I k*
· Lift torso away from right elbow, *I l*,
  widening across shoulder girdle

Exit

· Stabilize right big toe mound
· Deepen left outer heel pressure
· Inhaling, lift left femur and
  straighten right leg to
  Parsva Hasta Padasana
· Turn right leg in, *Uttitha
  Hasta Padasana*, and heel-
  toe feet to *Tadasana*
· Repeat to the second
  side, right heel to wall

Challenge

1. Right knee goes beyond ankle
2. Right groin binds
3. Left inner knee pain
4. Buttocks fall backward, right
   knee collapses inward
5. Lumbar pain, SI joint discomfort

Response

1. *Exit* the pose. Re-*Enter*
   with a wider stance.
2. Lighten right heel pressure when
   moving into *Virabhadrasana
   II*, and again when extending
   to *Parsvakonasana*.
3. Deepen outer heel pressure
   and lift inner femur. Allow left hip
   to roll forward slightly, and turn
   left toes away from wall 30°-45°.
   Lift left heel up wall 2-3", *I m*.
4. Increase external rotation
   while folding right leg.
   See also Synthesize.
5. Turn left foot inward more and
   roll left ilium forward. Minimally
   gather back iliums while drawing
   front iliums toward each other,
   I n-o. Also see Solution 3.

Parsvakonasana develops the thighs, opens the hips, increases ankle and spinal mobility, and introduces twisting and side extension. It also promotes healthy digestion, elimination, and pelvic organ health by stimulating pelvic/abdominal circulation.

Contact Points

Feet, forearm + thigh

External Supports

Wall, mat

Essence of Form

Lateral torso extension, leg abduction, knee flexion; arms and legs externally rotated

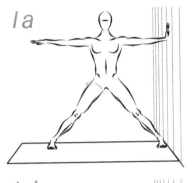

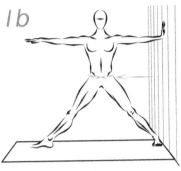

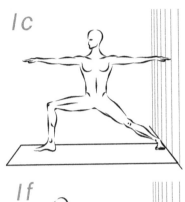

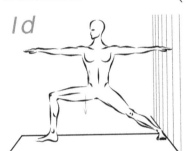

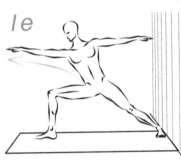

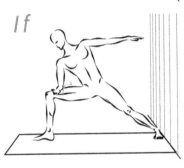

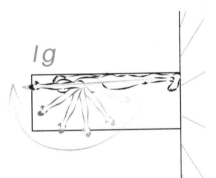

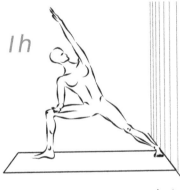

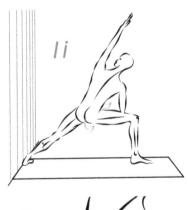

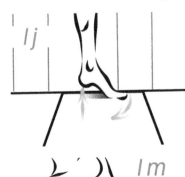

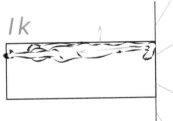

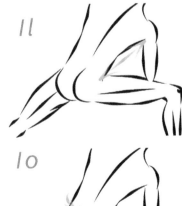

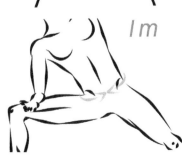

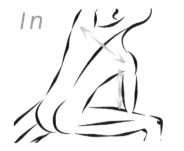

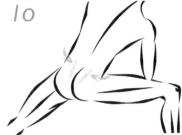

Uttitha Parsvakonasana
Extended Side-Angle Pose

Explore

Learn + Practice

After Anjaneyasana, before deep Twists, early in Standing series

Linked Poses

Anjaneyasana, Marichyasana A, Parivritta Janu Sirsasana

Safety Factors

Same as Simplify with lesser knee risk; shoulder injury (back arm)

Prepare

- Mat's short end to wall
- Set chair on mat, 2.5'-3' from wall, chair seat facing left side of mat
- Place block in front of chair, to the left, *ll a*

Enter

- Sit sideways on chair, right buttock and thigh on chair, torso facing away from wall, *ll b*
- Draw front iliums toward each other
- Extend left leg back, in *Anjaneyasana*, heel to wall, *ll c*
- Tuck right sitting bone toward chair's edge
- Keeping right thigh parallel to chair seat edge, externally rotate right thigh, turning torso and left leg to the left, *ll d*
- Externally rotate left thigh, *ll e*
- Bring outer left heel to wall, left sole to floor
- Pushing into outer left heel, lift left inner femur
- Without collapsing right thigh inward, exhale and extend torso over right thigh, hand to block on the inside of right foot, *ll f*
- Wrap left hand behind torso, catching chair's backrest, *ll g*

Sustain

- All *Sustain* actions from *Simplify*
- Continually slide right buttock toward chair's edge
- Descend right femur, lighten right sitting bone pressure
- Press right arm against inner right thigh
- Without untucking buttock, widen upper right femur away from pubis
- Move left side ribs toward the mid line, *ll h*
- Holding chair back with left hand, pull gently and twist torso toward ceiling, *ll i*

Exit

- Internally rotate left leg, lifting left heel, *ll j*
- Turn torso to face right leg in *Anjaneyasana*, *ll k*
- Bend left leg, sweeping it directly downward and forward, *ll l*
- Do not swing left leg out to the side
- Pressing feet into the floor and hands into thighs, inhale to *Tadasana*, *ll m*
- *Prepare* for the second side, turning the chair to face the other way before *Entering*

Challenge

1. Chair seat is too high or too low
2. Right knee collapse
3. Buttocks slide backward

Response

1. If buttocks descend below knee, build up chair seat height with blankets or flat foam blocks. For more height, sandwich 4 blocks (one for each chair leg) between folded mat and place chair on top, *ll n*. If chair is too high, build up blocks or wooden planks under both feet.

Solutions 2 + 3 are related:

2. Lengthen right inner femur forward and outer hip crease backward. Resist right thigh laterally while transitioning from *Anjaneyasana* to *Parsvakonasana*.
3. Place a mat on chair seat. Tuck right buttock while *Entering* and while *Sustaining* the pose. Place a bolster between chair back and outer thigh/buttock and rest torso back into bolster, *ll o*.

Using the support of a chair in Parsvakonasana deepens the pose and facilitates a longer hold without having to strain. This allows the twist to unfold and allows time to explore the finer aspects of the pose, how it affects the femurs, pelvis, and spine.

Contact Points

Feet, buttock/femur, forearm/hand

External Supports

Wall, mat, chair, block(s) Bolster

Essence of Form

Lateral torso extension, leg abduction, knee flexion; legs externally rotated, back arm internally rotated

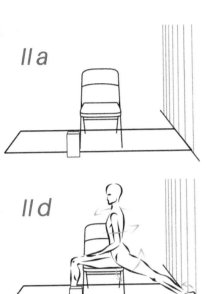

II a

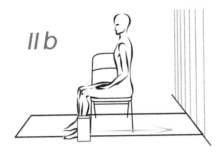

II b

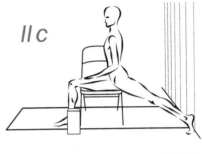

II c

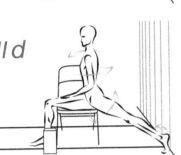

II d

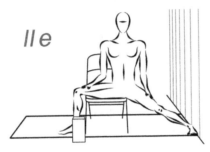

II e

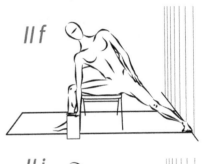

II f

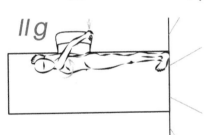

II g

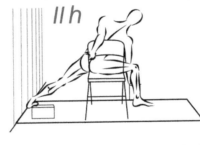

II h

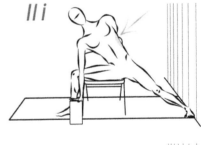

II i

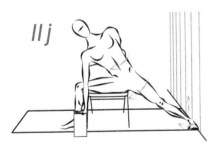

II j

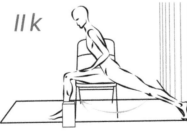

II k

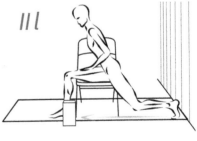

II l

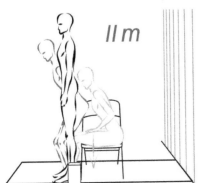

II m

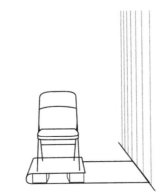

II n

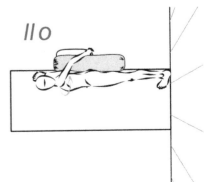

II o

Supta Parsvakonasana
Supine Extended Side-Angle Pose

Nourish

Learn + Practice

Learn after Simplify if possible, but can also be done when recovering from illness or injury

Linked Poses

Uttitha Parsvakonasana,
Supta Padangusthasana B,
Supta Baddha Konasana,
Supta Virasana

Safety Factors

Vertigo; safest option for joint injuries; prop well to avoid torque & over-stretch

Prepare

- Mat parallel to wall, about 18" away from it
- Follow *Enter* instructions to determine prop placement
- *Exit* and place blocks where left heel and left femur will be supported, *III a*
- If the right foot + thigh, left buttock, torso, + arm, and head do not contact floor, set up additional supports, *III b*

Enter

- Lie on right side with torso parallel to wall, pelvis 18"-2' from wall, legs bent, *III c*
- Bring right foot to wall, leg bent at 90°, *III d*
- Support lower right leg with right arm, or rest arm to the side
- Extend left leg, bringing left foot to wall
- Rest left thigh and heel on supports, *III e*, use additional supports if necessary
- Roll torso open to face ceiling, *III f*
- Extend left arm laterally or overhead, *III g-h*
- Ensure no limb is floating or unsupported — use additional supports if necessary

Sustain

- Similar to *Simplify + Explore*, plus:
- Without hyperextending knee, press left femur toward floor, *III i*
- Roll left back pelvis away from floor, *III j*
- Resist right greater trochanter into floor, lifting right front ilium toward ceiling
- Rest back torso into floor
- Slide right shoulder toward wall
- Lengthen from right ilium to right armpit and roll right side ribs toward ceiling as left shoulder blade descends toward floor, *III k*
- Keep head neutral or turn toward left arm if comfortable

Exit

- Stay for 3-15 minutes, provided there is no joint pain
- Roll torso, pelvis, and left leg toward wall
- Sweeping left leg directly toward wall (not swinging it toward the ceiling first), bring both legs together
- Roll onto right side
- Pressing into hands, come up from the side to seated
- *Prepare* for and repeat to the left side

Challenge

1. Torso is too far from wall or perpendicular to it, resembling *Virabhadrasana B*, *III l*
2. Right knee pain
3. Right side torso shortens, restricting lower abdominal breath
4. SI joint/lumbar pain

Response

1. Begin closer to wall and do not shift away from it while *Entering*. Ensure torso is parallel to wall before positioning legs.
2. Support outer right thigh and foot. Bring foot slightly higher than knee. Support back of left torso and arm to turn torso toward wall until right leg abduction is not so extreme as to cause pain.
3. Bend left leg, foot to floor. Pressing into left foot, lift pelvis and tuck right buttock flesh away from armpit. Keeping buttock tucked, re-extend left leg, *III m-n.*
4. *First refer to Solutions 2 + 3.* Wedge blocks under left back ilium and support left ribcage with folded blankets, *III o.* Bring left foot higher and support left femur well.

Parsvakonasana is one of many poses that can be practiced supine. Doing so helps those recuperating from severe illness or injury to develop strength, mobility, and resilience. This variation is well worth spending the time to support well and find comfort in.

Contact Points

Back, right buttock, right arm, head, feet

External Supports

Varies. Mat, wall, up to 6 blocks, several blankets, bolster(s), weights

Essence of Form

Reclining. Lateral torso extension, leg abduction, knee flexion; arms and legs in passive external rotation

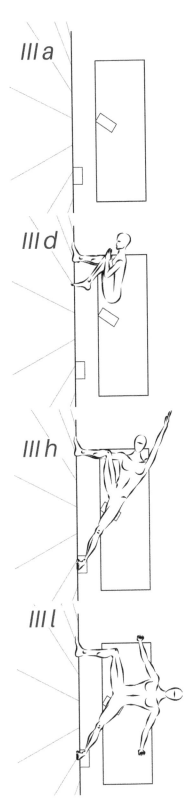

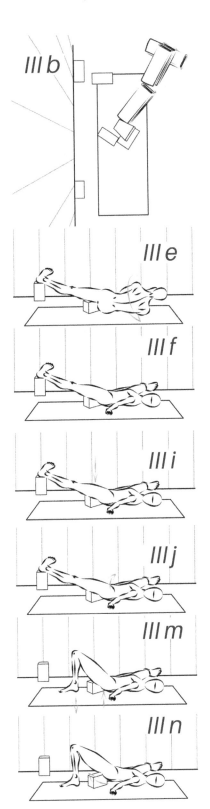

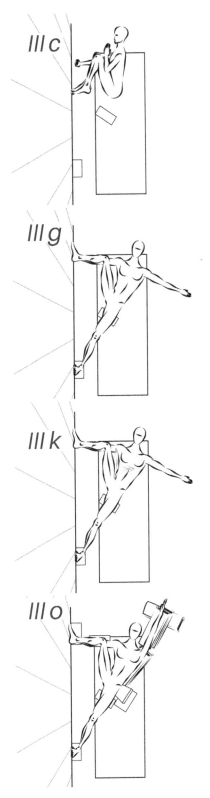

Uttitha Parsvakonasana
Extended Side-Angle Pose

Synthesize

Learn + Practice

Once Simplify is understood clearly, before deep hip openers

Linked Poses

Uttitha Trikonasana, Ardha Chandrasana, Marichyasana A, Parivritta Janu Sirsasana

Safety Factors

Groin injury, SI joint discomfort, hypertension, disc degeneration

Prepare

- Mat away from wall, free of obstructions
- Set blocks at each side of mat's long edge
- Stand in *Tadasana*, at the middle of mat

Enter

- Bending the legs, step or jump to *Uttitha Hasta Padasana*, *IV a*
- Gather front iliums and draw pubis in and up
- Resist heels laterally and descend back pelvis
- Continue as for *Simplify* through *Parsva Hasta Padasana* to *Virabhadrasana B*, *IV b*
- Keeping left outer heel heavy, lift left inner arch and femur
- Lift pelvis up off femur heads
- Draw outer right hip crease backward, folding at right hip crease
- Reach right arm and torso over right leg
- Place right hand on block or floor to inner side of right leg, *IV c*
- Sweep left arm forward then overhead, lengthening from heel to fingertips, *IV d*

Sustain

- Keeping heel pressure, bend left leg, *IV e*
- With left leg bent, tuck right buttock strongly
- Maintain tucked right buttock, pressing left femur backward to re-straighten leg
- Lift left front ilium as left leg extends, *IV f*
- Continue Actions from *Simplify + Explore*
- Without lifting pelvis, draw right tibia head inward, *IV g*
- Soften sternum inward and broaden behind it
- Revolve each section of the right side torso toward the ceiling while countering the left side torso toward the floor, *IV h*

Exit

- As for *Simplify*, deepening left outer heel pressure to lift into *Parsva Hasta Padasana*
- Turn legs and feet to *Parsva Hasta Padasana* on the left and repeat left
- After *Exiting* from the second side, return to *Uttitha Hasta Padasana* and step or jump to *Tadasana*

Challenge

1. Torso pitches forward and rolls downward
2. Torso leans back and lower ribs flare outward
3. Neck and shoulder strain

Response

1. Re-affirm all back leg actions, and lengthen right inner thigh more deeply while doing so. *Enter* facing the wall, 12-18" away from it or sit on chair, facing the backrest, *IV i-j*. Press left hand into wall (or chair backrest), rolling left torso backward (in chair, right hand pulls backrest gently).
2. Press left femur back and recede left groin. Soften front ribs downward and lift back ribs away from back pelvis. Practice with back to wall, moving bottom back ribs toward wall before shoulders.
3. Externally rotate right arm, fingertips facing backward on block, *IV k*. Roll outer left armpit forward as arm extends or keep left hand on hip. Push left hand into wall, *IV l*. Keep head neutral, or turn head toward floor.

Like Trikonasana, Parsvakonasana is essential in understanding the fundamental aspects of many intermediate and advanced poses. When practicing with minimal supports, try to find the spatial and kinesthetic awareness encouraged at earlier stages.

Contact Points

Feet, hand

External Supports

Mat, 2 blocks
Wall, chair

Essence of Form

Lateral torso extension, leg abduction, knee flexion; arms and legs externally rotated

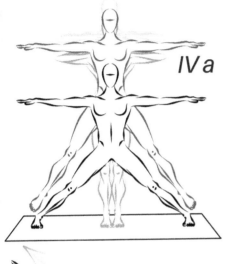

IVa

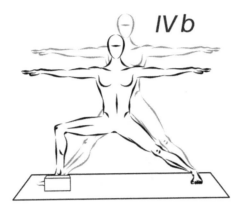

IVb

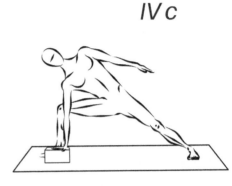

IVc

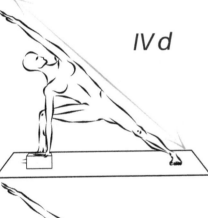

IVd

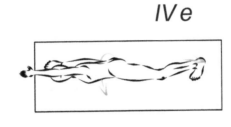

IVe

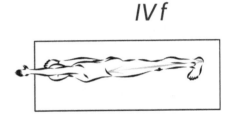

IVf

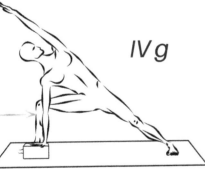

IVg

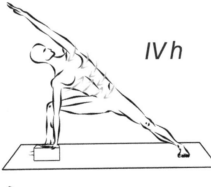

IVh

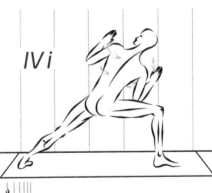

IVi

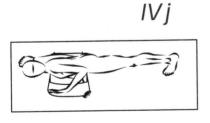

IVj

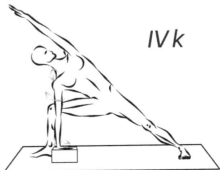

IVk

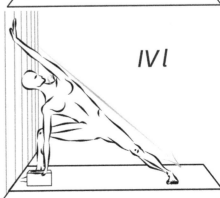

IVl

Parsvottanasana
Intense Trunk Extension Pose

Learn + Practice

After Uttanasana and Supta Padangusthasana A, before Standing Twists

Linked Poses

Uttanasana, Trikonasana, Virabhadrasana A + C, Parivritta Trikonasana, Janu Sirsasana

Safety Factors

Hamstring injury, SI joint dysfunction; use care with knee injuries

Prepare

· Set mat's short end to wall

Enter

· Stand facing wall in *Tadasana* with feet hip width apart, *I a*
· Bring hands to hips and step right foot forward, 18"-2' from wall
· Right foot and leg in neutral rotation
· Pressing into right big toe mound, step left foot 3-4' back and externally rotate left leg 45°, *I b*
· Gather front iliums and resist heels laterally
· Pushing into left outer heel, soften pubis in and up
· Without losing left leg rotation, lift left hip and draw left hip forward
· Increasing pressure through right big toe mound, roll right outer hip backward and down
· With both legs firm, lift pelvis up and over femur heads, folding forward
· Place hands on wall at chest, waist, or hip height, *I c*
· Pressing hands into wall, extend pelvis symmetrically backward, *I d*

Sustain

· Continue leg and pelvis actions from *Enter*
· Push diagonally from right greater trochanter to right big toe mound
· Without hyperextending legs, firm thighs and lift both kneecaps
· Extend outer left heel away from back pelvis
· Without dropping left pelvis or internally rotating left leg, roll left hip toward wall
· Articulate left femur rotation within left hip joint
· Pressing hands to wall, lengthen side torso symmetrically, *I e*
· Keep both hips equidistant from wall

Exit

· Increase left outer heel pressure
· Firming both legs, inhale and lift torso upright, bringing hands back to hips
· Step left foot forward and right foot back to *Tadasana*
· Repeat to the left
· Practice *Wall Push*, *I f* (*Ardha Uttanasana*, *Simplify*) between sides and repetitions

Challenge

1. Left knee torque, thigh collapse
2. Right leg hyperextension
3. Right groin binds
4. Pelvis doesn't square

Response

1. Decrease external rotation to 15° or 30°, but rotate from the hip joint. Differentiate external thigh rotation from pelvic action, *I g*. Once learned, gradually increase thigh rotation.
2. Wedge a block behind right calf, *I h*. Resist right tibia head forward. Emphasize firming the thigh by lifting the kneecap up rather than pushing the knee back. Lift pelvis more clearly while folding and while in the pose. Push left heel more heavily downward.
3. Lighten heel pressure or lift heel completely while *Entering*. Keeping groin soft, descend heel while *Sustaining*. *See also Explore; Nourish, Response 1.*
4. Pelvis will usually not be completely square. Do not force. Push back pelvis away from both feet, lifting off femur heads. *See also Response 1.*

Combining elements of Uttanasana, Virabhadrasana A, and Trikonasana, Parsvottanasana is preparatory to Virabhadrasana C and Parivritta Trikonasana. Although a Standing Forward Bend, it emphasizes length in the trunk and side torso.

Contact Points

Feet, hands

External Supports

Mat, wall
Block

Essence of Form

Folding pelvis symmetrically over asymmetrical leg action; front leg neutral, back leg external, arms neutral

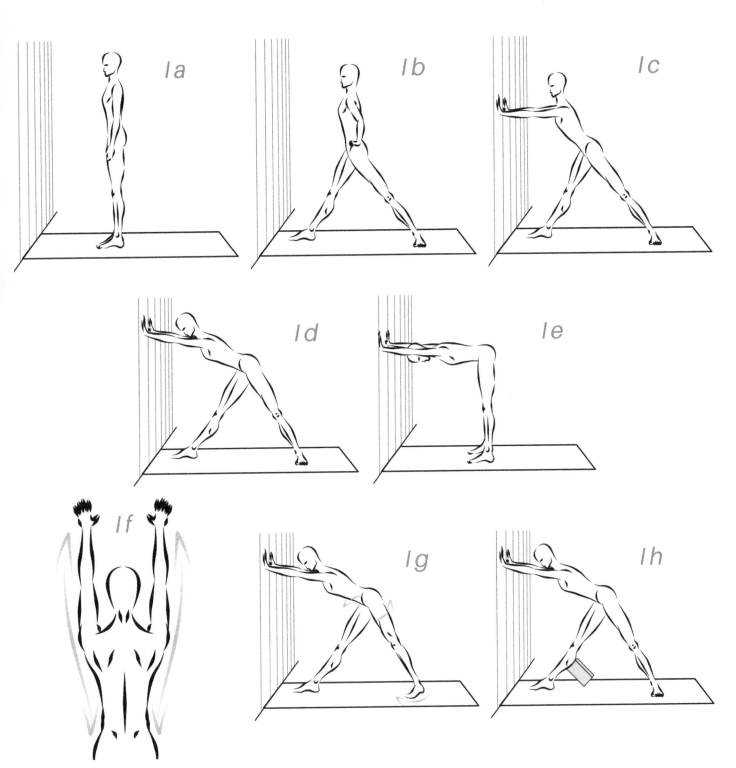

Parsvottanasana
Intense Trunk Extension Pose

Learn + Practice

Same as Simplify, once develop some familiarity with the chair before practicing

Linked Poses

Uttanasana, Trikonasana, Virabhadrasana A + C, Parivritta Trikonasana, Janu Sirsasana

Safety Factors

Hamstring injury, wrist or hand injury, be careful chair does not tip

Prepare

- Set mat's short end against wall
- Turn chair upside down, chair seat's lip and back of chair on floor, chair legs up
- Set chair on mat with chair back against wall and legs pointing away from it, *ll a*
- Protect heel by folding mat's far end over underside of chair seat if necessary, *ll b*

Enter

- Place hands on chair's back legs and stabilize with hands to prevent tipping, *ll c*
- Step right foot forward, stepping into chair's underside, *ll d*
- Right leg in neutral rotation with foot mid line parallel with chair seat edges
- Keeping chair stable with hands and pressing into right foot, step left leg back 3-4'
- Practice first with left leg and foot neutral, then externally rotate, *ll e*
- Gathering front iliums and softening pubis inward
- Continue folding pelvis over femur heads and lower hands to chair's crossbar

Sustain

- Maintain leg and pelvis actions from *Simplify*
- Equalize pressure through all 4 corners of right foot
- Push pelvis back and up away from right foot
- Roll left ilium forward, lifting away from left outer foot, *ll f*
- Pressing into hands, lengthen pelvis and side ribs away from each other, *ll g*
- Extend along both sides of torso from hips to armpits
- Without shortening back body and emphasizing side torso length extend from pubis to sternum

Exit

- Increase left outer heel pressure and gather front iliums
- With legs firm, walk hands to chair leg bottoms
- Neutralize left leg, lifting heel
- Stabilizing chair with hands, step right foot back to left foot distance
- Step left foot into chair, repeating to the left
- When finished, step left foot out of chair and step both feet forward

Challenge

1. Left inner arch collapse
2. Overstretch in left calf and/ or Achilles tendon
3. Overstretch in right hamstring and/or calf
4. Chest collapse

Response

1. Press into outer left foot. Reduce external rotation in left leg (adjust foot accordingly). Abduct big toe. Circularly roll left inner arch toward outer heel.
2. Reduce stance width. Calf/ Achilles tendon should be challenging but not in excess of 45-60° dorsi flexion.
3. Reduce chair angle with blocks under chair seat, *ll h*. Prepare with calf stretches, *ll i-j*. Practice *Simplify*, *Supta Padangusthasana*, and *Adho Mukha Svanasana*, *Simplify + Explore*.
4. Pressing into hands, lift back rib cage. Emphasize back and side body length over folding capacity. Resist hands backward and engage triceps to extend chest forward. Draw heads of upper arm bones toward shoulders.

Parsvottanasana uniquely lengthens both the hamstrings and groins due to the opposing leg actions. It is closely related to Janu Sirsasana, sharing many similar elements, particularly articulating the hip and femur movements in the back leg as the pelvis folds forward.

Contact Points

Feet, hands

External Supports

Wall, mat, chair
2 blocks

Essence of Form

As for Simplify, additional dorsi flexion; back leg in neutral rotation, then external, arms in external rotation

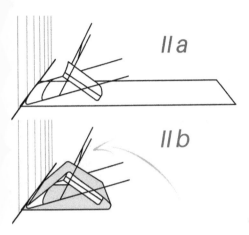

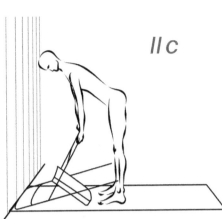

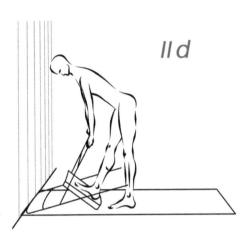

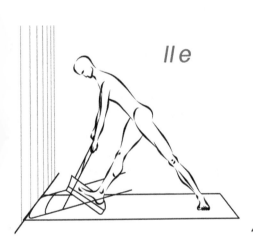

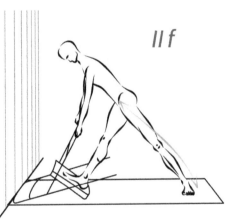

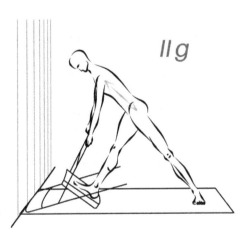

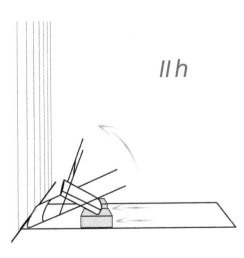

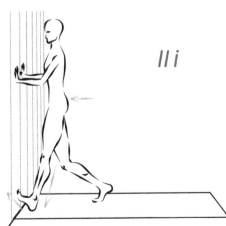

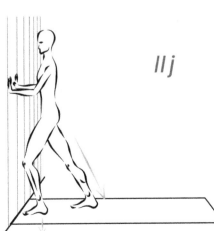

Intense Trunk Extension Pose — Explore

Learn + Practice

Once Simplify is stable, after Trikonasana and Anjaneyasana

Linked Poses

Uttanasana, Trikonasana, Virabhadrasana A + C, Parivritta Trikonasana, Janu Sirsasana

Safety Factors

As for Simplify; take particular care with hamstring injury and shoulder injury or laxity

Prepare

- Set chair 3.5-4.5' from wall, without a mat

Enter

- Stand between wall and chair, hands on hips
- Step left foot back, bringing outer heel to wall, foot and leg turned out 45-60°, *III a*
- Anchoring left outer heel to wall, step right foot forward, 3-4' from wall, foot between front chair legs, *III b*
- Firming right thigh, push diagonally from right greater trochanter to big toe mound
- Keeping left outer heel pressure and external left thigh rotation, level pelvis
- Using left heel pressure, lift left hip up and over femur head to initiate fold
- Exhaling, continue folding forward, lifting the pelvis over the femurs
- Keeping torso length, place hands under shoulders on chair seat, palms wide, *III c*
- Lift sternum away from pubis
- Pressing left outer heel backward, slide chair forward, extending arms and torso, *III d*

Sustain

- Continue actions from *Simplify + Explore*
- Deepen hip creases, drawing inner and outer right groin equally backward
- Recede left groin as hip lifts over femur
- Draw back of pubis in and up
- Press upper femurs back as arms extend forward
- Integrate all actions from left outer heel through to fingertips

Exit

- Stabilizing the legs, slide chair back to bring the chair and hands under shoulders
- Pressing hands into chair seat, lift chest, *III e*
- With torso long, press into the outer left heel and place hands on hips, *III f*
- Further deepening left heel pressure, descend the back pelvis to bring torso upright on inhalation, *III g*
- Turn right leg and torso to the left into *Uttitha Hasta Padasana*
- Step or jump the feet to *Tadasana*, then repeat with the left leg forward and right heel to wall

Challenge

1. Lifting pelvis over femur action not clear
2. Left pelvis drops
3. Right leg hyperextension
4. Chest/shoulder collapse

Response

1. *Prepare* on a sticky mat. Place folded chair's legs on either side of right foot or further forward depending on leg length. Bring chair back against pubis. Stabilize chair with hands, lean into chair and lift pelvis over chair. Use pubis as fulcrum and soften groins away from chair pressure, *III h.*
2. Increase outer left heel pressure, lift left inner arch and emphasize rotating from left upper femur. Without narrowing space between thighs, hug outer thighs toward mid line.
3. *See Simplify, Response 2.* Flex right foot and resist heel backward as torso extends forward.
4. Pressing down through hands, lift back ribcage. Draw upper humeri into shoulder joint. Widen shoulder girdle and draw forearms toward each other.

By sliding a chair away from the back leg in Parsvottanasana, the defining side torso length is reinforced. It also teaches the kinetic connection through the entire body from back heel to hands, balancing mobility and stability through the principle of anchor and extension.

Contact Points

Feet, hands

External Supports

Wall, chair
Mat

Essence of Form

As for Simplify, with arm and torso extension

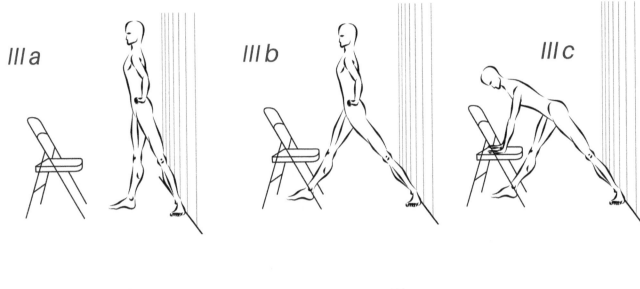

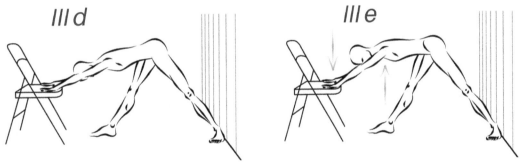

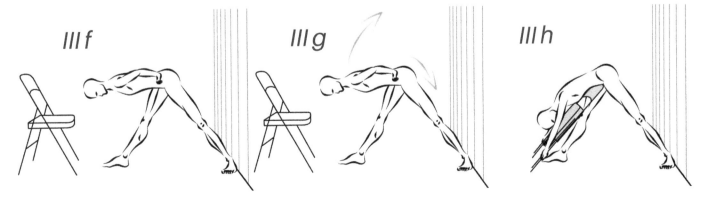

Parsvottanasana
Intense Trunk Extension Pose

Synthesize

Learn + Practice

After Simplify + Nourish; after some shoulder opening

Linked Poses

Virabhadrasana A + C, Janu Sirsasana, Marichyasana A, Salamba Sarvangasana

Safety Factors

Same as Simplify; shoulder, elbow or wrist injury

Prepare

· Set mat away from walls

Enter

· Stand at mat's center in *Tadasana*
· Step or jump to *Uttitha Hasta Padasana*, arms extended, *IV a-b*
· Exhaling, clasp opposite elbows behind back, *Paschima Baddha Hastasana, IV c*
· Turn left leg in and right leg out to *Parsva Hasta Padasana, IV d*
· Pushing left outer heel into floor, continue turning pelvis until torso faces right foot, *IV e*
· Using left heel pressure, lift pelvis hip up and femurs, folding torso forward, *IV f*

ॐ *If shoulders are injury-free, bring arms to Paschima Namaskara instead of clasping elbows:*

· In *Uttitha Hasta Padasana*, externally rotate arms, turning palms upward, *IV g*
· Exhaling, swiftly bend elbows and internally rotate arms, joining the palms behind back, *IV h*
· Lift and widen chest before folding forward over legs, *IV i*

Sustain

· Continue *Sustain* actions from *Simplify*, *Explore*, and *Nourish*
· Circularly roll skin from front shoulder over the top toward the back, releasing trapezium
· Broaden shoulder girdle and extend arms from inner chest to outer shoulders
· Draw upper humeri backward
· Lift front armpits and extend inner elbows down and forward
· In *Paschima Namaskara*, press index finger and thumb mounds together, drawing outer hands into upper thoracic spine

Exit

· Stabilize right big toe mound and firm right thigh
· Increasing left outer heel pressure, lengthen sternum forward
· Using left outer heel pressure, descend back pelvis and inhale, bringing torso upright, *IV j*
· Turn right leg inward and left leg out to *Parsva Hasta Padasana* on the left side and repeat to the left
· When finished, step or jump from *Uttitha Hasta Padasana* to *Tadasana*

Challenge

1. Leg hyperextension
2. Shoulders round forward
3. Length lost when folding past horizontal
4. Torso twists at deeper fold

Response

1. Without the support of the hands and arms, hyperextension is a deeper *Challenge. See Responses from Simplify + Nourish.* If still a *Challenge*, ensure knees do not internally rotate. Often hyperextension accompanies internal rotation at the lower leg. Counter this tendency by lifting the arches and externally rotating the lower leg slightly.
2. Widen chest by resisting shoulders and elbows away from each other.
3. When folding beyond horizontal, contact right leg with right side of abdomen, then bottom ribs, then chest, then head.
4. Observe which side is shortening and without increasing twist, lengthen the shorter feeling side. Guide the torso's mid line forward as though practicing *Uttanasana*.

In addition to lengthening the groins and hamstrings while increasing hip mobility, Parsvottanasana also introduces shoulder extension with internal rotation through Paschima Namaskara. This combination of leg and arm movements makes it an essential Twists preparation.

Contact Points

Feet, hands
Elbows

External Supports

Mat

Essence of Form

As for Simplify, posterior arm extension, elbow flexion; internal arm rotation

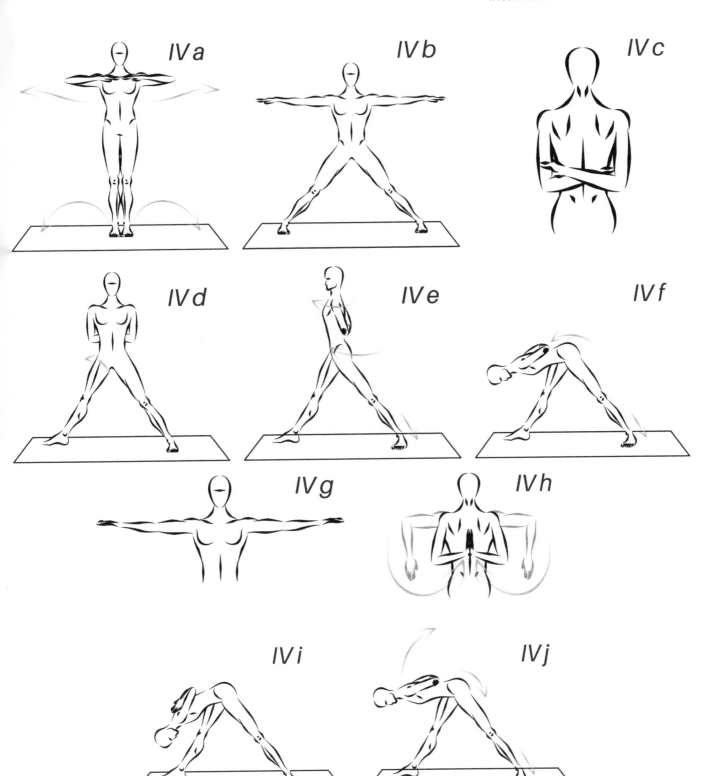

IVa

IVb

IVc

IVd

IVe

IVf

IVg

IVh

IVi

IVj

Dandasana Urdhva Hastasana
Staff Pose with Arms Raised

Simplify

Learn + Practice

Introduce early, before Seated Forward Bends, with or before Supta Padangusthasana A + B

Linked Poses

Virasana, Upavistha Konasana, Adho Mukha Svanasana, Uttanasana

Safety Factors

Lower back strain; do not raise arms if hypertense

Prepare

- Mat's short edge to wall
- Set chair on mat facing wall, 3/4 of a leg's length from it, *I a*

Enter

- Sit at chair edge, with legs bent and feet flat on floor
- Have feet and thighs hip-width apart, *I b*
- Without collapsing knees inward, manually roll inner thigh flesh downward
- Press hands to chair seat, beside pelvis, *I c*
- Tilt pelvis to neutral, sitting on the front sitting bones and moving L4 + L5 inward
- Keeping pelvis neutral, extend right leg, then left, pushing balls of feet into wall and heels into floor away from back pelvis, *I d*
- Ensure foot and leg mid lines are parallel, feet together or hip-width apart
- Resist heels laterally and gather front iliums, descending inner femurs
- Keeping femurs descending and without protruding front ribs, inhale, raising arms to *Urdhva Hastasana, I e*

Sustain

- Descend and widen inner back femurs
- Soften pubis in and up
- Lengthen inner thighs from pubis to big toe mounds
- Broaden soles of feet, activate arches
- Equalize pressure through all 4 corners of feet
- Lift front iliums up away from descending femurs
- Without hardening abdomen or tilting pelvis backward, descend lower front ribs, *I f*
- Lift bottom back rib cage, *I g*
- Lengthen through arms, extending side torso
- Descend chin slightly and ascend occiput, *I h*

Exit

- Keeping torso length, exhale and lower arms
- Bend the legs and bring feet flat to floor
- Pressing feet into floor, inhale to standing

🕉 *When lumbar can be kept neutral throughout, Prepare + Enter with blocks at wall to raise feet, I.4*

Challenge

1. Pelvis tilts backward and lumbar rounds
2. Groins bind and femurs lift
3. Front ribs protrude
4. Chest collapse

Response

1. Manually internally rotate thighs, using hands to drag back thigh flesh laterally outward. Raise chair's back legs on blocks, tilting the seat's angle forward, *I i.* Add height on chair seat under pelvis to reduce hip flexion and strain on hamstrings.
2. Tie a strap behind chair's front legs and around upper thighs, *I j.* Press hands into chair back to increase traction on upper femurs and lift chest. Can also be done with legs through chair as in *Response 3.*
3. Turn chair around and bring legs through chair back. Sit at edge so that chair back presses lightly against front ribs. Soften ribs away from chair contact and lift chest, *I k.* Without rounding lumbar, descend back pelvis and ascend back ribs.
4. *See Responses 2 + 3.*

Most Seated Poses begin in Dandasana as a foundation, similar to how Tadasana is the root of Standing Poses. Accurately tilting the pelvis in Seated Poses is often challenging. Sitting on a chair helps establish the neutral pelvis while minimizing required hamstring length.

Contact Points

Sitting bones, upper back femurs, heels, balls of feet, hands

External Supports

Mat, chair, block, wall
Strap, block

Essence of Form

Hip flexion, leg extension, arm extension; arms and legs neutral

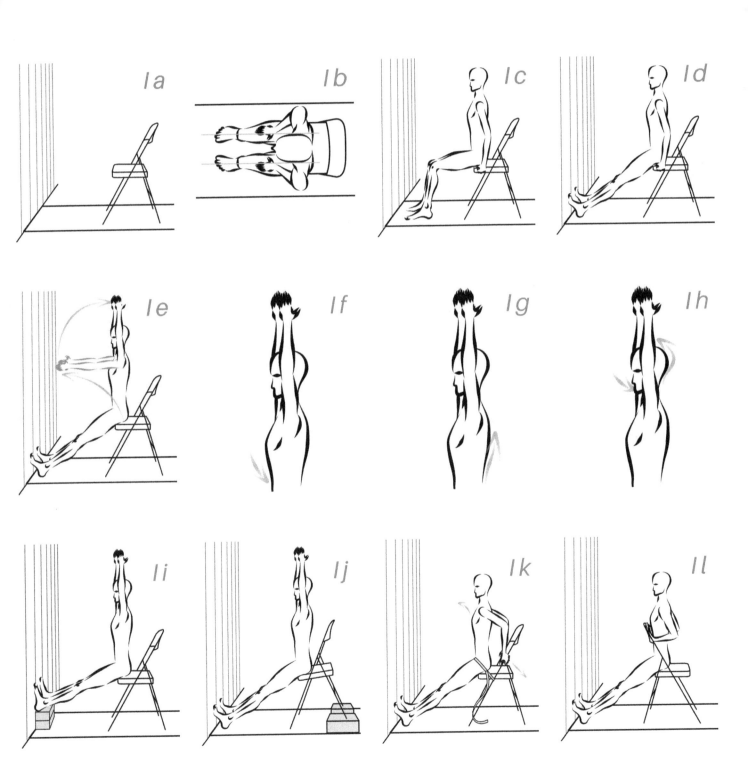

Learn + Practice

After Simplify, once lumbar curve can be retained with feet on blocks

Linked Poses

All Seated Poses, Adho Mukha Svanasana, Urdhva Prasarita Padasana

Safety Factors

Hamstring injury; keep feet apart if pregnant, back to wall without arm lift if hypertense

Prepare

- With mat's short end to wall, lie on right side
- Roll onto back and extend legs up the wall
- If lumbar flattens into floor, move away from wall until L4 + L5 move inward
- Measure the distance between sitting bones and wall, fill gap with blocks, *II a*
- This determines sitting height: set height one leg's distance from wall
- Set additional blocks beside seat height to support palms, *II b-c*

🕉 *Can also be practiced keeping legs up wall*

Enter

- Sit on height from *Prepare* and extend legs, feet pressing into wall away from back pelvis, *II d*
- Manually drag back thigh flesh outward and descend inner thighs
- Adjust buttock flesh as well, moving it diagonally out and backward
- Keeping neutral lumbar and descending front ribs, raise arms to *Urdhva Hastasana*, *II e*

Sustain

- Continue all actions from *Simplify*
- Extend the heels away from the calves, calves away from back thighs, *II f*
- Widen the backs of each thigh
- Extending through big toe mounds, and spread the toes laterally
- Recede and broaden inner groins, moving the femurs away from the pubis
- Descend sitting bones heavily, lifting upper sacrum + lower lumbars up and forward
- Release top buttocks away from back rib cage and away from mid line, *II g*
- With inner femurs descending, lift torso upward
- Lengthen side torso from hips to armpits and continue through arms
- Extend from sacrum to occiput

Exit

- Hold 5-10 breaths
- Keeping torso length, lower arms and rest hands beside or behind pelvis
- Hold an additional 5-10 breaths
- Bend the legs and release

Challenge

1. Leg hyperextension
2. Knee pain
3. Groin tightness
4. Mid-upper back discomfort, pelvis falls back

Response

1. Place a rolled blanket beneath calves. Resist tibia heads upward as femurs descend, *II h*.
2. *See Response 1*. Ensure inner knees are not collapsing as inner thigh flesh descends. Hold a block between the thighs and/or strap the big toes and resist outward, *II i*.
3. Add height under pelvis, or angle support to tip pelvis forward, *II j*, so that hip flexors do not have to overwork. Press femurs downward with a stick and lift pelvis away from pressure, *II k*.
4. Increase stamina and capacity with shorter hold repetitions. Practice with back to wall, *II l*, or with bolster against wall and blocks to support hands, *II m*, for deeper chest opening before *Nourish*. *See also Response 1 from Synthesize*.

Once a neutral spine can be established and maintained while seated on a chair, increase the challenge by lowering the sitting height. This variation explores how to determine the appropriate sitting height based on hamstring and pelvis capacity in preparation for other Seated Poses.

Contact Points

Sitting bones, back femurs, feet

External Supports

Mat, wall, blocks, foam blocks, blankets

Essence of Form

As for Simplify; legs internally rotated, arms externally rotated

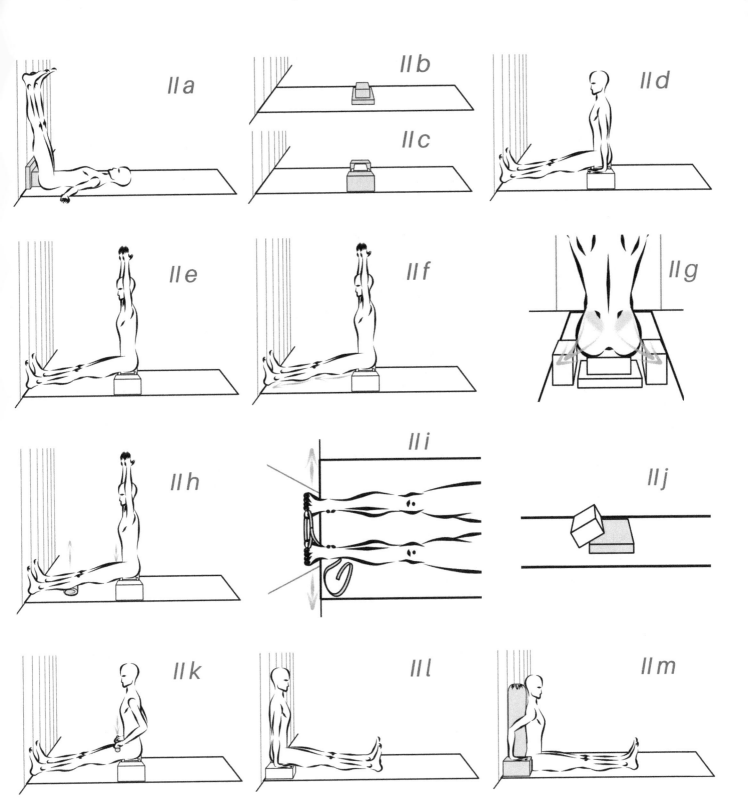

Learn + Practice

After Adho Mukha Svanasana,
Before Viparita Dandasana
and Back Bends

Linked Poses

Viparita Dandasana,
Viparita Karani, Ustrasana,
Intermediate Back Bends

Safety Factors

As for Explore; support
hands on blocks beside
pelvis if hypertense

Prepare

- Mat's short end to wall
- Set chair on mat, back to wall
- Place sitting height in front of chair, under chair lip; use minimal height possible
- Put one bolster on chair seat, *III a*
- Place folded blanket on bolster for additional head support

Enter

- Sit in front of chair, with back rib cage against chair lip at bottom shoulder blade level, *III b*
- Press feet away from back pelvis and extend legs to *Dandasana*
- Gather front iliums and resist heels laterally
- Descend inner femurs
- Without lifting femurs and keeping back rib contact, inhale and raise arms to *Urdhva Hastasana, III c*
- Lifting torso, reach hands up and back to touch wall
- Bending elbows, walk hands down wall to catch chair back with hands
- Draw elbows toward each other and lengthen elbows upward, lifting chest, *III d*
- Exhaling, keep chest lift and rest head back on bolster

Sustain

- Engage and maintain *Sustain* actions from *Simplify + Explore*
- Rest back body into chair lip and bolster
- Gently pull chair with hands, increasing chair lip pressure against mid-back
- Lengthen sternum from bottom to top
- Widen upper shoulder blades
- Deepen inner armpits while wrapping outer armpits forward
- If capacity allows, walk hands toward chair seat

Exit

- Resting head, release hands from chair and hold head with hands, *III e*
- Inhaling, lift head to neutral
- Bring hands to floor beside pelvis
- Pushing into hands, inhale and lift chest, coming upright to seated
- Sit upright until extreme sensations dissipate

☀ *This variation can be practiced in all seated poses, particularly Upavistha Konasana, Baddha Konasana, and Virasana, III f-h*

Challenge

1. Inability to reach chair
2. Chair tips back or chest collapses
3. Shoulder pain
4. Neck discomfort
5. Tingling in arms or hands

Response

1. Tie strap to backrest in *Prepare*. Gradually walk hands along strap until hands reach chair in *Enter*, *III i*. Bend legs and lift pelvis to catch chair, then slowly descend pelvis, *III j*. Practice *II m, Explore,* first. *See also Response 2.*
2. Move pelvis further back. Increase sitting height until chair lip contacts mid- to lower shoulder blades, *III k*. Lift armpit chest up and over chair lip rather than just straight back.
3. Resist upper humeri back and out, gathering elbows inward, *III l*. Soften trapezius.
4. Increase head support. *See Response 3.*
5. Pad chair lip with folded mat. Come out until tingling dissipates. *See Responses 3 + 4.*

Upashrayi Dandasana introduces a supported Back Bend to open the chest. It is beneficial when recuperating from illness, during times of stress or physical strain, and during pregnancy. Modify by supporting the hands beside the pelvis if the overhead extension is too extreme.

Contact Points

Legs, sitting bones, back ribs

External Supports

Wall, mat, chair, blocks, bolster, blanket
Strap, blocks, folded mat, additional blankets

Essence of Form

As for Simplify; armpit/chest extension with elbow flexion; legs neutral toward internal, arms external

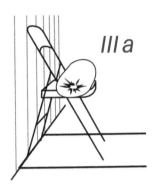

III a

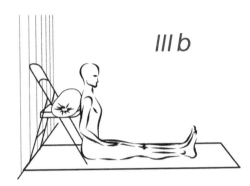

III b

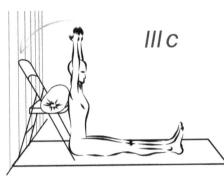

III c

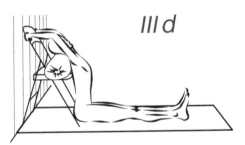

III d

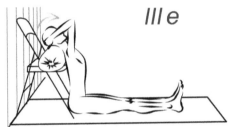

III e

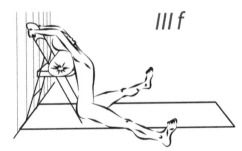

III f

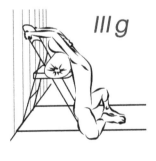

III g

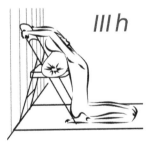

III h

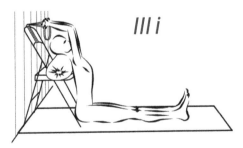

III i

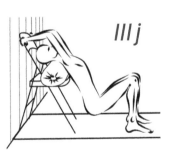

III j

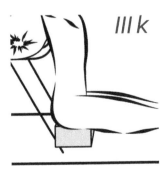

III k

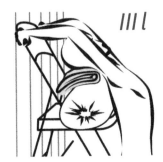

III l

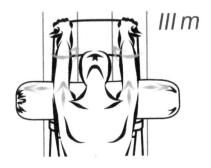

III m

Dandasana
Staff Pose

Synthesize

Learn + Practice

Once *Nourish* is integrated, before seated Forward Bends

Linked Poses

Halasana, Viparita Karani, Purvottanasana, Phalakasana

Safety Factors

Same as *Simplify, Explore,* and *Nourish;* lumbar disc problems

Prepare

- Place sitting height on mat, determined by *Explore*
- If possible, reduce height without losing neutral pelvis
- Set additional support for upper femurs
- If hands do not reach floor when seated, place additional blocks beside pelvis

Enter

- Sit on height with legs bent, feet flat on floor
- Lean slightly forward and move sitting bones backward, *IV a*
- Roll inner thigh flesh downward, dragging back thighs outward, *IV b*
- Extend legs, pushing feet away from back pelvis
- Place hands beside pelvis on floor or blocks
- Pushing into hands, lift sitting bones up off support, *IV c*
- Descend upper femurs and make contact with support, then lower sitting bones, *IV d*
- Pressing hands and back femurs down, lift trunk
- Without straining throat or tongue, lift sternum and occiput, lower chin toward chest

Sustain

- Apply *Sustain* actions from *Simplify* + *Explore*
- Descending and widening inner back femurs, also descend outer back femurs
- Keep weight centered on back heel, neither rolling toward inner nor outer heel
- Widen across the shoulder blades and draw the lower shoulder blades forward
- Soften behind abdominal wall
- Lift and broaden the diaphragm, creating space for the abdominal organs
- Lift and widen the front collarbones while descending the posterior collarbones
- Broaden across the back of the neck and deepen the cervical curve inward
- Soften the throat and sense organs

Exit

- Continue to *Paschimottanasana* or other seated poses, and return to *Dandasana*
- Roll the legs into external rotation, then bend the legs and release the pose

Challenge

1. Pelvis rolls back, leg action unclear
2. Femur collapse, abdominal breath restriction
3. Shoulder restriction, chest collapse

Response

1. Tie a loose strap below the pelvic rims. Thread 2nd strap through pelvic strap, with strap's end pulling toward the torso. At the foot end, secure a block with a half-hitch, *IV e*. Bend the legs to tighten 2nd belt, *IV f*. Pushing feet into the block, extend both legs, *IV g*. Also applicable to *Explore + Nourish*.
2. Hold a block between thighs and strap legs, *IV h*. Have 2 assistants with belts: loop belts around upper inner thighs. Assistants press feet against greater trochanters and lower femurs and symmetrically pull straps, *IV i*.
3. Strap around the shoulders, below the humerus heads and resist outward, *IV j*. Partner presses down on acromion from behind. Lift acromion up into partner's resistance, *IV k*.

All variations of Dandasana help develop strength and endurance in the spinal muscles, particularly when sitting height is minimal and the back is unsupported. This classical variation also introduces Jalandhara Bandha, used in Pranayama and all Sarvangasana-family poses.

Contact Points

Sitting bones, femurs, hands

External Supports

Blocks, folded blanket
2 straps

Essence of Form

Hip flexion, leg extension, neck flexion; slight internal arm rotation, legs neutral

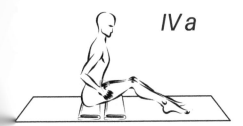

IVa

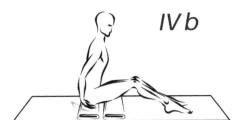

IVb

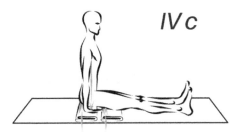

IVc

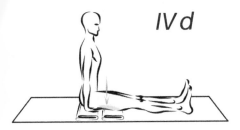

IVd

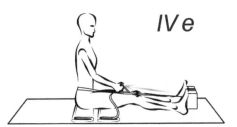

IVe

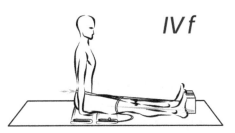

IVf

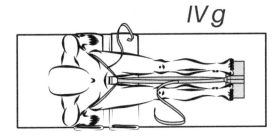

IVg

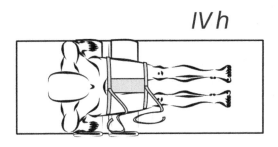

IVh

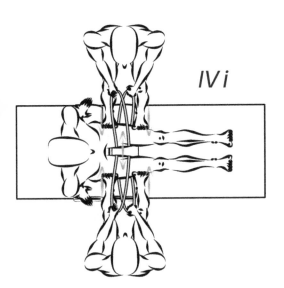

IVi

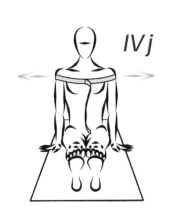

IVj

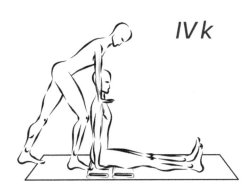

IVk

Upavistha Konasana
Seated Wide-Angle Pose

Learn + Practice

*Before narrow Forward
Bends and Seated Poses*

Linked Poses

*Supta Padangusthasana B,
Prasarita Padottanasana,
Dandasana, Baddha Konasana*

Safety Factors

*Groin, hamstring, or
adductor injury*

Prepare

- Place mat's short end to wall
- Ensure wall is clear 3-4'
  to each side of mat

Enter

- Lie on right side, toward
  mat's right edge with torso
  perpendicular to wall, legs bent
- Bring the buttocks to the wall
- With sitting bones against
  wall, roll onto the back, and
  extend legs up wall, *I a-b*
- Reach both sitting bones
  equally into wall, creating
  a neutral lumbar curve
- Symmetrically contact sacrum
  against floor and extend
  legs away from back pelvis,
  reaching through heels
- Gather front iliums
- Pressing left heel into wall,
  lift right leg and abduct
  45°-60° from mid line, *I c*
- Repeat with the left leg, *I d*,
  bringing legs equally away
  from body's mid line, *I e*

🕉 *For holds longer than a
minute, Prepare with a second
mat, long edge against wall.
Place chairs on each side to
support legs in Enter, I f.*

Sustain

- Firm the thighs and extend
  backs of legs, reaching heels
  away from back pelvis
- Maintain a neutral lumbar curve
- Lengthen big toe mounds
  away from inner groins
- Spread toes and deepen groins
- Press backs of thighs into wall
- Neutralize leg rotation, internally
  rotating if legs turn outward
- Resist heels laterally and
  roll front iliums toward
  opposite inner thighs
- Soften pubis inward
  and toward navel
- Release abdomen and
  breathe naturally

Exit

- Place hands against outer
  thighs, using them to draw
  the legs back together, *I g*
- Exhaling, bend legs
  and roll to the right
- Pressing left hand into the floor,
  inhale and press to seated
- Once *Enter* movements are
  smooth, reverse for *Exit*
- If holding less than a
  minute, repeat 4-6 times
- During repetitions, alternate
  leading leg for each set

Challenge

1. Lower back flattens into the floor
2. Buttocks do not touch the wall
3. Legs externally rotate
4. Legs do not straighten
5. Head tilts backward,
   throat tension

Response

1. Internally rotate thighs. Extend
   pubis toward the wall. Support
   lumbar with blanket folded
   3-4" wide. Move further from
   wall. Ensure sitting bones
   retain contact point by
   filling space with blocks.
2. If lumbar is not flattening,
   roll to the right and bring
   buttocks closer to the wall.
   Re-*Enter* the pose. Fill any
   remaining gap between wall
   and buttocks with blocks.
3. Grip right upper thigh firmly
   with the hands and manually
   internally rotate it. Holding
   this rotation, adjust the
   left leg the same way.
4. Push both feet actively away
   from the back pelvis. Tie straps
   from the pelvis to each foot, *I h.*
   See *Prasarita Padottanasana.*
5. Support head with
   folded blankets

Practicing Upavistha Konasana supine with legs up the wall reduces strain on the groins and lower back, emphasizing the pelvic floor breadth, hip mobility, and lateral abdominal space inherent to the pose. Use care not to overstretch the inner thighs as gravity draws the legs down.

Contact Points

Back of pelvis, ribcage, and skull, sitting bones

External Supports

Mat, wall, blocks
Additional mat, 2 chairs, 2 straps, blankets

Essence of Form

Leg abduction and hip flexion; arms and legs in neutral rotation

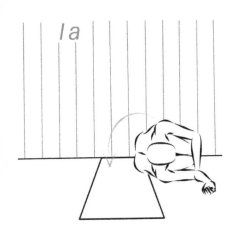

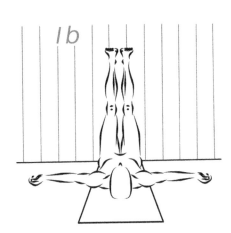

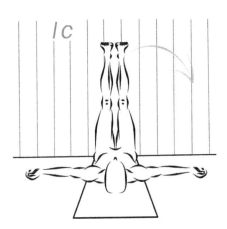

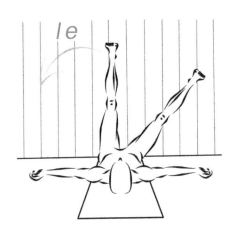

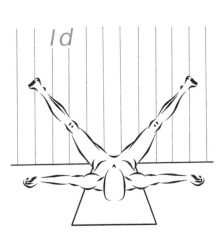

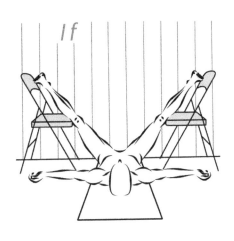

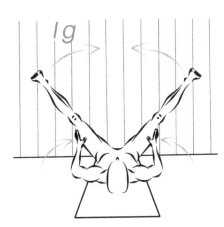

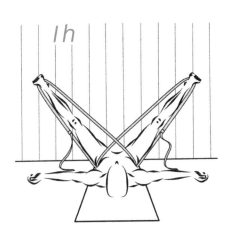

Seated Wide-Angle Pose — *Simplify*

Learn + Practice

Before narrow Forward Bends, after *Prasarita Padottanasana*

Linked Poses

Lateral Standing Poses, *Dandasana, Baddha Konasana, Supta Padangusthasana B*

Safety Factors

Groin, hamstring, or adductor injury

Prepare

- Place mat away from walls and obstructions
- If blocks were used between buttocks and wall in *Simplify*, set same support near mat's long edge
- Place blocks beside support for hands
- Use at least one folded blanket under pelvis

Enter

- Sit on support in *Dandasana*, extending legs perpendicular to mat's long edge, *II a*
- Descend heels and femurs
- Bring hands to floor or blocks on either side of back pelvis
- Pressing into the hands, lift the chest and lean torso slightly back into the hands
- With left leg stable, lengthen right heel away from back pelvis and lift right leg
- While lifted, abduct right leg 45°-60° from the mid line, do not open to the maximum, *II b-c*
- Stabilizing right leg, lengthen, lift, and abduct left leg 45°-60°, *II d*
- Abduct legs symmetrically, with line between heels parallel to mat's long edge

Sustain

- Extend legs, reaching both heels away from back pelvis
- Neutralize leg rotation, *II e*
- Keep both thighs firm throughout
- Move L4 + L5 inward, bringing the sacrum to vertical
- Lengthen the inner thighs from pubis to big toe mounds
- Roll onto the front sitting bones and descend them symmetrically
- Descend inner thighs toward the floor
- Without lifting inner thighs, descend upper outer thighs as well
- Release buttock flesh away from back ribs
- Lift both sides of torso equally from hips to armpits

Exit

- Maintain full leg extension
- Lengthen and lift right leg
- Adduct right leg to *Dandasana*, further lengthening leg to lower
- With the right heel stable, lengthen, lift, and adduct left leg back to *Dandasana* also
- Repeat *Enter* and *Exit* 6-10 times, alternating which leg moves first

Challenge

1. Lumbar collapses backward
2. Front ribs poke forward
3. Knee hyperextension
4. Inner knee pain

Response

1. Increase pelvic support and sit higher. Draw front iliums diagonally to opposite inner thighs. Descend the pubis lifting upper sacrum forward, into the body and increasing pelvic tilt. Increase internal rotation in both thighs.
2. Without dropping chest, lift back ribs and slide them backward. Soften the belly and differentiate pelvic tilt from ribcage action.
3. Support with rolled blankets, *II f*. Press calves and heels down, resist tibia heads up, *II g*.
4. Broaden the upper femurs away from each other. Without externally rotating, descend the upper outer thighs more fully.

❀ *Challenges 1 + 2 are related: rest against a bolster at the wall, II h. Loop straps around the feet. Turn palms up and draw L4 + L5 inward while resting back ribs into bolster, II i*

Once mobility is found in the hips supine, sitting upright in Upavistha Konasana lengthens the inner thighs, broadens and tones the pelvic floor, and strengthens the spine. Moving in and out of the pose by lengthening and lifting the legs strengthens the groins and abdomen.

Contact Points

Sitting bones, back femurs, heels, hands

External Supports

Folded blanket
Blocks, blankets

Essence of Form

Leg abduction with hip flexion; arms and legs in neutral rotation

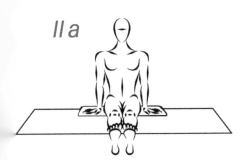

II a

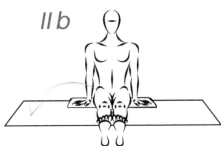

II b

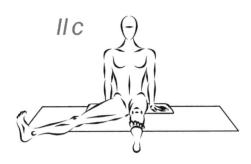

II c

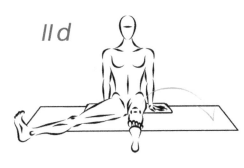

II d

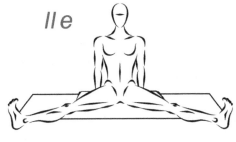

II e

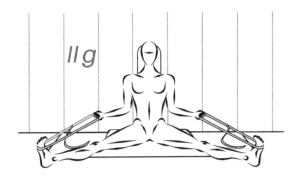

II g

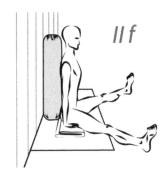

II f

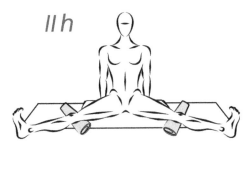

II h

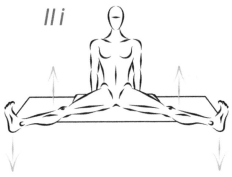

II i

Upavistha Konasana
Seated Wide-Angle Pose

Nourish

Learn + Practice

After Explore, once transitions are smooth and lumbar is neutral

Linked Poses

Baddha Konasana, Janu Sirsasana, Prasarita Padottanasana

Safety Factors

As for Simplify + Explore; do not raise the arms for hypertension

Prepare

- *Prepare as for Explore*

Enter

- Sit in *Dandasana*
- Bring hands to floor or blocks, behind pelvis
- Lean slightly backward on hands, keeping spine erect
- Lengthening heels away from back pelvis, lift both legs simultaneously and open them 90°-120°, *III a-b*
- Lower heels symmetrically and in line with each other
- Press hands down beside pelvis
- From hand pressure, lift pelvis off floor, *III c*
- Exhaling, descend femurs and contact backs of thighs to floor before sitting bones, *III d*
- Once seated, interlock fingers and turn palms outward, fully extending arms in front of chest
- Without protruding bottom front ribs, lift extended arms overhead, *III e*
- Push heels of hands and index finger mounds up

☙ *This arm variation is called Parvatasana or Urdhva Baddhanguliyasana*

Sustain

- Continue *Simplify + Explore Sustain* actions
- Keep kneecap centers facing the ceiling with legs in neutral rotation
- Pushing through big toe mounds, extend inner thighs more fully than inner thighs
- Spread the toes and draw the outer feet toward outer pelvis
- Extending through the heels, broaden across the back thighs
- Descend upper back femurs
- With femurs descending, lift hips and torso and lengthen equally along side torso through armpits to palms
- Descend inner shoulder blades

Exit

- Keep the legs long, firm, and stable
- Without losing torso lift, release interlock and lower arms
- Lean back on to hands
- Extending the legs away from the back pelvis, inhale and lift both legs back to *Dandasana*
- Repeat 6-10 times
- Each repetition, change dominant hand when interlocking fingers

Challenge

1. Lumbar collapse
2. Index finger side of hand drops and elbows bend in *Urdhva Baddhanguliyasana*
3. Mid and upper back strain

Response

1. Without internally rotating, press inner thighs toward floor. Broaden upper inner femurs. Move both iliums towards the pubis. Increase siting height if necessary to tilt pelvis forward and remove strain on hip flexors.
2. Extend arms away from inner shoulder blades, pressing index finger mounds upward and descending little finger mounds. Fully extend arms before raising, and only raise arms to the extent they can be kept straight
3. Support pelvis and descend femurs to create spinal length, rather than lifting from the floating ribs. Broaden between shoulder blades. Bring arms slightly forward and emphasize opening armpit angle. *See Explore, Responses 1 and 2.*

Developing the leg movements from Explore by lifting both legs simultaneously further strengthens the groins, spine, abdomen. Urdhva Baddhanguliyasana lengthens the torso, keeps the shoulders and wrists supple, counteracts kyphosis, and may help elevate mood.

Contact Points

Sitting bones, backs of femurs, back of heels, hands

External Supports

Mat, blanket, blocks

Essence of Form

Leg abduction, hip flexion, arm extension with interdigitation; arms and legs neutral

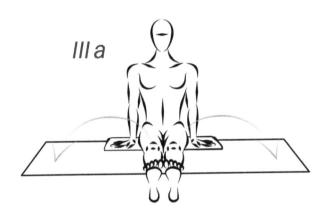

III a

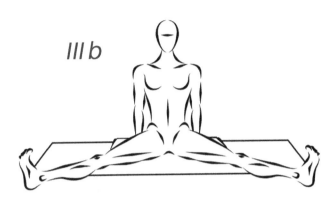

III b

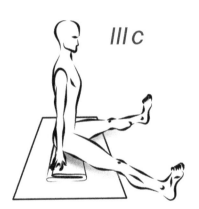

III c

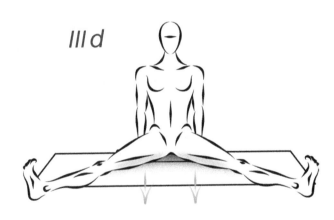

III d

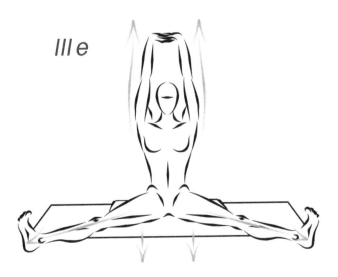

III e

Upavistha Konasana
Seated Wide-Angle Pose

Synthesize

Learn + Practice

*After Explore + Nourish;
before deep Forward Bends*

Linked Poses

Deep Forward Bends, Janu
Sirsasana, Baddha Konasana,
Paschimottanasana

Safety Factors

*As for Nourish; use care for
knee, hip, and hamstring
injuries; do not strain*

Prepare

· *Prepare* as for *Explore*

Enter

· Sit in *Dandasana* and bring legs
  to *Upavistha Konasana*, as for
  described in *Explore* or *Nourish*
· Press femurs downward, making
  maximum contact with floor
  from femurs to heels, inner back
  thighs to outer back thighs
· Lift lumbar spine up and out of
  the pelvis, moving upper sacrum
  and lower lumbar spine inward
· Without protruding front
  ribs, inhale and extend
  arms upward, *IV a-b*
· Descending femurs,
  symmetrically lift front iliums
· Reaching upward through arms
  and torso, fold forward 30°, *IV c*
· Without losing length from
  pubis to sternum, lower
  hands to the floor, *IV d*
· Gather front iliums toward
  each other, between femurs
· Descend pubis, then navel,
  then sternum, then forehead
· Walk hands forward while
  folding, and extend arms
  forward at last stage *IV e-g*
· Support head and torso for
  holds longer than 1 minute

Sustain

· Spread the toes, continuously
  widening the soles of feet
· Broaden space between
  femurs and pubis
· Lift and gather front iliums away
  from femurs on each inhalation
· On exhalations, further
  descend femurs
· Guide iliums toward opposite
  inner thighs, *IV h*
· Without lifting inner thighs,
  descend outer buttocks to
  neutralize leg rotation
· Extend big toe mounds away
  from inner groins, drawing outer
  feet toward outer pelvis, *IV i*
· Pressing hands into floor extend
  inner groins backward
· Keeping inner groins moving
  back, pull hands backward to
  lengthen sternum forward

Exit

· Keeping legs long and stable,
  walk hands under shoulders
· Pressing into hands, descend
  back pelvis and slowly come
  up to seated on inhalation
· Exhale back to *Dandasana*
  as for *Explore* or *Nourish*
· For longer holds, place hands
  to outer thighs and manually
  gather legs to *Dandasana*

Challenge

1. Groins bind when folding forward
2. Chest collapse, excessive
   spinal roundness
3. Knee hyperextension
4. Inner knee pressure

Response

1. Sit on more height. Press
   hands down into upper front
   thighs and lift iliums off femurs
   before folding. Soften thighs
   and buttocks to release
   groins. Keeping groins and
   buttocks soft, re-firm thighs.
2. Reduce fold and lift torso,
   lengthening from pubis to
   sternum. *See Response 1.*
3. If sitting on a height, support
   calves and femurs. Without
   bending legs, press heels down
   and resist tibia heads up.
4. Place blocks against inner
   thighs, just above knees.
   Push blocks into inner thighs
   with hands or elbows and
   pull femurs away from block
   pressure. Resist heels inward.

⚜ *For Responses 3 + 4, descend
outer knees slightly without
externally rotating thighs*

The pelvic space created by a wider leg angle in Upavistha Konasana often makes the action of tilting the pelvis over the femurs in Seated Forward Bends more accessible. For many, it may be the first extended-leg Forward Bend. It is also a good foundation for learning Seated Twists.

Contact Points

Femurs, heels, sitting bones (only when upright)

External Supports

Wall, mat, blanket

Essence of Form

Leg abduction, deep hip flexion; arms and legs neutral

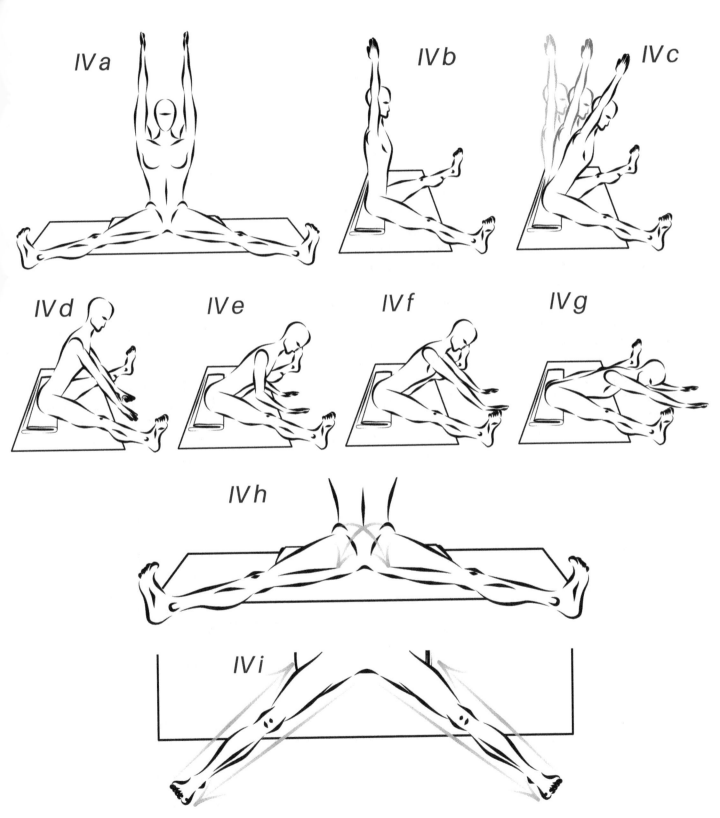

IVa

IVb

IVc

IVd

IVe

IVf

IVg

IVh

IVi

Baddha Konasana
Bound Angle Pose

Learn + Practice

Among the earliest poses to learn; before Seated and lateral Standing Poses

Linked Poses

Trikonasana, Parsvakonasana, Virabhadrasana B, Upavistha Konasana, Janu Sirsasana

Safety Factors

Groin, hamstring, adductor, or knee injury; use care with hip replacement

Prepare

· Mat's short end against a wall

Enter

· Lie on right side near right long edge of mat, spine perpendicular to wall
· Bring buttocks against wall, *Ia*
· Roll onto the back, swinging legs up the wall, *Ib*
· Contact back pelvis symmetrically against the floor, moving L5 + L4 inward
· Lengthen legs, pushing heels away from back pelvis
· From the tops of thighs, exhale and externally rotate the legs, *Ic*
· Keeping legs externally rotated, fold the legs one at a time, bringing heels to perineum *Id-e*
· Release thighs toward wall, without force *If*
· Rest the arms beside torso, palms up
· Alternate leading leg with each repetition when *Entering*

❀ *Once movement is smooth an comfortable, Enter and Exit as for Synthesize (but supine) to strengthen groins*

Sustain

· Keeping balanced contact through back pelvis, lengthen both sitting bones to the wall
· Press heels symmetrically against each other
· Extend femurs away from back pelvis
· Gather front iliums
· Widen greater trochanters laterally, broadening inner groin space
· Without losing lumbar curve, descend the bottom back ribs
· Keeping bottom back ribs descending, lift and broaden collarbones, descending outer shoulder blades toward floor
· Soften the abdomen
· Rest abdominal organs

Exit

· Bring hands to the outer thighs and manually draw the legs together
· Extend the legs up the wall and rest for a few breaths
· Exhaling, bend the legs and roll to the right
· Pressing the hands into the floor, come up from the side to seated on an inhalation

Challenge

1. Buttocks do not reach the wall
2. Thighs pull toward armpits
3. Significant asymmetry
4. Head tilts backward

Response

1. Before rolling onto the back, move closer to the wall. If the buttocks do not reach wall, fill the gap with blocks until sitting bones make firm contact, *Ig*.
2. Bring pelvis away from wall until the thighs release away from armpits and free the respiratory diaphragm. Fill the gap between wall and sitting bones with blocks as for *Response 1*.
3. First ensure pelvis is makes balanced contact both against floor and wall. With the pelvis level, draw less restricted thigh toward you and then release both thighs symmetrically away from each other. Equalize heel pressure, and lengthen both femurs before releasing toward wall.
4. Use a folded blanket under the head so the forehead slopes downward, *Ih*. Using hands, manually drag occiput away from shoulders.

Baddha Konasana is a fundamental pose that stretches the adductors, releases the groins, and helps relieve stiffness in the hips and hamstrings. Practicing it supine reduces strain on the hip flexors, which often overwork to keep the pelvis upright when seated.

Contact Points

Feet, sitting bones, back pelvis, back ribcage, shoulder blades, back of skull

External Supports

Wall, mat, blocks
Blanket, bolster, additional blocks

Essence of Form

Knee flexion with leg abduction; legs externally rotated, arms neutral

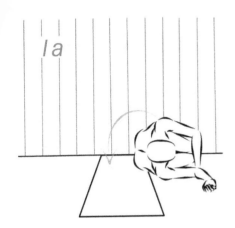

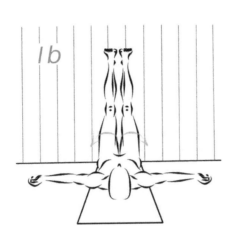

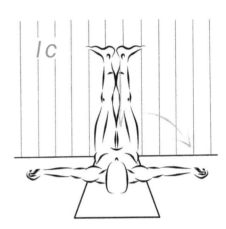

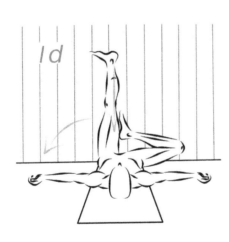

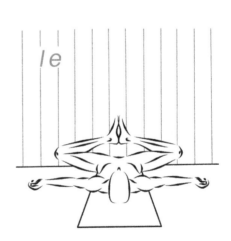

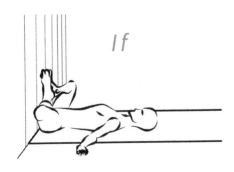

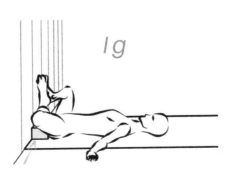

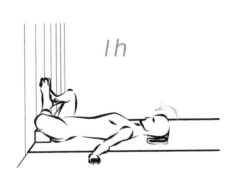

Bound Angle Pose — Simplify

Baddha Konasana
Bound Angle Pose

Explore

Learn + Practice

*Before Standing Poses and
Seated Forward Bends*

Linked Poses

*Lateral Standing Poses,
Janu Sirsasana, Upavistha
Konasana, Padmasana*

Safety Factors

*Groin, hamstring, adductor, or
knee injury, hip replacement*

Prepare

· Mat's short edge to wall
· If a block was used between
  buttocks and the wall in *Simplify*,
  set that height against the wall
· Place a rolled mat or blanket
  in front of sitting height,
  to elevate the heels

Enter

· Sit in *Dandasana*,
  back to a wall, *II a*
· Lengthening left leg away
  from back pelvis, fold right leg,
  placing the right foot on the floor
· Bring both thumbs to the pit
  at the back of right knee, *II b*
· Sliding the thumbs downward,
  bifurcate the calf, *II c-d*,
  while drawing right heel
  toward right buttock
· Keeping right leg folded,
  abduct right thigh, releasing
  it to the side, *II e*
· Fold the left leg in the
  same manner, *II f-g*
· Place the rolled mat or blanket
  under heels, *II h*, inner feet
  sloping down from heel to toe
· Sit higher if thighs are
  above hip creases, *II i*

Sustain

· Balance sacrum against
  the wall and sitting bones
  against floor or block
· Without losing heel contact,
  pull heels away from each
  other to release groins
· Keeping groins soft, re-
  pressurize heels
· Lengthen femurs away from
  back pelvis to an imaginary
  point far in front of feet, *II j*
· Lift and lengthen both sides of
  the torso to release diaphragm
· Without hardening abdomen,
  draw front ribs inward,
  back ribs upward
· Soften shoulders and
  rest back into wall
· Contact wall with both outer
  shoulder blades equally

Exit

· Place both hands
  under the thighs
· Using the hands, manually
  lift both thighs evenly
· Extend the legs to *Dandasana*
· Hold for 3-5 minutes or repeat
  6-10 times for shorter holds
· Alternate which leg
  moves first for *Enter*

Challenge

1. Numbness or tingling in the feet
2. Knee pain when folding the leg
3. Strain in outer knee
   or inner thighs
4. Overstretch of the inner thighs
5. Chest collapse

Response

1. Use a softer support under
   the pelvis and feet, widen
   groins. Release from pose
   until numbness dissipates.
   Return to pose for short holds,
   progressively increase hold
   time as circulation improves.
2. Ensure calf flesh does not roll
   excessively inward or outward.
   Often, thigh flesh rolls out while
   calf rolls in, torquing knee.
   Place a folded strap in the knee
   crease, fold to the outer knee.
   After abducting the leg, pull
   the strap ends upward and
   outward, separating them, *II k*.
3. Support under thighs with
   blocks, *II l*. Increase ankle
   support. *See Response 2*.
4. Deepen groin space by widening
   upper femurs away from pubis.
5. Place a foam block or folded
   blanket behind the ribs, *II m*.

classically, this fundamental pose is practiced seated. Baddha Konasana is the base of all lateral poses, involving both external rotation and abduction. It develops the space and mobility required for Standing Poses and may be learned at any level.

Contact Points

Sitting bones, outer thighs, outer feet, back pelvis, back ribs, shoulder blades

External Supports

*Wall, mat, blocks, rolled mat or blanket
Foam block*

Essence of Form

Knee flexion, leg extension and abduction; legs in external rotation, arms neutral

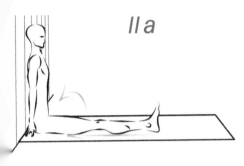

II a

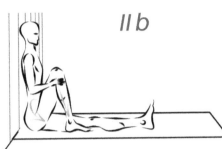

II b

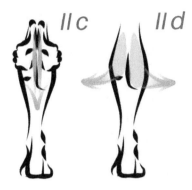

II c   *II d*

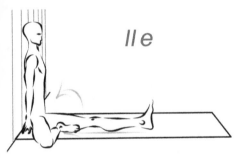

II e

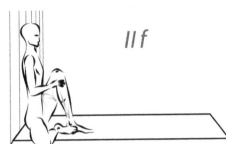

II f

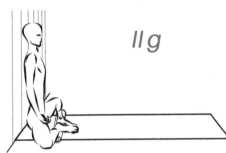

II g

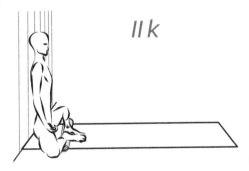

II k

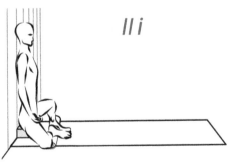

II i

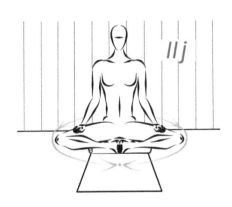

II j

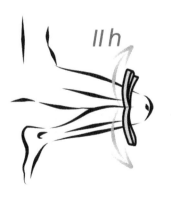

II h

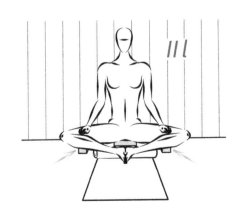

II l

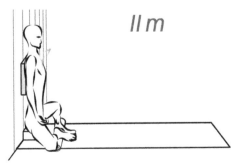

II m

Supta Baddha Konasana
Supine Bound Angle Pose

Nourish

Learn + Practice

Learn as soon as possible; practice at the beginning or end of sequences

Linked Poses

Baddha Konasana, Supta Virasana, Savasana B, Ekapada Rajakapotasana

Safety Factors

Groin, hamstring, or lower back injury; support thighs generously for hip replacement

Prepare

- Mat away from wall and obstructions
- Set bolster lengthwise on mat, folded blanket across its head end
- Roll a blanket and place it 12-15" in front of bolster
- Place blocks on either side of mat between bolster and rolled blanket, *III a*
- Have a buckled strap nearby

Enter

- Sit 3-8" in front of bolster
- Bring legs to *Baddha Konasana, Entering* as for *Explore, III b*
- Loop strap around the back pelvis, below pelvic rims, *III c*
- Keep buckle away from skin, strap's end pulling toward pelvis
- Pass loop over inner thighs, under ankles, and over feet, *III d*
- Tighten strap snugly, drawing feet close to perineum
- Support thighs on blocks, and heels on rolled blanket
- Ensure insteps slope downward
- Press hands into bolster's end, compressing it, *III e*
- Exhaling, lie back over the bolster and rest head on blanket, forehead sloping down

Enter

- Lift pelvis and manually slide buttock flesh toward heels to decompress lumbar, *III f*
- Lower pelvis to floor
- Rest the arms comfortably to the sides with palms upturned, *III g*

Sustain

- Release inner thighs away from strap contact
- Soften abdomen and buttocks
- Recede inner groins, resting outer thighs into the supports
- Observe the respiratory diaphragm's lateral movement
- Reduce tension in the eyes, lips, jaw, tongue, face, and throat
- Rest in the natural breath

Exit

- Place hands beside the bolster's lower end, palms down, *III h*
- Keeping the belly soft and without twisting, lead with the chest while pushing into the hands to lift the torso
- Once seated, loosen the strap and extend the legs

Challenge

1. Lower back discomfort
2. Shoulders push forward as arms rest, or numbness in the hands and arms
3. Blocks cut sharply into thighs
4. Feet and legs go numb or tingly

Response

1. *Prepare* with either a slightly larger or smaller gap between pelvis and bolster. Angle bolster upward with additional blocks, reducing back bend. Use less height, such as foam blocks or folded blankets. Elevate feet and lower legs on lateral bolster, back against the floor, *III i*. To *Exit III i*, roll to the right and push up from the side to seated.
2. Support hands and forearms, *III j*, so that humeri are not drawn so sharply backward. Lengthen collarbones away from sternum, soften outer upper chest.
3. Angle the blocks, *III k*, or use blankets to support thighs.
4. Loosen strap slightly and increase thigh support; use a softer support under the pelvis and feet. Practice *III i*.

Supta Baddha Konasana is a quintessential Restorative Pose. It increases blood flow to the abdomen, pelvis, and back, and is soothing to the digestive organs. It is usually also calming to the senses and nervous system, and is an excellent pose to begin or finish a practice in.

Contact Points

Pelvis, outer thighs, outer feet, back rib cage, back of skull

External Supports

Bolster, 2 blankets, strap, 2 blocks
Additional blankets + blocks

Essence of Form

Knee flexion, leg abduction, back extension; legs in external rotation, arms in slight external rotation

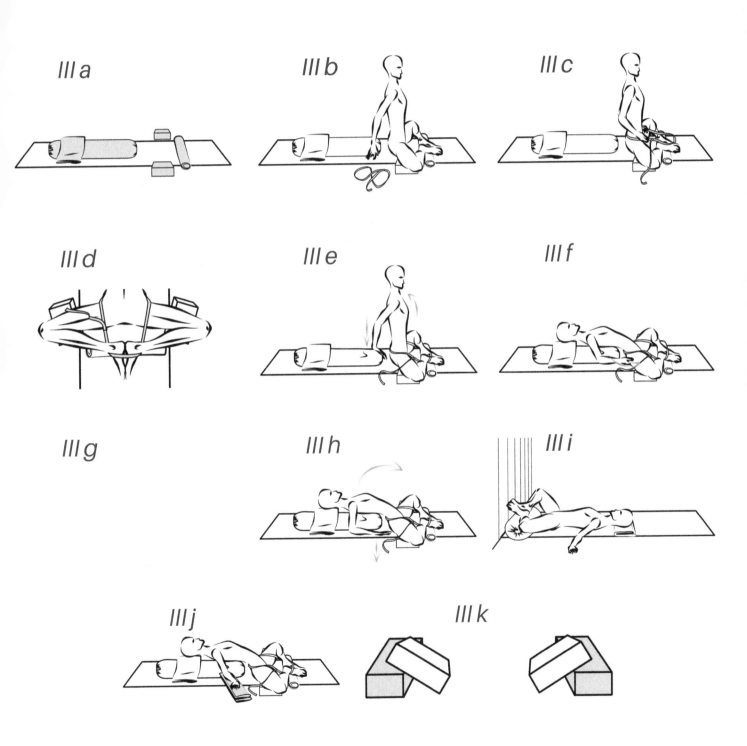

III a

III b

III c

III d

III e

III f

III g

III h

III i

III j

III k

Baddha Konasana
Bound Angle Pose

Synthesize

Learn + Practice

In conjunction with Standing Poses, well before deep hip openers and Padmasana

Linked Poses

Virasana, Sukhasana, Janu Sirsasana, Mandukasana, Mulabhandasana, Padmasana

Safety Factors

Groin, hamstring, or lower back injury; do not practice block variations with hip replacement

Prepare

· *Prepare as for* Explore
· Have an extra block nearby

Enter

· Sit on height in *Dandasana*
· Pushing heels away from back pelvis, lengthen the legs
· Lean back slightly on hands and reach through right heel to lengthen and lift right leg, *IV a*
· Bend the right leg, bringing heel toward the perineum onto the rolled blanket and release the thigh to the side, *IV b*
· Keeping the right leg position, repeat with the left leg, *IV c-d*
· Place a block between the feet, heels pressing against block's faces, *IV e*

❧ *For a deeper experience, and if capacity allows:*

· Remove block from between heels
· Provided thighs remain below hip creases with L4 + L5 moving forward, reduce sitting height and lower pelvis
· Repeat with heels against block sides, then the ends, *IV f-g*
· *Enter* without use of hands

Sustain

· Without losing skin contact against block, draw heels away from block
· Broaden greater trochanters laterally, increasing inner groin space
· Descend inner groins, creating neutral rotation
· Roll front iliums to opposite inner thighs
· Soften space behind pubis and in front of sacrum
· Ascend back ribs and descend front ribs, then lift and broaden collarbones

Exit

· Maintain the left leg position
· Without lifting the right thigh, lift the right heel clear off the floor, *IV h-i*
· Extend the right leg to the side, *IV f-j*
· Once right leg is extended, bring to *Dandasana* and lower the heel, *IV k*
· Repeat with the left leg
· Alternate which leg leads when *Entering* and *Exiting*
· Once *Enter* and *Exit* movements are smooth, move both legs simultaneously

Challenge

1. Femur and hip actions are unclear
2. Groins bind from leg movements in *Enter* and *Exit*
3. Pelvis tips backward and inner thighs grip

Response

1. Tie a strap from below the right ilium to the left knee, the same on the other side. Ensure the buckles are on the outer thighs with the strap ends pulling toward the pelvis. Lengthen femurs away from back pelvis into straps' resistance, *IV l.*
2. Return to *Simplify*, practicing the movement with legs up the wall instead. Without collapsing chest, lean torso backward more during leg movements.
3. Lean back on hands to release adductors. Without re-engaging adductors, descend pubis and return torso to upright. With a partner, bring strap as low as possible across back pelvis, over inner thighs. Partner presses feet into shins and leans backward, pulling strap ends downward to tilt pelvis. Keep this action as partner releases, *IV m.*

As the basis for all lateral and externally rotated poses, Baddha Konasana is deeply related to Virasana in that all poses can be categorized as being related to either as their foundations. Understanding these two poses deeply will yield fruit as the practice advances.

Contact Points

Sitting bones, outer thighs, outer feet, hands

External Supports

Supports used for Explore, block, rolled mat
2 straps, assistant

Essence of Form

Knee flexion, leg extension and abduction; legs neutrally rotated, arms neutral

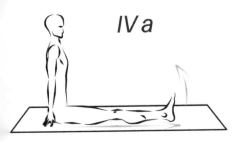
IVa

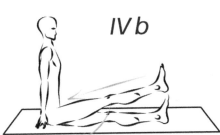
IVb

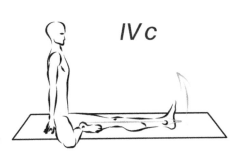
IVc

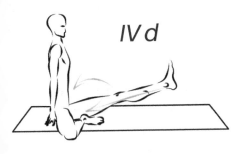
IVd

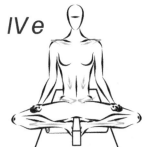
IVe

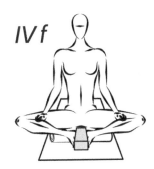
IVf

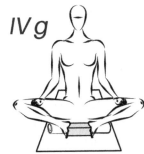
IVg

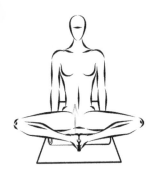

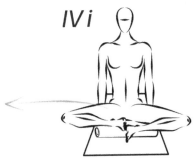
IVi

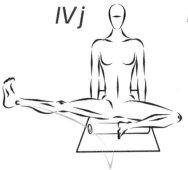
IVj

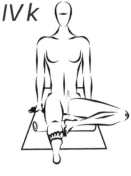
IVk

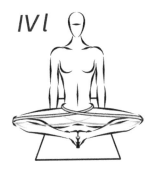
IVl

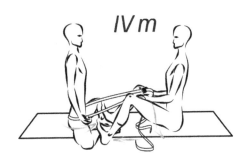
IVm

Bound Angle Pose — Synthesize

Virasana
Heroic Pose

Simplify

Learn + Practice

Learn in the first few classes and practice before Seated Poses and simple Back Bends

Linked Poses

Tadasana, Dandasana, Anjaneyasana, Back Bends

Safety Factors

Knee and ankle strain

Prepare

- Place mat at or away from wall, depending on poses that follow
- Have one or two blocks nearby

Enter

- Kneel on mat, outer knees no wider than greater trochanters, tops of feet on floor, *l a*
- Lean forward and lift buttocks off heels, touching head to floor or block, *l b*
- Without separating knees, place feet hip-width apart, slightly internally rotating thighs
- Ensure feet point directly backward, foot mid lines in line with tibias
- Place thumbs in pit at back of each knee
- Sliding thumbs backward, bifurcate calves (inner calves in, outer calves out), *l c*
- Sit between heels as thumbs slide back, *l d*
- Use block(s) under sitting bones if they do not touch floor, or if there is knee discomfort
- Settle weight heavily into sitting bones
- Rest hands on thighs, *l e*, or practice arm position variations, *l f-h*

Sustain

- Anchor tops of the feet into floor and spread the toes
- Press sitting bones equally downward
- Gather the lower femurs and front iliums
- Gently resist upper femurs outward
- Soften pubis in and up
- Descend inner thighs and soften inner groins
- Draw upper sacrum, L4 + L5 forward
- With sitting bones heavy, lift side torso from pelvis to armpits
- Soften front ribs inward
- Kept the head neutral, with neck and shoulders soft

Exit

- Walk hands forward along mat, lifting pelvis off floor or support and come to all fours position
- Exhaling, press into hands and lift thighs backward to *Adho Mukha Svanasana*, *l i*
- Alternatively, extend each leg back one at a time to open backs of knees, *l j*
- Step to standing or continue to next pose

Challenge

1. Inner or outer knee pain
2. Front or top of knee discomfort
3. Back of knee pain
4. Ankle discomfort

Response

1. Rise up on both shins. Rotate top thigh in direction of discomfort. Keeping rotation, lower pelvis. Alternatively, lift one knee at a time and grasp with hand. Turn knee skin toward pain, *l k-l*. Ensure feet point directly back to minimize knee torque.
2. Lift skin from under knee up and forward. Pad knees and shins with blanket or double mat thickness. *See Response 3.*
3. Increase sitting height. Fill back of knee space with folded blanket or rolled washcloth. *See also Explore.*
2. Lean sideways and lift ankle/top of foot skin out from underneath. Fill gap between ankle and floor with washcloths or folded straps, *l m*. Sit on 2-6 folded blankets, fold at ankle crease, feet hanging off edge, *l n*. Do not turn feet outward to avoid strain, *l o*.

One of four essential Seated Poses, Virasana reduces swelling and excess tension in the legs. It stretches the quadriceps and opens the front of the ankles, and is an essential preparation for Back Bending Poses. It is also a neutralizing rest pose appropriate for meditation and Pranayama.

Contact Points

Tops of feet, tibias, sitting bones

Mat, blocks

External Supports

2-6 blankets, strap, washcloth, additional blocks

Essence of Form

Hip and knee flexion, plantar extension; legs internally rotated, arms neutral

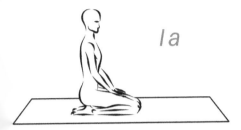
Ia

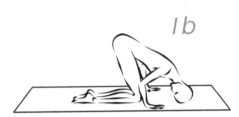
Ib

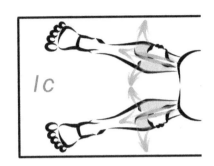
Ic

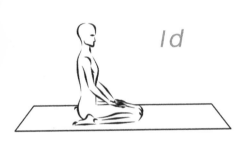
Id

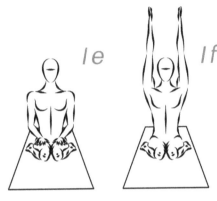
Ie If Ig Ih

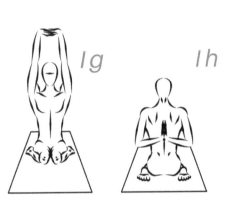

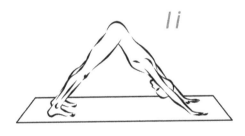
Ii

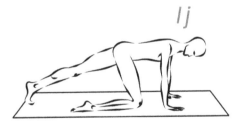
Ij

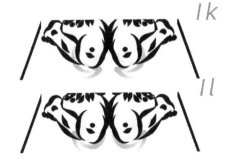
Ik

Il

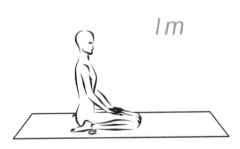
Im

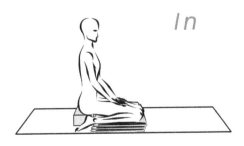
In

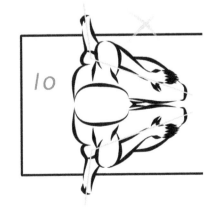
Io

Virasana
Heroic Pose

Learn + Practice

Usually learned after *Simplify*, but can be learned and practiced before

Linked Poses

Supta Padangusthasana A, Uttanasana, Back Bends, Paschimottanasana

Safety Factors

Knee and ankle strain; use care with extremely sensitive calves and hamstrings

Prepare

- Set block on mat, with an extra block nearby
- Roll stick inside a mat or blanket

Enter

- Sit in *Virasana* as for *Simplify*: if sitting on the floor, support pelvis on block, *ll a*
- Lifting pelvis, place stick between calves and hamstrings, 1-2" from sitting bones, *ll b*
- Descend pelvis; ensure sitting bones are well supported — add second block if sitting bones do not descend or stick's pressure is too intense
- As thighs and pelvis settle, roll stick away from sitting bones in $1/2$-1" increments, *ll c*
- Bring stick no further than 2" from pit of knees
- Increase or decrease pelvic support to capacity as stick position changes

ॐ *When reasonable, remove stick padding and reduce sitting height*

Sustain

- Continue *Sustain* actions from *Simplify*
- Neutralize pelvis, aligning the pubis and front iliums on the same vertical plane
- Use stick contact as feedback to soften calves and hamstrings
- Descend femurs into stick support as calves and hamstrings soften
- Broaden calf and hamstring flesh, further bifurcating both muscle groups
- Draw outer ankles inward
- Without splaying knees, lengthen inner femurs away from pubis
- Release upper buttock flash away from spine and pelvic rims

Exit

- Hold for 30 seconds to a minute at each stick position or until hamstrings and calves release, according to capacity
- Lift pelvis and remove stick
- Sit in *Virasana* without stick for an additional 1-3 minutes
- Reduce sitting height if possible
- Walk hands forward and exhale to *Adho Mukha Svanasana*, *ll d*

Challenge

1. Overwhelming sensation from stick pressure
2. Knee compression
3. Knee torque

Response

1. Increase padding around stick, or remove stick and use rolled mat alone. Ensure pelvis is well supported, reducing weight on stick. Keep pelvis neutral, not tilting forward or back to avoid sensation. Keep stick at less sensitive spots and move it more gradually.
2. Without the stick, *Enter* with straps looped in the pit of each knee. Place a block on the left thigh. Hold left leg strap with left hand, palm up, and press forearm into block. Pushing down on block with elbow/forearm, pull up on strap to create traction. Repeat with the right side, *ll e*.
3. Adjust knees as described in *Simplify*. Do not move stick as close to knees, or use two sticks so that the knee plane is not torqued, *ll f*.

…irasana softens the calves and hamstrings through compression. In this variation, compression …focused more acutely by using a stick. People with very tight calves and hamstrings may …enefit from practicing this variation of Virasana before extended-leg Forward Bends.

Contact Points

Tops of feet, tibias, femurs, sitting bones

External Supports

Mat, block, stick, additional mat or blanket
Strap, additional blocks

Essence of Form

Hip and knee flexion, plantar extension; legs internally rotated, arms neutral

II a

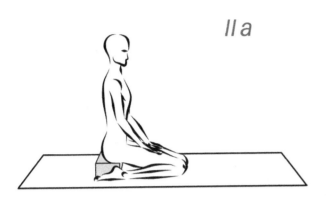

II b

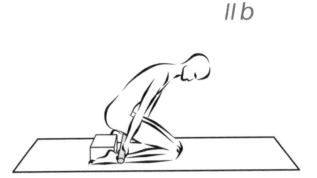

II c

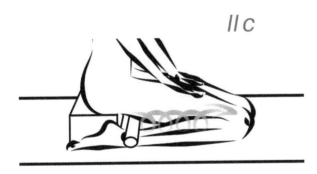

II d

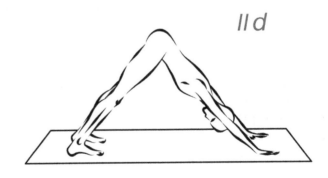

II e

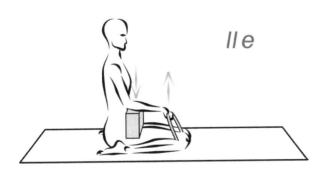

II f

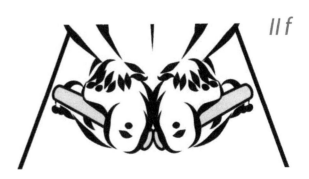

Learn + Practice

After Simplify, before deep Back Bends, also useful before Standing Poses

Linked Poses

Supta Tadasana, Anjaneyasana, Parsvakonasana, Back Bends

Safety Factors

Lower back strain; groin, quadricep, or knee injury

Prepare

- Place a bolster lengthwise on mat with a folded blanket at head end, *III a*
- Set *Virasana* sitting height in front of bolster
- If sitting height is significant, elevate bolster at a downward angle from head to pelvis
- Have a strap nearby

Enter

- Sit 1-3" in front of bolster in *Virasana*, *III b*
- Adjust knee and ankle skin as necessary
- Strap lower thighs, femurs parallel to each other
- Place hands on soles of feet or on floor behind pelvis
- Inhaling, descend femurs and lift pelvis slightly off floor
- Drawing back pelvis forward, lift back rib cage upward
- Exhaling, lie back on bolster, *III c*
- Slide buttock flesh away from bolster
- Manually draw mid-back flesh away from spine
- If head tilts backward, increase support
- Rest arms beside torso, palms face up, *III d*

Sustain

- Settle upper femurs away from front thighs
- Gather front iliums and soften pubis inward
- Draw lower femurs toward each other, and abduct upper femurs
- Descend inner femurs and soften groins
- Lift front iliums away from upper femurs
- Lengthen back femurs away from back pelvis
- Release back pelvis away from back ribs
- Rest and widen back ribs into bolster, softening abdomen
- Soften throat and sense organs

Exit

- Keeping abdomen soft, place hands on soles of feet
- Without twisting, press into hands and inhale to seated, *III e*
- Sit upright in *Virasana* for a few breaths
- Remove strap and walk hands forward
- Exhaling, press to *Adho Mukha Svanasana*

- ॐ *Can also be practiced with legs extended, III f*

Challenge

1. Knee or ankle discomfort
2. Lower back discomfort
3. Femurs lift
4. Sacroiliac joint pain
5. Chest collapse

Response

1. *See Simplify + Explore Solutions.*
2. Often psoas/quadricep tightness. Support bolster at sharper incline, either with chair, *III g*, or blocks *III h*. Practice *Ardha Supta Virasana*, *III i*, with left leg in *Virasana* first, then right. Do *Anjaneyasana, Simplify*, and quadricep stretches, *III j* before practicing.
3. Apply weight to femurs, *III k*. Pass strap over top thighs, under front ankles, doubling strap ends over upper thighs to buckle, *III l*.
4. Tie strap just below iliums, pulling front ilium of pain side toward opposite front ilium, *III m*. Deepen internal rotation and keep groins receding.
5. Support bolster under chest, *III n*. Add slant board or rolled blanket at shoulder blades, moving shoulder blades inward, *III o*.

Supta Virasana is both a deeply Restorative Pose and an excellent preparation for Back Bends. Its action on the femurs may aid digestion and help settle the nervous system. Lengthen the groins and quadriceps before learning, and once learned practice early in sequences.

Contact Points

Tops of feet, tibias, back pelvis, back ribs, back of skull

External Supports

Mat, bolster, strap, blanket
Chair, blocks, bolster, blankets, slant board

Essence of Form

Hip + spine extension, knee flexion with adduction; legs internally rotated, arms passively external

III a

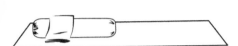

III b

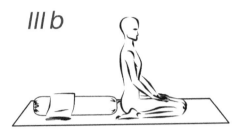

III c

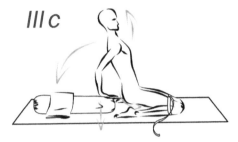

III d

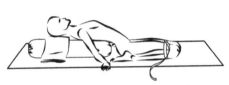

III e

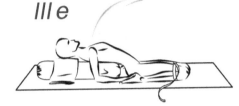

III f

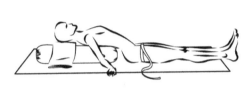

III g

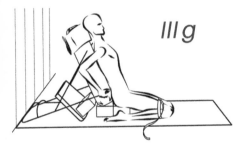

III h

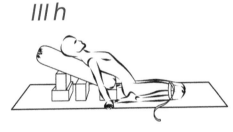

III i

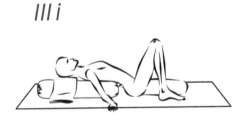

III j

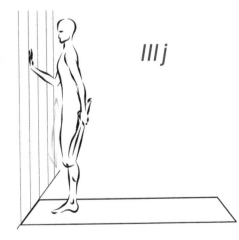

III k

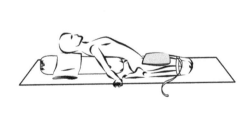

III l

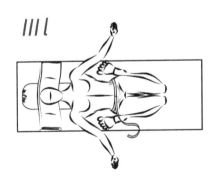

III m

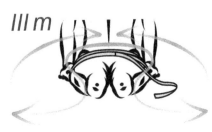

III k

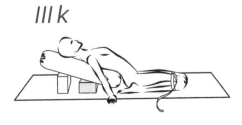

III l

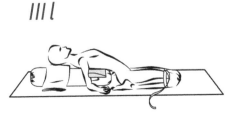

Adho Mukha Virasana
Forward-Bending Heroic Pose

Synthesize

Learn + Practice

*After Uttana Balasana,
Before Trianga Mukhaikapada
Paschimottanasana*

Linked Poses

*Uttana Balasana,
Trianga Mukhaikapada
Paschimottanasana,
Krounchasana, Malasana*

Safety Factors

*Knee and ankle strain,
disc problems, hip injury
or replacement*

Prepare

- Set sitting height for *Virasana*
- Place a chair or blocks 2-3'
  in front of sitting height

Enter

- Sit facing chair in *Virasana, IV a*
- Descend upper femurs
- Keeping femurs descending, raise
  arms to *Urdhva Hastasana, IV b*
- Lift pelvis up and over thighs,
  increasing internal thigh
  rotation to fold forward
- Deepening groins, symmetrically
  fold iliums up and over femurs
- Fold to capacity, keeping
  lumbar spine moving inward
  with minimal effort
- Catch chair with hands or rest
  hands and elbows on floor, *IV c-d*
- Rest forehead on chair
  seat or blocks
- Ensure forehead skin is sliding
  downward, toward nose

Sustain

- Continue *Virasana* actions
  from *Simplify + Explore*
- Descend lower outer
  buttocks while lifting
  sacrum up and forward
- Move spine inward and
  broaden back body flesh
  away from mid line
- Release neck muscles
  away from occiput
- Slide forehead skin down
  face toward nose
- Soften throat and tongue

Exit

- Pressing hands into floor,
  inhale to seated
- Sit in *Virasana* for a few breaths
- Walk hands forward and exhale
  to *Adho Mukha Svanasana*

Challenge

1. Legs externally rotate
2. Knee pain
3. Groin compression
4. Numbness or tingling
   in legs and feet
5. Sitting bones lift

Response

1. Manually internally rotate
   femurs before *Entering*. Tie
   strap across back pelvis,
   around inner thighs, and behind
   upper thighs, *IV e*. Pull strap
   ends outward when folding.
2. *See Response 1 and Responses
   in Simplify + Explore*. Loop
   straps in knee creases, loops
   forward. Have a partner
   gently pull loops, creating
   traction, *IV f*. Also applicable
   to *Simplify* and *Nourish*.
3. Practice *Uttana Balasana*,
   with crossed sticks or metal
   bars (for weight) in groins.
   Lift iliums up and over sticks.
   Strap thighs as described
   in *Nourish, Response 2*.
4. Place soft support under tops of
   feet and tibias. Descend femurs,
   softening and deepening groin
   spaces, assuring circulation
   through femoral arteries.
   See also Response 5.
5. Increase sitting height and
   decrease forward fold. Set
   block behind pelvis, with
   folded mat on back pelvis.
   Place weight over mat on
   back pelvis, partly supported
   by block, *IV g*. Have assistant
   press thumbs or stick down
   into upper front femurs, *IV h*.

Bending forward in Virasana accentuates the groin deepening action of all the pose's variations. This variation may help to reset the sacrum between the iliums, and the femurs within the hip joints. It also helps descend the femurs in preparation for deeper Forward Bends.

Contact Points

Tops of feet, tibias, sitting bones, forehead

External Supports

Mat, blocks, chair
Straps, mat, sandbag, assistant

Essence of Form

Hip and knee flexion, leg adduction; legs internally rotated, arms neutral

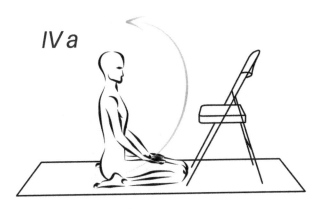

IV a

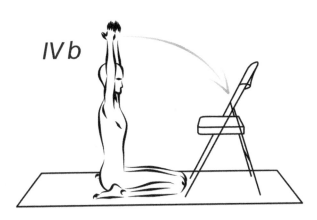

IV b

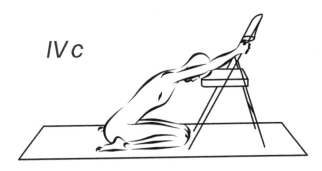

IV c

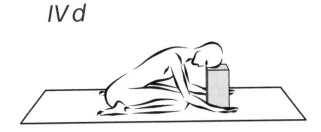

IV d

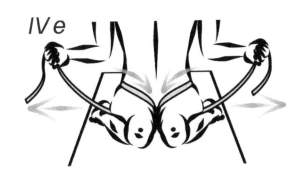

IV e

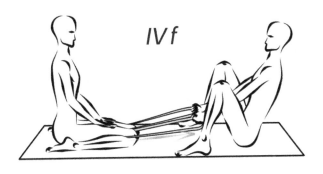

IV f

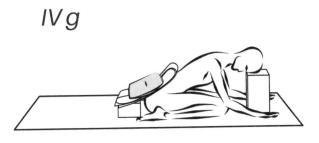

IV g

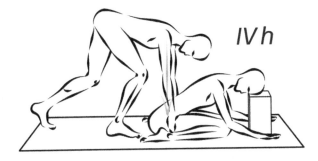

IV h

Paschimottanasana
Intense Back-Body Stretch

Learn + Practice

Once Uttanasana is accessible and lumbar is stable in Dandasana

Linked Poses

Supta Padangusthasana A, Uttanasana, all deep Forward Bends

Safety Factors

Hamstring injury, low blood pressure; bring feet hip-width apart (or wider) if pregnant

Prepare

- Set mat's short end to wall
- Place chair on mat, chair's back against wall
- Have a bolster within reach

Enter

- Sit at chair's edge with feet flat on floor, *I a*
- Extend legs away from back pelvis to *Dandasana*, legs in neutral rotation, *I b*
- Place bolster lengthwise on thighs, close to lower abdomen, *I c*
- Softening hip creases, release femurs down and away from front iliums
- Pressing hands into bolster, lift torso up and over thighs *I d*
- Lay torso over bolster, extending torso forward as back body releases, *I e*
- Contact bolster first with lower abdomen, then lower rib cage, and lastly the chest
- Once torso is fully supported, rest head and arms on bolster, *I f*

ༀ *See Dandasana for additional ways to work. When pelvis tilts easily, Prepare blocks to elevate feet*

Sustain

- Keeping legs fully extended, push feet away from back pelvis and descend upper femurs
- Resist tendency to externally rotate legs
- Continue lifting pelvis up and over femurs, initiating any further length
- Extend lumbar spine out of pelvis, lifting sacrum, L4 + L5 in toward front body
- Soften abdomen and receive bolster's pressure against it
- Extend bottom ribs and top hip crests away from each other
- Lengthen side body from hips to armpits
- Release spinal muscles away from mid line
- Descend forehead skin toward the nose
- Soften the face, throat, and back of neck

Exit

- Exhaling, place hands under shoulders on bolster, *I g*
- Gather front iliums and resist heels downward
- Pushing into hands, descend back pelvis and inhaling, lift torso to seated

Challenge

1. Chair lip's pressure causes hamstring pain
2. Legs fall into external rotation
3. Torso does not contact bolster or fold is too deep
4. Difficulty breathing through nose, or face discomfort against bolster

Response

1. Though uncomfortable, pressure may help manage hamstring injury. Pad chair edge with sticky mat. Elevate chair's back legs on blocks so it doesn't cut so deeply into thighs.
2. Strap thighs or big toes together, or hold a block between thighs. *Enter* with chair facing wall, feet pressing into wall, *I h*.
3. Use two bolsters, either crossing or stacking them, *I i-j. Prepare* with blocks beside legs, press into blocks and extend torso, *I k. See also Response 3.*
4. Avoid turning head. Rest forehead on crossed forearms or use a folded blanket under the forehead and/or chest, *I l.*

Paschimottanasana releases tension along the back-body chain from soles to brow. It can be quite challenging, especially if there is significant hamstring restriction. Learning it on a chair eases the transition from standing to seated, utilizing gravity to create a mechanical advantage.

Contact Points	External Supports	Essence of Form
Sitting bones, back of heels	*Chair, bolster, wall 2nd bolster, blocks*	*Hip flexion with leg extension, arm and shoulder extension; arms and legs neutrally rotated*

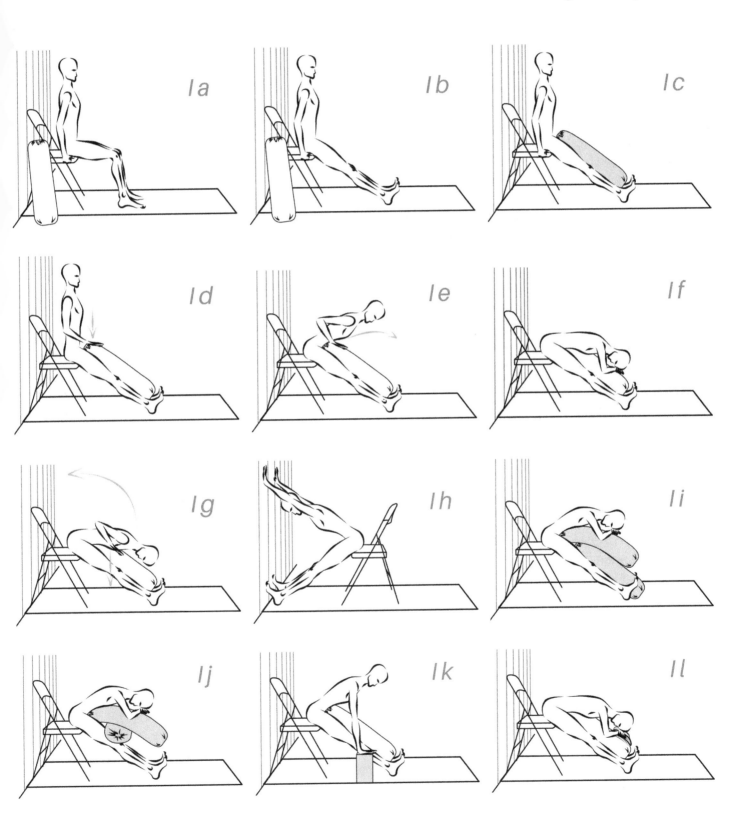

Paschimottanasana
Intense Back-Body Stretch

Explore

Learn + Practice

Once raised leg reaches 90° or greater with ease in *Supta Padangusthasana A*

Linked Poses

Uttanasana, Dandasana, Supta Padangusthasana A, deep Forward Bends

Safety Factors

As for Simplify; depression, lower back strain or disc herniation

Prepare

- Mat's short end to wall
- Set sitting height against wall, determined from *Dandasana*, *Explore*
- Place additional supports for under thighs and/or calves as necessary

Enter

- Sit on height against wall in *Dandasana*, *II a*
- Extending legs away from back pelvis, stabilize inner thighs toward floor
- Gathering front iliums, resist heels laterally
- Softening abdomen, draw pubis in and up
- Place hands on wall beside waist, with fingertips pointing downward and elbows bent, *II b*
- Pressing hands downward and backward, lift torso up and out of pelvis
- Keeping torso extension, lift pelvis up and over thighs to fold forward, *II c*
- Without collapsing chest, tuck chin slightly downward, lengthening back of the neck
- If arms fully extend, walk hands up wall, *II d*

Sustain

- Continuously extend legs, pushing heels away from back pelvis
- Spreading the toes, draw outer ankles inward
- Descending inner thighs toward floor, broaden the back of each leg
- Soften and deepen inner groins, moving inner upper femurs away from each other
- Extend from pubis to sternum, lengthening front torso
- Resist upper humeri outward, broadening collarbones laterally
- Widen upper shoulder blades and extend occiput away from mid-upper back
- Keeping the chest lifted, release throat and jaw

Exit

- Hold 10-15 breaths
- Keeping torso length, place hands beside legs
- Pressing into hands, descend back pelvis and inhale to seated, *II e*
- Sit upright in *Dandasana*, and let legs roll into external rotation before releasing, *II f*

Challenge

1. Hands do not reach wall, push not generated
2. Chest collapse
3. Groins bind upward
4. Chin juts forward, neck tension

Response

1. Place blocks at wall, beside pelvis. Ensure blocks are high enough that hands are at or above pelvic rims. Press heels of hands down into blocks to lift torso, *II g*. After folding, use blocks as arm extensions, pressing blocks directly back into wall to lengthen torso, *II h*.
2. Externally rotate arms slightly. Adjust hand height at wall to lift chest optimally. Without moving hands, resist hands toward ceiling to extend chest forward.
3. Use a stick against the upper thighs, *II i*. Push stick into thighs instead of pushing wall. Pressing femurs down, lift pelvic rims up and away from femurs to fold forward.
4. Lift up before folding. Lead with chest rather than chin. If neck tension is due to arm extension, keep elbows slightly bent.

eeping the torso extended is one of the main challenges of Paschimottanasana. Pressing
he hands back into the wall while folding helps maintain this length while also reducing
train on the hip flexors, which tend to overwork when the posterior chain is limited.

Contact Points

Sitting bones, backs
of heels, hands

External Supports

Wall, pelvic supports
Blocks, strap

Essence of Form

Hip flexion, leg and torso
extension, posterior arm
extension; arms and legs
neutrally rotated

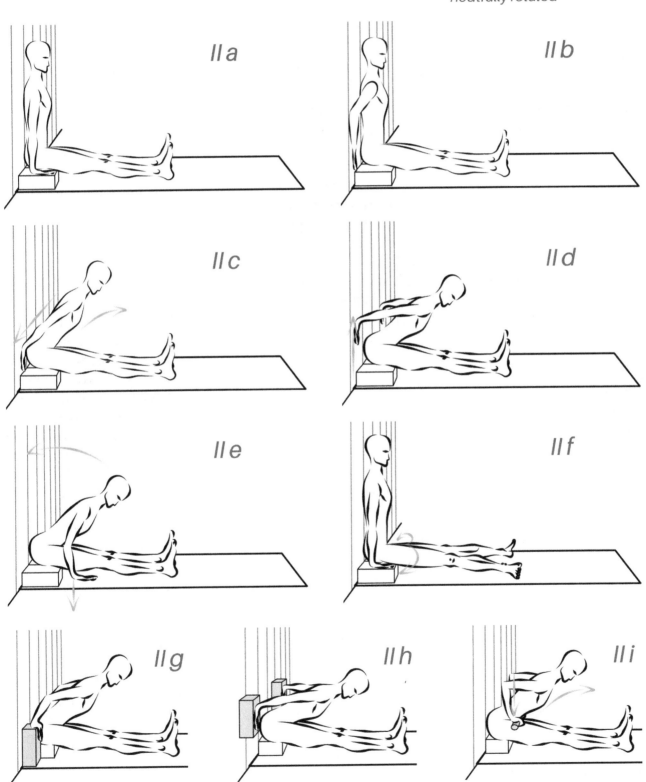

II a

II b

II c

II d

II e

II f

II g

II h

II i

Learn + Practice

After Explore and Salabhasana,
before Halasana and
deep Forward Bends

Linked Poses

Back Bends and Forward Bends

Safety Factors

As for Explore, use extra
care with hamstring, groin,
or lower back injury

Prepare

- Use minimal sitting height
  and place folded blanket to
  support upper femurs, *III a*

Enter

- Sit as described in *Dandasana*,
  Synthesize, establishing
  leg and pelvis actions
- Pressing femurs downward,
  inhale and raise arms to
  Urdhva Hastasana, *III b*
- Lengthening side torso, lift
  pelvis up and over femurs and
  fold forward on exhalation
- Without rounding lumbar, catch
  big toes with first 2 fingers,
  palms facing each other, *III c*
- Bend elbows slightly,
  resisting torso backward
- Do not pull torso toward legs

Sustain

- Engage leg and pelvis *Sustain*
  actions from *Simplify* + *Explore*,
  as well as *Dandasana* actions
- Keeping elbows slightly bent,
  lift torso up and away from
  thighs, lengthening spine, *III d*

Sustain

- Engaging paraspinal muscles,
  move spine inward and
  widen back body, *III e*
- Broaden the diaphragm and lift it
  uniformly out of the pelvic girdle
- Keeping back ribs voluminous,
  soften the xyphoid process
  inward and lift upper sternum
- Without protruding front
  ribs, draw bottom shoulder
  blades forward, *III f*
- Keep head and neck neutral,
  chin neither lifted nor tucked

Exit

- Hold up to 1 minute
- Keeping torso length and
  paraspinal muscle engagement,
  release toe hold and press
  hands to floor beside legs, *III g*
- Pushing hands and heels into
  floor, descend back pelvis
  and inhale to *Dandasana*
- Rest in *Dandasana* up to an
  additional minute, similarly
  engaging paraspinals, *III h*

- ॐ *Once spinal muscles are
  strengthened, extend arms
  overhead and press thighs
  down, inhaling to upright, III i*

Challenge

1. Hands do not reach feet
   unless spine rounds
2. Lumbar discomfort and/
   or SI joint pain
3. Mid- and upper back fatigue

Response

1. Use a chair, with soles of feet
   braced against back rung. Hold
   sides of chair's seat or backrest,
   III j. When possible, deepen
   by adding blocks between
   soles and chair rung, *III k*. Loop
   strap around soles of feet with
   forearms crossed to open
   chest, *III l*. Take enough length
   that spine does not round. Do
   not pull torso toward feet.
2. Do not pull torso forward.
   Rather, resist torso backward
   and decrease hip flexion.
   Observe asymmetry and
   fold only while both halves
   of pelvis fold symmetrically.
   When symmetry is lost, reduce
   hip flexion on freer side.
3. Descend femurs more
   heavily. Mid- and upper back
   muscles often overwork when
   foundation is lost. Draw bottom
   ribs backward and descend
   elbows, releasing trapezium.

Paschimottanasana can both be used to release or strengthen the spinal muscles, depending on the actions engaged within the pose. Here, a Back-Bending action is engaged within the Forward Bend in order to strengthen the spine first, before releasing it in Synthesize.

Contact Points

Back thighs, sitting bones

External Supports

2 blankets or other
pelvic support
Chair, blocks, strap

Essence of Form

Hip flexion, leg and arm
extension, spinal extension;
arms and legs neutrally rotated

III a
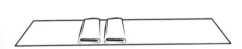

III b
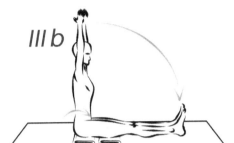

III c
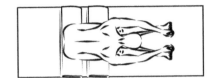

III d
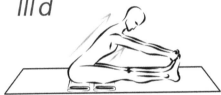

III e
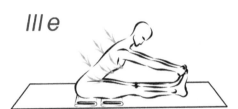

III f
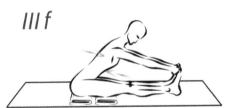

III g
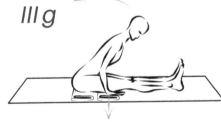

III h
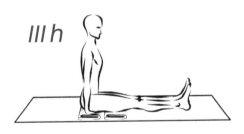

III i
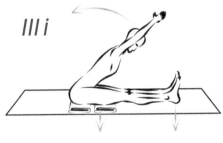

III j
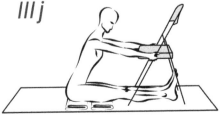

III k
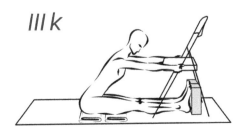

III l
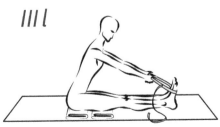

Paschimottanasana
Intense Back-Body Stretch

Synthesize

Learn + Practice

Once lumbar concavity is no longer challenging, after Nourish

Linked Poses

All deep Forward Bends, Uttana Balasana, Halasana

Safety Factors

Slipped disc, hamstring or groin injury, knee hyperextension

Prepare

· Set sitting height as for *Nourish*
· For holds longer than 1 minute, use additional support for head, either blocks or a chair
· If using head supports, place them 2-3' in front of sitting height

Enter

· Sit in *Dandasana, IV a*
· With femurs and pelvis stable, inhale and raise arms to *Urdhva Hastasana, IV b*
· Descending femurs, inhale and lift pelvis up and over femurs, tilting forward 30-45° or until L4 + L5 can no longer lift inward, *IV c*
· Keeping spinal length, lower arms and rest hands beside legs, palms down, *IV d*
· With arms passive, extend chest forward, from pubis to sternum
· Without tilting pelvis backward, keep torso length and release torso, rounding spine slightly, *IV e*
· If using head support, rest forehead and elbows on chair seat, *IV f*, or forehead on blocks with hands to floor beside legs, *IV g*

Sustain

· Broaden backs of legs, making maximum contact with floor from inner to outer back thigh
· Release buttock flesh away from pelvic rims
· Keep lifting back ribs away from back pelvis, even with rounded spine
· Maximize front body length from pubis to sternum and minimize spinal roundness
· Extend side torso from hips to armpits
· Release spinal muscles laterally
· Lengthen back of neck, drawing chin slightly toward chest
· Soften throat, lips, jaw, tongue, and eyes

Exit

· Stay for 1-3 minutes
· Bend elbows and bring hands under shoulders or to chair seat
· Lengthen legs, pushing heels away back pelvis
· Descending femurs and back pelvis, press into hands and inhale to seated
· After long holds, bring hands to back of thighs to assist bending the legs one at a time

Challenge

1. Hamstring injury
2. Groin injury
3. Groins bind, femurs lift
4. Chest collapse, mild depression

Response

1. Reduce fold until there is no discomfort. Place stick behind both thighs at point of injury (even if only injured on one side). Press femurs into stick, widening hamstrings against support, *IV h-i.*
2. *Enter* with feet slightly wider than hip-width, creating space in groins (also applicable when practicing while pregnant). If necessary, externally rotate legs while folding, then internally rotate legs to neutral once pelvis is folded. Resist heels laterally and gather front iliums.
3. Once pelvis tilts well, raise heels on blocks, letting femurs drop down out of pelvis, *IV j.*
4. Extend arms, keeping armpits open. If using chair, hold chair back, *IV k.* If using blocks, elevate hands on blocks as well, *IV l.*

Contact Points

Back of legs, sitting bones
Forehead

External Supports

2 blankets, blocks, chair
Additional blocks, stick

Essence of Form

Hip flexion, leg extension, mild spinal flexion; legs in neutral rotation, arms in passive internal rotation

IV a

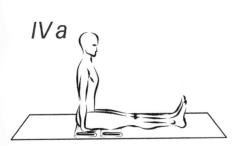

IV b

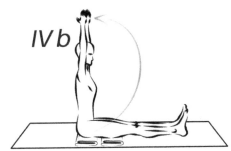

IV c

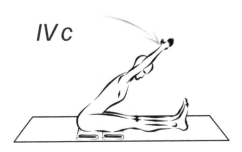

IV d

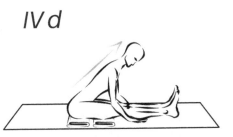

IV e

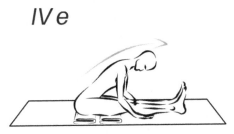

IV f

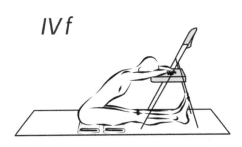

IV g

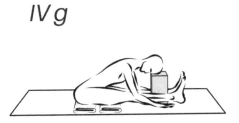

IV h

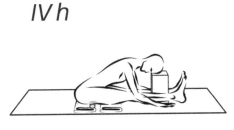

IV i

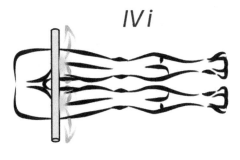

IV j

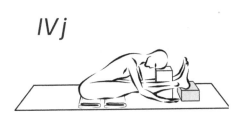

IV k

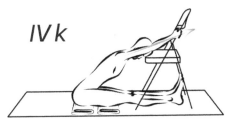

IV l

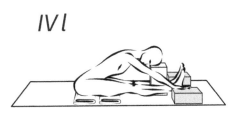

Learn + Practice

After Dandasana and Baddha Konasana, before Twists; after lateral Standing Poses

Linked Poses

Trikonasana, Parsvakonasana, Virabhadrasana A, Parsvottanasana, Twists

Safety Factors

Groin, hamstring, adductor, or knee injury

Prepare

- Set mat's short end to wall
- Have blocks nearby
- Place folded blanket at mid-mat to support head if desired

Enter

- Lie on right side near mat's right edge, spine perpendicular to wall, buttocks against it
- Pressing into left hand, roll onto the back and extend legs up the wall, *I a-b*
- Extend sitting bones equally into wall and balance sacrum
- Ensure spine is perpendicular to wall, L4 + L5 moving inward
- Lengthen legs, pushing heels away from back pelvis
- Resist heels laterally and gather front iliums
- Pressing left heel into wall, lengthen right leg and lift away from wall, *I c*
- Without lifting left inner thigh and keeping sacrum balanced against floor, bend right leg and draw right heel toward perineum, opening the thigh laterally, *I d*
- Right thigh may not touch wall
- Rest the arms beside torso, palms turned upward

Sustain

- Continue extending both sitting bones symmetrically toward wall, L4 + L5 lifting inward
- Reach left leg out of back pelvis
- Move left femur toward wall
- Press right heel against left inner thigh
- Using heel pressure and keeping left back pelvis heavy, lengthen right thigh laterally
- Do not force right leg toward wall or floor
- Rest abdomen and abdominal organs
- Soften the face, throat, and back of neck

Exit

- Hold 10-15 breaths
- Pressing into left heel and keeping right thigh moving toward wall, lift right heel, *I e*
- Extend right leg 30-45° to the side, *I f*
- Exhaling, bring right leg vertical, neutralizing rotation, *I g*
- Repeat, keeping right leg extended and bending left leg
- When finished, bend both legs and roll to the right
- Pressing the hands into the floor, inhale to seated

Challenge

1. Buttocks do not reach wall
2. Right thigh binds toward armpit
3. Left leg bends and/or externally rotates when moving right thigh
4. Left side of pelvis lifts
5. Head tilts back, throat tension

Response

1. Have buttocks as far away from the wall as necessary to have a neutral lumbar when legs are extended. Fill gap between wall and sitting bones with blocks, *I h.*
2. Tie a strap from left ilium to head of right knee, *I i.* Extend through right thigh into strap, then release thigh toward wall. Move further from wall and fill gap with blocks.
3. Keep attention on stabilizing the left leg, and initiate movement from that stability.
4. Roll right front ilium toward left inner thigh.
5. Support head with folded blanket. Manually adjust head, drawing occiput away from back ribs and descending forehead toward nose.

One of the first asymmetrical seated forward bends, Janu Sirsasana increases hip joint articulation. Learning it supine helps keep the pelvis balanced within the asymmetrical leg position. In this variation, active leg raises moving in and coming out of the pose help strengthen the groins.

Contact Points

Back pelvis, back ribs, shoulder blades, back of skull, sitting bones, back of heel, outer foot

External Supports

Mat, wall
Blanket, blocks, strap

Essence of Form

Leg extension, knee flexion with leg abduction; bent leg externally rotated, extended leg neutral, arms neutral

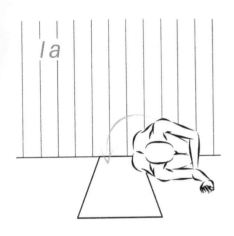

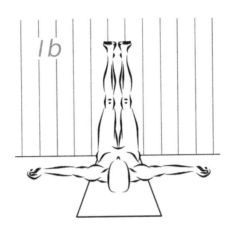

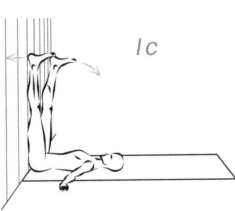

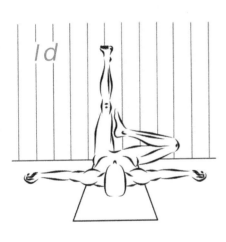

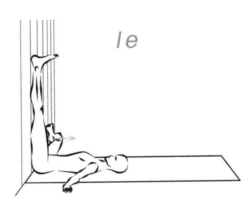

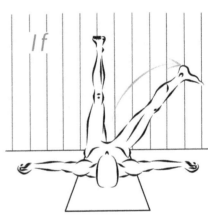

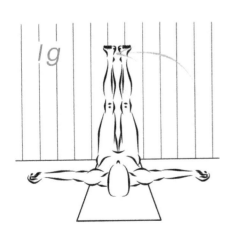

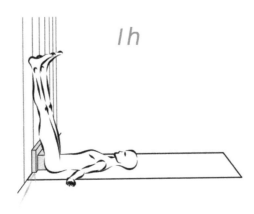

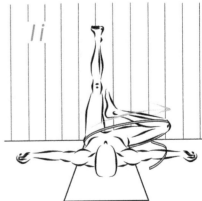

Janu Sirsasana
Head of the Knee Pose

Learn + Practice

After Simplify, once lumbar curve is maintained Dandasana, Explore

Linked Poses

Dandasana, Baddha Konasana, lateral Standing Poses, Twists

Safety Factors

As for Simplify, lower back strain, do not raise arms if hypertense

Prepare

- Mat's short end to wall
- Place pelvic supports a leg's length from wall
- Have an extra block nearby (optional)

Enter

- Sit in *Dandasana*, pushing feet into the wall
- Keeping left foot pressing firmly into wall, bend right leg and bring foot to floor, *ll a*
- Bring thumbs to pit at back of right knee, *ll b*
- Slide the thumbs down, bifurcating the calf while folding the right leg completely, *ll c*
- With the leg folded, abduct the leg and place sole of right foot against left inner thigh, *ll d*
- Draw right heel as close to the perineum as possible
- Descending left inner thigh, draw L4 + L5 inward, particularly on the right
- For a deeper hip opening, place block between inner left thigh and right sole, *ll e*
- Inhaling, raise arms to *Urdhva Hastasana*, *ll f*
- Extending through arms, lift torso out of pelvis

Sustain

- Equally pressurize 4 corners of left foot into wall, away from back pelvis
- Gather front iliums, resisting left heel laterally
- Soften pubis inward and away from wall
- Press right heel into left inner thigh (or block) using heel pressure to extend right femur
- Descend both femurs, lifting torso and pelvis
- Without rotating knee inward, descend left inner thigh completely
- Keeping inner thigh contact, descend left outer upper thigh
- Softly drawing front ribs inward, ascend bottom back ribs

Exit

- Hold 5-10 breaths
- Keeping torso lift and length, lower arms
- Using right hand, lift right thigh toward mid line, resting foot on floor, *ll g*
- Extend right foot to wall away from back pelvis and rest in *Dandasana*, *ll h*
- Repeat with the right foot to wall and bending left leg in

Challenge

1. Right leg binds upward, *ll i*
2. Right ankle pain
3. Right knee pain
4. Numbness or tingling in right leg or foot
5. Sacroiliac joint pain

Response

1. Raise sitting height so that right femur falls away from pelvis, *ll j*. Support right thigh and release inner thigh muscles, *ll k*.
2. Elevate right heel, *ll l*, bringing joint planes into agreement. Keep right inner thigh lifting.
3. Place a folded strap in knee crease, ends toward inner knee. Pull strap ends upward and outward, separating them, *ll m*. See also Responses 1 + 2.
4. Add soft support under right outer thigh and ankle. Elevate right thigh and descend inner femur away from inner thigh flesh.
5. Continue drawing front iliums toward each other, and visualize gathering back iliums to stabilize pelvis. Balance sacrum with back against wall. Do not practice *ll e*.

anu Sirsasana accentuates side torso length, which is beneficial in many poses, particularly Twists. his length can also be applied to symmetrical Forward Bends. Stabilizing the extended leg foot gainst a wall establishes connection and relationship between the extended and bent legs.

Contact Points

eet, back thigh, outer high, sitting bones

External Supports

Mat, wall, blocks, blankets
Strap, rolled blanket,
additional blocks

Essence of Form

Leg extension, knee flexion with leg abduction; bent leg externally rotated, extended leg neutral, arms neutral

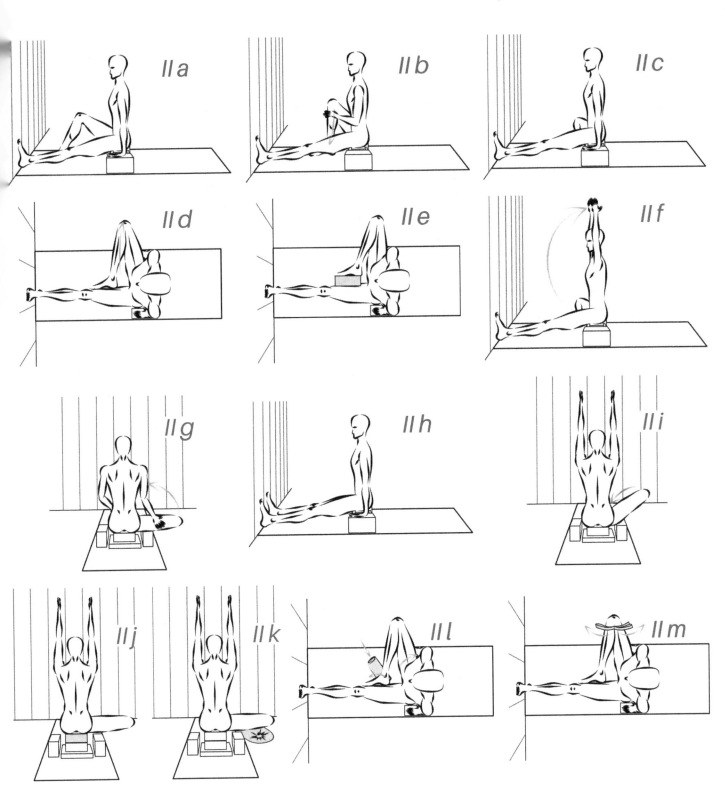

Maha Mudra
The Great Seal

Nourish

Learn + Practice

After Explore, in conjunction
with Standing Poses,
especially Parsvottanasana

Linked Poses

Parsvottanasana, Baddha
Konasana, Paschimottanasana,
Viparita Karani, Sarvangasana

Safety Factors

As for Simplify + Explore, be
cautious of leg hyperextension

Prepare

· Set sitting height on mat
· Have a looped a strap
  nearby and supports for
  bent leg as necessary

Enter

· Sit in *Dandasana*
· Place looped strap beside left
  lower leg for easy reach
· Follow *Enter* instructions
  for *Janu Sirsasana, Explore*
  (except without wall)
· With arms raised, exhale, lifting
  pelvis up and over femurs 30-
  45°, moving L4 + L5 inward, *III a*
· Keeping spinal length, loop
  strap around left sole, *III b*
· With hands through strap
  loops, externally rotate arms
  and turn palms upward, *III c*
· Inhaling, resist torso backward
  away from hands, lift spine
  up and out of pelvis
· Without pulling torso forward,
  create a slight back bend,
  lifting chin upward, *III d*
· Holding chest lift, gently
  tuck chin, *III e*

☸ *If reasonable, catch sides
  of left foot with hands,
  arms extended, III f*

Sustain

· Continually extend left leg,
  pushing through ball of big toe
· Pressing right heel into left
  upper inner thigh, lengthen right
  femur away from of pelvis
· Descending femurs, lift
  torso and maximize space
  between legs and torso, *III g*
· Continue resisting torso
  backward, drawing sacrum, L4
  + L5 symmetrically inward
· Bend elbows slightly and
  engage triceps, drawing lower
  shoulder blades forward
· Use shoulder blade action
  to lift and widen collarbones
  away from sternum
· Extend torso equally
  from hips to armpits
· Lengthen spine from
  sacrum to occiput, *III h*

Exit

· Continue to *Synthesize,* or:
· Keeping spinal length,
  exhale and place hands on
  either side of left leg, *III i*
· Pressing into hands, inhale
  to lift torso to seated, *III j*
· Extend right leg to *Dandasana*
· Repeat, folding left leg
  with right leg extended

Challenge

1. Right knee or ankle pain
2. Left femur binds upward
3. Left leg hyperextends,
   left heel lifts
4. Neck tension when lifting chin
5. Nausea/indigestion

Response

1. *See Solutions in Explore.*
2. Press stick or strap into left upper
   femur while folding forward.
   Externally rotate left leg before
   folding torso. Once folded,
   bring leg to neutral rotation.
   Increase sitting height and lift
   pelvis up and over femurs.
3. Broaden left calf as thigh and
   heel descend. Resist left heel
   downward and left tibia head
   upward. Support upper left calf.
4. Lengthen the strap. Deepen
   chest and shoulder blade action
   before lifting chin. Initiate back
   bending action from mid- and
   lower thoracic spine. Keep
   neck long and do not jut chin
   forward when lifting head.
5. Practice with chair, foot
   against chair rung, hands and
   forearms on chair seat, palms
   facing downward, *III k-l.*

Developing the groin strengthening action of Simplify, Maha Mudra gently tones the abdomen, stimulates pelvic organ circulation, and stretches the kidneys. It is a helpful recuperative pose after periods of inactivity due to illness, fatigue, or injury, and may help alleviate nausea.

Contact Points

Sitting bones, back of extended leg, outer side of bent leg, hands

External Supports

Mat, strap, sitting height
Stick, chair

Essence of Form

As for Explore, arm and torso extension; arms slightly externally rotated

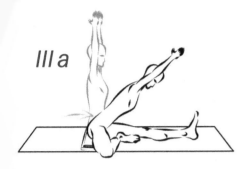

III a

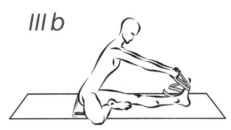

III b

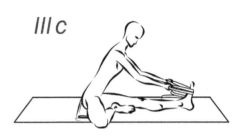

III c

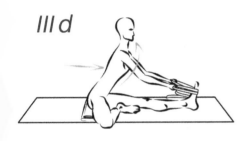

III d

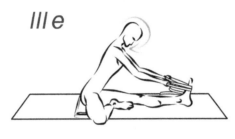

III e

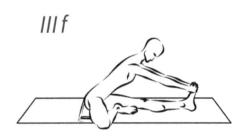

III f

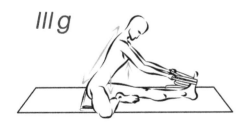

III g

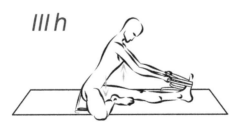

III h

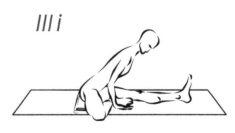

III i

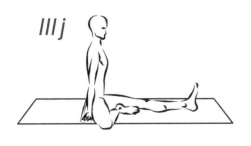

III j

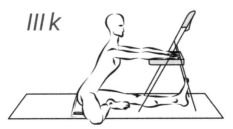

III k

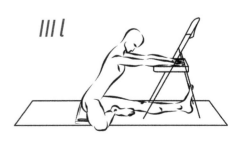

III l

Janu Sirsasana
Head of the Knee Pose

Synthesize

Learn + Practice

After Nourish, in conjunction with Standing Poses, Twists, and deep Froward Bends

Linked Poses

Parsvottanasana, Parighasana, Vrksasana, Marichyasana A, Parivritta Janu Sirsasana

Safety Factors

As for Simplify, Explore + Nourish; do not open leg wide for SI joint dysfunction

Prepare

- Place sitting height on mat
- For holds over 1 minute, set chair or block(s) in front of sitting height to support head

Enter

- Sit in *Dandasana*
- Exhaling, lean slightly back on hands, *IV a*
- Pressing left inner thigh and heel downward, extend and lift right leg, *IV b*
- Without lifting left inner thigh, fold and abduct right leg, heel to perineum, *IV c*
- Inhaling, raise arms to *Urdhva Hastasana*
- Exhaling, lift pelvis up and over femur heads, folding torso forward over left leg, *IV d*
- Rest hands and elbows on each side of or beyond left foot, palms face down, *IV e*
- For holds greater than 1 minute, rest forehead on chair seat or blocks, *IV f-g*

☸ *Once right thigh releases to the side with ease, abduct right leg further, turning pelvis 15-30° to the right and draw right heel to right groin, IV h*

Sustain

- Descend inner left thigh, bringing inner and outer back knee level
- Fold pelvis as symmetrically as possible, observing the right hip's tendency to roll back
- Spreading toes, press top of right foot and toe nails into floor
- Lengthen right femur away from back pelvis
- As right femur lengthens laterally, draw right ilium toward left inner thigh, articulating right hip and femur, *IV i*

Exit

- Exhaling, bring hands under shoulders
- Descending back pelvis, press hands into floor and inhale to seated, *IV j*
- For shorter holds, lean backward on hands
- Keeping right thigh descending, lift right heel and extend right leg laterally, *IV k*
- With right leg extended, adduct right leg to *Dandasana, IV l*
- For longer holds, use right hand to lift right leg, then slowly extend right leg to *Dandasana*
- Repeat to the second side

Challenge

1. Left leg externally rotates while folding
2. Left femur binds upward
3. Left outer hamstring tightness
4. Right ilium falls backward
5. Front torso length is lost

Response

1. Emphasize keeping left inner thigh descending toward floor through all steps of *Enter*.
2. Support left femur and press into support. Elevate left heel on block and let upper left femur fall toward the back thigh, *IV m*.
3. Release left leg into external rotation. Lean to the left, lifting right thigh and sitting bone. Roll onto outer left thigh and fold torso to the left and over left leg. As right thigh releases, roll back to neutral, descending right thigh and returning left leg to neutral rotation, *IV n-o*.
4. *See Response 3.* Draw right front ilium leftward.
5. Practice with back to wall, hands pushing wall, *IV p. See Paschimottanasana, Explore*.

Forward bending in Janu Sirsasana continues from Maha Mudra, deepening some of the recuperative effects on the pelvis, spine, and organs. Supporting the head while releasing the spine and torso forward often calms the nervous system, initiating a restorative response.

Contact Points

Sitting bones, back of extended leg, outer side of bent leg and foot, hands

External Supports

Mat, blocks and/or blankets
Block, chair, wall, additional blocks and/or blankets

Essence of Form

As for Nourish; arms neutral

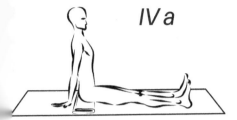
IV a

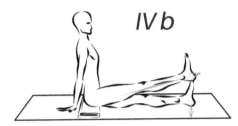
IV b

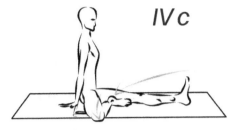
IV c

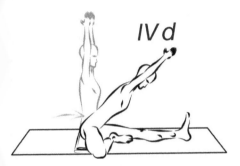
IV d

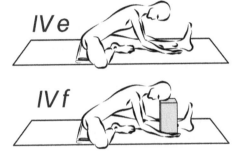
IV e

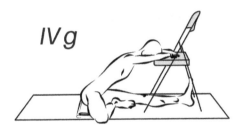
IV g

IV f

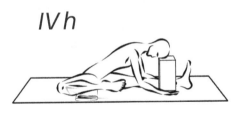
IV h

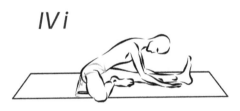
IV i

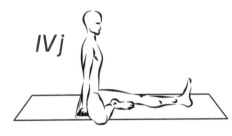
IV j

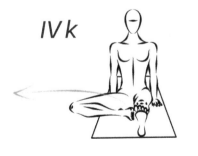
IV k

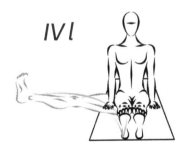
IV l

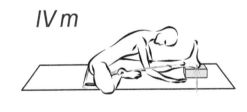
IV m

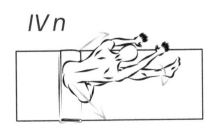
IV n

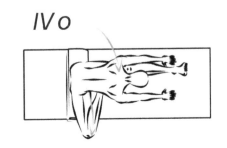
IV o

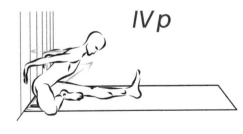
IV p

Trianga Mukhaikapada Paschimottanasana
Three Limbs Facing One Intense Back-Body Stretch

Learn + Practice

After Virasana and Dandasana, before Ardha Supta Virasana and intermediate Twists

Linked Poses

Virasana, Dandasana, Anjaneyasana, Krounchasana, Parighasana, Marichyasana A

Safety Factors

Lower back strain, sacroiliac discomfort, knee and/or ankle strain

Prepare

- Set sitting height for *Dandasana*
- If using a blanket, set right edge 4-6" from mat's mid line or place it lengthwise, *I a-b*
- Have an additional block or blanket nearby

Enter

- Sit in *Dandasana*
- Keeping left leg extended, bend right leg and bring foot flat to floor, *I c*
- Place thumbs in pit of right knee, *I d*
- Dragging thumbs downward, bifurcate calf fold leg completely and bring heel to right sitting bone, *I e*
- Bring left hand to the floor beside left pelvis
- Supporting weight on left hand, lean to the left and lift right sitting bone, *I f*
- Without abducting right leg and keeping knee joint fully closed, bring right leg to *Virasana*
- Point right foot directly backward and descend right sitting bone, *I g*
- Keeping sitting bones stable, inhale and raise arms to *Urdhva Hastasana, I h*

Sustain

- Anchor top of right foot, spreading toes
- Draw right outer ankle inward
- Lengthen backs of femurs away from of back pelvis
- Gather front iliums and draw lower femurs inward
- Resist upper femurs outward
- Soften pubis in and up
- Move L4 + L5 inward
- Release excess hip flexor tension and settle femurs
- Symmetrically descend both sitting bones
- Lift trunk up and out of pelvis

Exit

- If raising arms, keep torso length and lower arms on exhalation, *I i*
- Anchoring top of right foot, bend left leg and place left foot flat on floor, *I j*
- Lean slightly forward, lifting pelvis off support
- Remove pelvic support and pass right foot under pelvis, externally rotating right leg, *I k*
- Once right foot clears pelvis, lower pelvis and extend both legs in *Dandasana*
- Repeat, folding left leg with right leg extended

Challenge

1. Ankle pain
2. Knee pain
3. Knee torque when taking leg back
4. Folded leg sitting bone lifts

Response

1. Keep femur close to mid line when taking foot back. Lift foot completely and point toes before drawing foot back. Do not wing foot out laterally, *I l.* Alternately, enter pose from lunge, placing right knee to floor then sitting back, *I m-n.*
2. Adjust knee and thigh skin toward pain as in *Virasana.* Use folded strap or washcloth in knee pit to create space. *See Responses 3 + 4.*
3. Increase pelvic support. Manually drag ankle skin laterally, out from under top of foot. Fill gap between ankle and floor with spacer, such as a rolled cloth or towel. Use a blanket under right tibia, *I o.*
4. Raise sitting height until both sitting bones descend symmetrically. *See also Nourish, Response 1.*

This pose combines Paschimottanasana and Virasana. Due to the asymmetry, it can be more accessible for those who have difficulty in Virasana, though moving in and out of the pose can present other risks. Be especially mindful of this when Entering and Exiting the pose.

Contact Points

Sitting bones, back of extended leg, bent leg shin, top of foot

External Supports

Mat, blanket or block,
Block, blanket, strap, washcloth

Essence of Form

Leg extension, knee flexion with adduction, arm extension; legs internally rotated, arms neutral

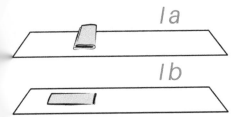

Ia

Ib

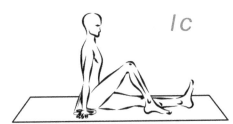

Ic

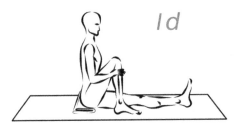

Id

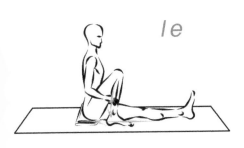

Ie

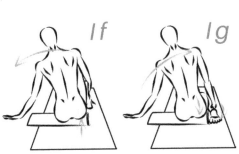

If

Ig

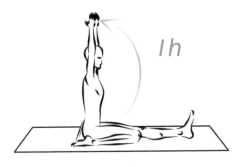

Ih

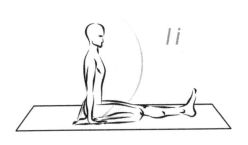

Ii

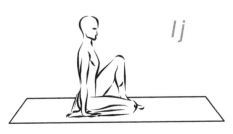

Ij

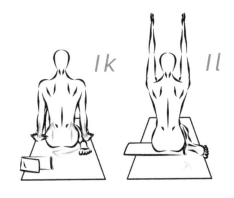

Ik

Il

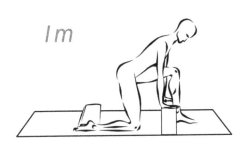

Im

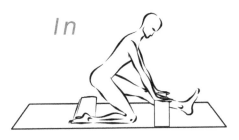

In

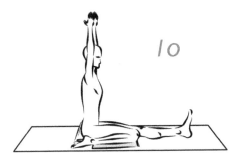

Io

Learn + Practice

After Simplify, when learning deeper Forward Bends,

Linked Poses

Paschimottanasana, Virasana, Krounchasana, Virabhadrasana C

Safety Factors

Same as Simplify; if pregnant, practice Janu Sirsasana instead

Prepare

- Mat's short end to wall
- Set 2 blocks on end and sides together against wall, *II a*
- Place sitting height in front of blocks
- If using a blanket, off-set it to the left as for *Simplify*

Enter

- Sit in *Dandasana*, with back pelvis against vertical blocks, *II b*
- Shift to the left and fold right leg as for *Simplify, Enter*
- Descend both inner femurs and extend through left leg
- Bring hands to wall, fingertips pointing down, elbows bent, *II c*
- Pressing down through hands, lift torso up and out of pelvis
- With torso lifted, push backward through hands and fold torso forward over left leg, *II d*
- If back pelvis loses block contact, place hands beside legs and lift pelvis slightly
- Once pelvis is lifted, scoot backward, making symmetrical contact against blocks
- Replace hands to wall
- Press hands into wall to keep chest lifted and torso long while continuing to fold forward

Sustain

- Engage leg and pelvis actions from *Simplify, Sustain*
- Fold pelvis symmetrically over legs, as though both legs were in *Dandasana, II e*
- Descend both inner thighs
- Soften right groin and descend right femur, extending through back of right femur
- Push left big toe mound away from pubis as pubis recedes
- Lift sternum away from pubis, lengthening front body
- Extend side torso from hips to armpits
- Soften front ribs inward and lift back ribs away from back pelvis
- Release trapezium and broaden space between shoulder blades

Exit

- Release hands from wall, bringing hands to floor under shoulders
- Inhaling, push into hands and lift torso upright, *II f*
- Lift pelvis and extend legs to *Dandasana* as described in *Simplify, Exit*
- Repeat, folding left leg with right leg extended

Challenge

1. Pelvis tilts leftward
2. Left leg externally rotates
3. Right femur lifts, groin binds
4. Hands do not reach wall

Response

1. Press more firmly through left hand, pushing weight toward right sitting bone to equalize, *II g*. Use more height under left buttock.
2. *See Response 1*. Manually rotate left thigh inward before folding. Draw both thighs toward each other, as external rotation and abduction are often related. *See also Responses in Nourish + Synthesize*.
3. *See Responses 1 + 2*, groin often binds to compensate for weight shifting leftward. Press stick against right thigh, lifting pelvis up and over right thigh to fold, *II h*.
4. Use blocks as arm extensions, pressing blocks directly back into wall, *II i*.

ॐ *See also Paschimottanasana, Explore*

Contact Points

Sitting bones, back of extended leg, bent leg shin, top of foot

External Supports

Mat, sitting height +
2 blocks, wall
Blanket, strap, washcloth

Essence of Form

Leg extension, knee flexion with adduction, hip flexion, torso extension; legs internally rotated, arms neutral toward external

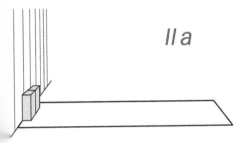

II a

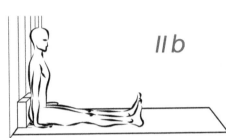

II b

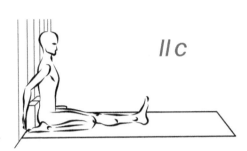

II c

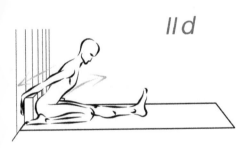

II d

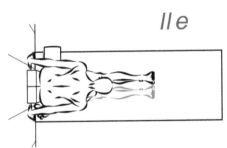

II e

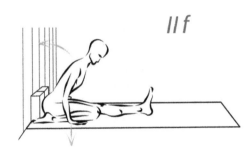

II f

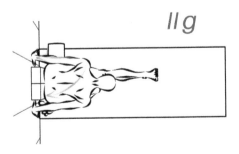

II g

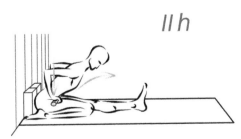

II h

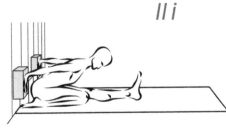

II i

Learn + Practice

Once pelvis folds with symmetry in Explore, before asymmetrical Back Bends

Linked Poses

Maha Mudra, Krounchasana, Supta Padangusthasana A, all Eka Pada Back Bends

Safety Factors

Same as Simplify + Explore, Exit as for Simplify if there is any knee concern

Prepare

- Place sitting height on mat, off-set to the left
- Set chair in front of sitting height

Enter

- Sit in *Dandasana*, feet against chair rung, *III a*
- Fold right leg as for *Simplify*, *Enter*
- Inhaling, raise arms to *Urdhva Hastasana*
- Lifting pelvis up and over femur heads, exhale and fold symmetrically forward, *III a*
- Fold to capacity, only as far as pelvic symmetry can be maintained
- Keeping spinal length, catch chair seat sides or chair legs with hands, arms extended, *III c-d*
- Inhaling, resist torso backward away from hands, lift spine up and out of pelvis
- Drawing shoulder blades forward, inhale to lift chest and chin into a slight back bend, *III e*
- Keeping slight back bend, lengthen back of skull upward and tuck chin toward chest, *III f*

🕉 *To deepen, Prepare with block against chair rung, III g, or use stick against foot, III h*

Sustain

- Engage leg and pelvis actions from *Simplify + Explore, Sustain*
- Continually lift chest and draw L4 + L5 inward
- Without pulling torso forward, pull chair seat with hands, drawing chair rung against foot
- Press left foot into chair rung, away from back pelvis
- Deepen both groins inward, extend inner femurs away from inner groins
- Soften lower abdomen, broadening back pelvis

Exit

- Strongly press right foot and left heel down
- Inhaling, lift torso symmetrically to seated
- Pass right foot under pelvis as in *Simplify*, or:
- Lean to the left, lifting right sitting bone
- Keeping the right leg completely folded, and without turning foot, ankle, or knee, use right hand to lift right leg directly up and forward
- Place right foot flat on the floor, then extend to *Dandasana*
- Repeat to the other side

Challenge

1. Pelvis rolls leftward, left leg externally rotates
2. Hamstring injury
3. Left leg hyperextension

Response

1. Wedge blocks or a folded blanket along outer left thigh to prevent thigh from rolling outward, *III i-j. See also Synthesize.*
2. Do not fold forward. Place a stick between folded leg calf and hamstring, *III k,* and/or behind extended leg hamstring. Soften and widen hamstrings against stick pressure as right buttock descends. This also helps right buttock descend once stick is removed. When *Exiting*, clasp hands behind right hamstring and resist femur into hands while extending leg to *Dandasana, III l.* Practice both sides, even if injury is only on one side.
3. Resist left tibia head upward as heel and femur descend. Support upper left femur and/or upper left calf, *III m.* Observe and resist tendency to internally rotate from lower femur.

As an asymmetrical pose, Trianga Mukhaikapada Paschimottanasana is preliminary to deep Twists. It also increases mobility in the ankles, balances external hip rotation, and can help correct flat feet. This variation may reduce hyperacidity and aid digestion, especially when recovering from illness.

Contact Points

Sitting bones, back of extended leg, bent leg shin, top of foot

External Supports

Mat, sitting height, chair Sticks, blocks, foam blocks, blankets

Essence of Form

As for Simplify + Explore, with neck flexion; legs internally rotated, arms neutral toward external

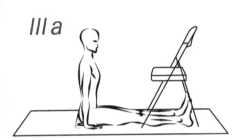
IIIa

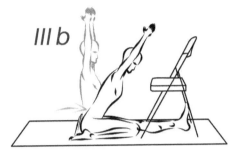
IIIb

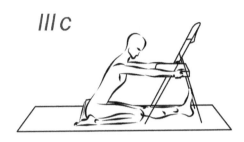
IIIc

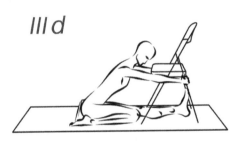
IIId

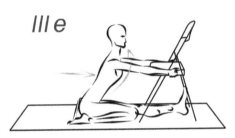
IIIe

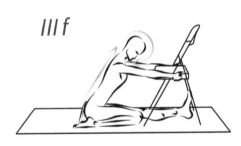
IIIf

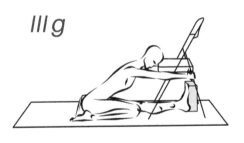
IIIg

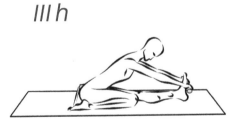
IIIh

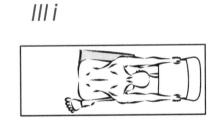
IIIi

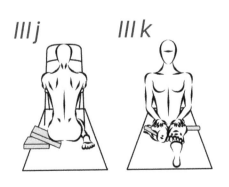
IIIj   IIIk

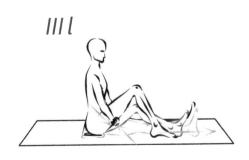
IIIl

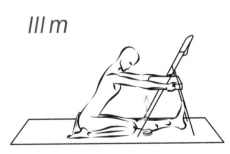
IIIm

Trianga Mukhaikapada Paschimottanasana
Three Limbs Facing One Intense Back-Body Stretch **Synthesize**

Learn + Practice

Learn after Simplify, before Twists and deep Back Bends

Linked Poses

Marichyasana A, Virasana, Upavistha Konasana, Krounchasana, Parighasana

Safety Factors

As for Simplify, Explore + Nourish; groin injury

Prepare

- Place sitting height on mat
- Use head support (chair or blocks) for holds longer than 1 minute

Enter

- Sit in *Dandasana*, then fold right leg as for *Simplify*
- Anchoring right tibia, lengthen and lift left leg, abducting to *Upavistha Konasana, IV a*
- With left leg abducted, inhale and raise arms to *Urdhva Hastasana, IV b*
- Lifting pelvis up and over femur heads, exhale and symmetrically fold forward to capacity
- Once folding capacity is reached, keep torso length and lower hands to floor, slightly to the right of mid line, *IV c*
- Pushing into hands, maintain pelvic fold and draw left leg back to *Dandasana, IV d*
- Bring hands to either side of left tibia lengthen torso sides equally, *IV e*
- Exhale to rest forehead on chair seat or blocks, rounding the spine slightly, *IV f*

Sustain

- Engage *Sustain* actions from *Simplify, Explore, + Nourish*
- Pressing left hand forward, descend outer right buttock
- Descending outer right buttock, decrease left hand pressure
- Without shortening right side waist, soften right groin inward as buttock descends
- With right outer buttock and inner groin descending, extend right side torso

Exit

- Exhale and bring hands to floor below shoulders
- Pushing left heel and right tibia downward, minimally gather back iliums and Press into hands, inhaling to seated
- Extend right leg to *Dandasana* as for *Explore* or *Nourish*
- Alternatively, lean slightly forward onto hands and lift pelvis, bending left leg, *IV g*
- Pass left foot under pelvis, extending legs to *Adho Mukha Svanasana, IV h-i,* or vinyasa (*see Urdhva Mukha Svanasana, Synthesize*)
- Repeat to the second side

Challenge

1. Ribcage shifts leftward
2. Lower abdominal breath restriction
3. Inner left groin binds
4. Right femur pulls back

Response

1. Lengthen right side ribs away from right inner groin. Resist left heel laterally, drawing left side ribs inward.
2. Keep left leg in *Upavistha Konasana* and gradually reduce abduction over time. As leg adducts, resist left heel laterally to keep lower abdominal breath free. Strap around right thigh and pull laterally while folding, *IV j.*
3. *See Responses in Explore + Nourish.* Elevate left heel on block, bringing more wight to right sitting bone and reducing over-effort in left leg, *IV k.*
4. *Prepare* facing a wall, with 3-4 blocks within reach. After folding right leg, place blocks between the wall and end of right femur, *IV l.* Extend femur into blocks while folding.

For some, internal rotation may cause tension in the groins and narrow the lower pelvic space, restricting the capacity to Forward Bend. Entering the pose with the extended leg abducted may help address this common problem, allowing the pelvis to fold more deeply.

Contact Points

Sitting bones, back of extended leg, bent leg shin, top of foot; forehead, hands

External Supports

Mat, sitting height, chair
Sticks, blocks, foam
blocks, blankets

Essence of Form

As for Simplify + Explore, with mils spinal flexion; legs internally rotated, arms neutral

IV a
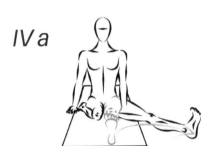

IV b
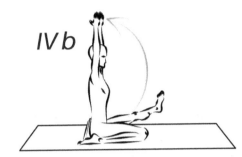

IV c
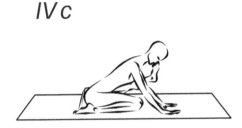

IV d
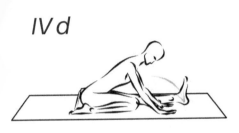

IV e
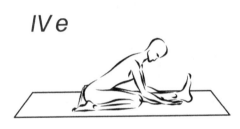

IV f
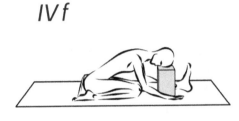

IV g
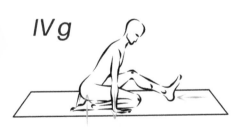

IV h
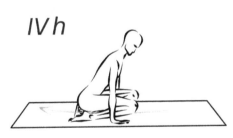

IV i
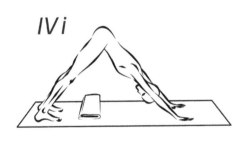

IV j
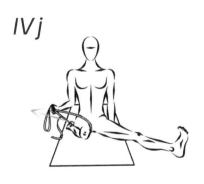

IV k
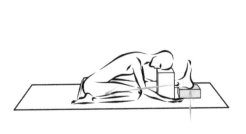

IV l
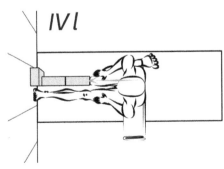

Uttitha Marichyasana A (*Forward-bending*)
Sage Marichy's First Pose, Standing

Learn + Practice

After Uttanasana and Anjáneyasana, before Seated variations of Marichyasana

Linked Poses

Uttana Balasana, Uttanasana, Anjaneyasana, Marichyasana A + C, Malasana

Safety Factors

Lower back strain, SI joint discomfort, hip replacement or joint hypermobility

Prepare

· Set chair's left legs on center mat
· Place blocks on mat edge in front of chair, *l a*

Enter

· Stand in *Tadasana* on long edge of mat, facing blocks with chair to the right, *l b*
· Line up big toes with chair's left front leg, standing 6-8" from it
· Step right foot up on chair seat, foot and thigh parallel to mid line, tibia vertical, *l c*
· Gather front iliums and resist heels laterally
· Press right hand into upper right thigh, thumb toward hip crease, *l d*
· Push right femur downward and lift right ilium up and away from right femur, *l e*
· Keeping left thigh firm, roll pelvis up and over femur heads and fold forward on exhalation, bringing torso below inner right thigh, *l f*
· Center left hip joint atop left heel
· Bring hands to blocks or clasp elbows, *l g*

ॐ *This variation is also sometimes called Ardha Uttanasana*

Sustain

· Stabilize both big toe mounds and spread toes
· Press upper left femur backward and resist left tibia forward
· Descending right femur, soften right inner groin
· Hug lower right femur toward the mid line and resist upper femur laterally
· Roll right ilium toward left inner thigh
· Soften right buttock flesh and let it descend away from back pelvis
· Soften abdomen and let torso to hang freely
· As torso lengthens, also allow head to hang without tension

Exit

· Stabilize hands on blocks
· Without lifting torso, step right foot off chair to *Uttanasana*, feet hip-width apart, *l h*
· Rest in *Uttanasana* for 5-10 breaths, *l i*
· Bending legs, place hands on thighs, *l j*
· Press hands into thighs and descend back pelvis, inhaling to lift torso upright, *l k*
· Repeat with left foot on chair

Challenge

1. Pelvic asymmetry
2. Groin binding
3. Dizziness or blood pressure drop upon standing

Response

1. Pelvic placement will change as right groin releases and femur drops. Allow pelvic shift, but keep left hip joint above left heel, keeping left leg vertical, regardless of pelvic position.
2. Before *Entering*, place strap across upper right thigh. Hold strap in each hand, pushing femur down, *l l*. Keeping femur descending, wrap strap under right thigh, holding both ends with right hand at outer thigh, pulling femur outward, *l m*. Pulling femur both down and outward, lift right ilium up and over right femur, directing it toward left inner femur while folding forward.
3. Rest forehead on wall or press heel of hand to forehead immediately after *Exiting*, sliding forehead skin downward. Lift torso to standing on an exhalation rather than inhalation.

The Marichyasanas are a broad family of asymmetrical poses in which one leg is in Malasana, or a squat-like position. Each variation takes the non-Malasana leg through all other possibilities. Standing upright in Marichyasana A facilitates freer movement in the legs, pelvis, and spine.

Contact Points

Feet, hands

External Supports

Mat, chair, 2 blocks
Strap, wall, additional blocks

Essence of Form

Leg extension and knee flexion, hip flexion, femoral abduction with leg adduction; arms and legs neutrally rotated

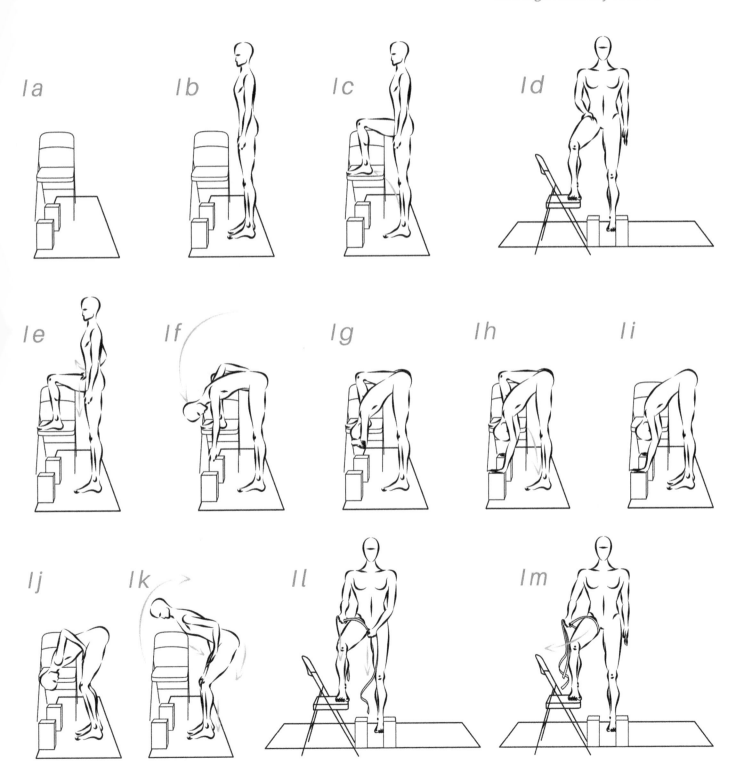

I a   I b   I c   I d

I e   I f   I g   I h   I i

I j   I k   I l   I m

Marichyasana A (Forward-bending)
Sage Marichy's First Pose

Learn + Practice

Once pelvis folds beyond 90° to standing leg in *Simplify*; Before twisting variations

Linked Poses

Marichyasana A (twisting), Marichyasana C, Anjaneyasana, Uttana Balasana, Malasana

Safety Factors

As for *Simplify*, do not wrap with neck or shoulder injury; open extended leg 45° if pregnant, *II l*

Prepare

- Set sitting height on mat; minimally use a folded blanket, *II a*

Enter

- Sit on height in *Dandasana, II b*
- Keeping left inner thigh descending, bend right leg and place thumbs in knee pit
- Drag thumbs from knee pit to Achilles tendon, bifurcating calf to fold leg completely, *II c*
- Without tipping upper sacrum backward, draw right heel close to right sitting bone, *II d*
- Set right foot wide enough that thigh is lateral to side torso, without externally rotating, *II e*
- Ascending bottom back ribs, inhale and raise arms to *Urdhva Hastasana, II f*
- Keeping torso length, lift pelvis up and over femur heads to fold forward, drawing L4 + L5 inward
- Fold to reasonable capacity and rest hands on either side of left leg, *II g*
- If possible, bring right armpit past right tibia, *II h*
- Use head support for holds greater than a minute, *II i*

Sustain

- Push through left heel and big toe mound, extending left leg away from back pelvis
- Roll left inner thigh toward floor
- Gather front iliums and resist heels laterally
- Soften pubis inward and upward
- With right sitting bone heavy, recede, broaden, and descend right inner groin
- Lengthen side torso equally from hips to armpits
- If right armpit moves beyond right tibia, resist arm back into tibia and tibia into upper arm
- Lift and widen collarbones away from sternum
- Keeping collarbone lift, internally rotate arms and clasp left wrist behind back with right hand, *II j*

Exit

- Stabilizing left leg and extended, minimally gather back iliums
- If binding, release bind and place hands under shoulders
- Pressing hands into floor, descend back pelvis and inhale to lift torso upright
- Extend right leg to *Dandasana*
- Repeat to the second side

Challenge

1. Sacrum tips backward as torso folds forward
2. Right sitting bone lifts
3. Abdominal compression, breath restriction

Response

1. Increase sitting height and reduce fold. Use a chair if necessary, with adequate hand support, *II k. See Solution 3. Practice Simplify.*
2. Raise left sitting bone and keep pelvis level throughout. Place right foot more lateral to mid line and increase internal rotation
3. Lean leftward, lifting right sitting bone. Roll right ilium and lower abdomen leftward, folding toward the floor. Lengthen right side torso. Without lifting torso, retain length and descend right sitting bone, sweeping torso back toward mid line. Widen left leg 45° before folding forward, *II l.*

ॐ *See also Paschimottanasana, Janu Sirsasana, and Trianga Mukhaikapada Paschimottanasana for additional ways to work in forward bends*

This pose shifts the bent leg femur both laterally and posteriorly without abducting the entire leg, which increases lateral hip joint space, helpful in deepening Twists and Forward Bends. Marichyasana A fosters lower abdominal breath and may aid in elimination.

Contact Points

Sitting bones, back of extended thigh, bent leg foot, hands

External Supports

Mat, blankets or bolster
Chairs, blocks

Essence of Form

Leg extension, knee flexion, hip flexion, arm extension; legs neutrally rotated neutral, arms internal when wrapping

II a

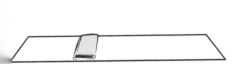

II b

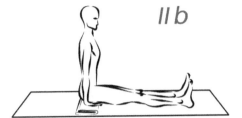

II c

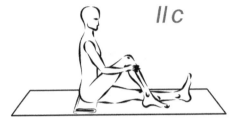

II d

II e

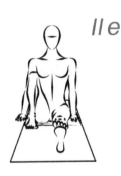

II f

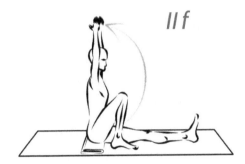

II g

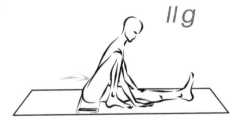

II h

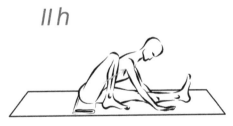

II i

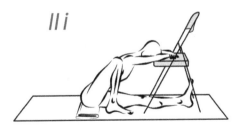

II j

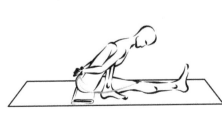

II k

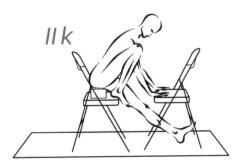

II l

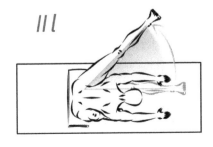

Learn + Practice

Learn after lunges, before closed twists or when closed Twists are contraindicated

Linked Poses

Trikonasana, Parsvakonasana, Janu Sirsasana, Marichyasana C, Bharadvajasana

Safety Factors

SI joint injury, lumbar disc problems, kyphosis, high blood pressure

Prepare

- Place bolster lengthwise on mat

Enter

- Sit on bolster's end in *Dandasana*, *III a*
- Without lifting left inner thigh, bend right leg, bringing foot flat to floor, *III b*
- Place thumbs at knee pit and broaden knee tendons while folding the leg completely
- Draw right heel toward right sitting bone, holding tibia with right hand
- Keeping torso length, lean back, exhale, and place left hand on bolster behind pelvis, *III c*
- Without lifting right sitting bone, inhale and raise right arm to *Urdhva Hastasana*, *III d*
- Exhaling, bend right elbow and bring right arm inside leg with forearm vertical, *III e*
- Bracing right arm against right leg, inhale to lengthen spine
- Keeping length, soften spinal and abdominal muscles before twisting leftward on exhalation
- At deepest twist, maintain twist and draw L4 + L5 inward, bringing torso upright, *III f*

Sustain

- Fully extend left leg away from back pelvis and descend left inner thigh
- Gather front iliums and resist heels laterally
- Continually descend right buttock and deepen right inner groin
- With a soft belly, turn the lower abdomen leftward, initiating twist from as low as possible, *III g*
- Resist right arm and right inner thigh against each other, *III h*
- Lift right collarbone away from right groin
- When deepening twist, repeat *Enter* cycle: lean back, lengthen, soften, twist, maintain twist, sit upright
- Keeping gaze level, turn head to the left

Exit

- Exhaling, lean back on left hand
- Leaning back, descend inner groins and inhale to untwist and bring torso upright
- Exhaling, extend right leg to *Dandasana*
- Repeat to the second side

Challenge

1. Right foot lifts when leg is folded
2. SI joint discomfort
3. Chest collapses when sitting upright
4. Neck discomfort when turning the head

Response

1. Use block or rolled blanket under right heel, *III i*.
2. Reduce overall twist. Broaden right inner femur away from mid line and roll right ilium over femur head, allowing pelvis to turn with twist. Move twist up toward thoracic spine.
3. Use a block or additional support under left hand, *III j*. Descend left femur heavily. Turn abdomen and rib cage rather than just shoulder girdle. *Prepare + Enter* with left side to wall and press hands into wall to twist, *III k*.
4. Turn head from mid-thoracic spine or not at all. Keep head in line with spine, neither tipping forward nor back. Turn head rightward for thyroid and hormonal imbalance, *III l*.

Twisting Marichyasana A is an open Twist where the bent leg does not cross the torso's mid line, thereby keeping the lower abdomen spacious. Particularly useful when abdominal compression is contraindicated, such as during pregnancy, abdominal cysts, and high blood pressure.

Contact Points

Extended leg, bent leg foot, sitting bones, hand

External Supports

Mat, bolster, Rolled blanket, block

Essence of Form

Leg extension, leg flexion, hip flexion, spinal twist; legs slightly internally rotated, arms externally rotated

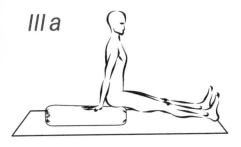
III a

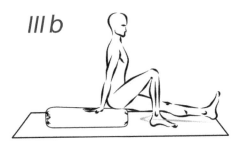
III b

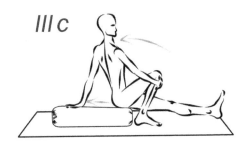
III c

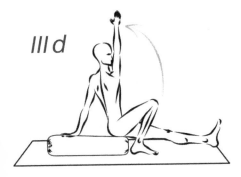
III d

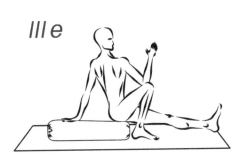
III e

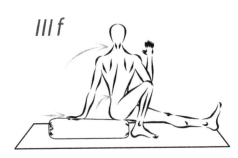
III f

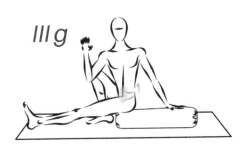
III g

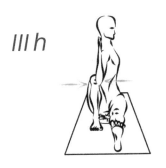
III h

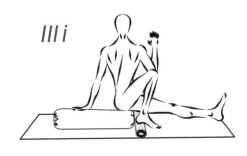
III i

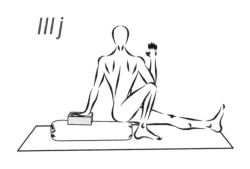
III j

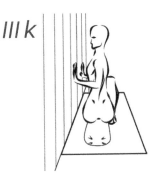
III k

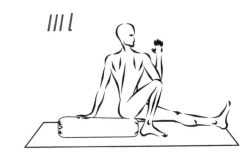
IIII l

Learn + Practice

Once Explore and Nourish are stable and done with ease Before closed and Forward-Bending Twists

Linked Poses

Trikonasana, Parsvakonasana, Janu Sirsasana, Marichyasana C, Bharadvajasana

Safety Factors

As for Nourish, do not bind with neck or shoulder injury; do not practice this variation if pregnant

Prepare

- Place sitting height on mat, minimally use a folded blanket, *IV a*

Enter

- Sit in *Dandasana, IV b*
- Keeping left leg extended, fold right leg, dividing knee tendons and bifurcating calf
- Draw right heel as close to buttocks as possible, stabilizing right heel into floor, *IV c*
- Place left hand on floor beside pelvis, *IV d*
- Lean leftward, bending elbow, lift right sitting bone and roll onto outer left thigh and hip, *IV e*
- Extend and turn torso to the left, bringing both hands to the left of pelvis on the floor, *IV f*
- Roll abdomen and right ilium to the left, *IV g*
- Maintain turning action to the left
- Keeping torso low toward floor, sweep right side torso around toward left leg, descending left inner thigh and right sitting bone, *IV h*
- Hook right armpit on right tibia and lean back into right leg, opening torso leftward, *IV i*

Sustain

- Keep leg and pelvis actions from *Explore + Nourish*
- Broaden soles of feet from inner foot to outer foot, widening back pelvis reciprocally
- From back pelvis width, lift L4 + L5 upward and inward, broadening chest and back ribs
- Widen and roll front collarbones upward
- Keeping collarbone lift, internally rotate arms, wrapping right arm around right leg and behind pelvis to clasp left wrist, *IV j*

Exit

- Keeping left leg stable, exhale and turn torso to face left leg, *IV k*
- Release bind if wrapping
- Keeping torso low, reverse *Enter* instructions: sweep torso to the left, lifting right sitting bone, *IV l*
- Place hands under shoulders
- Pressing into hands, descend right sitting bone and inhale to push torso upright,
- Untwist and extend right leg to *Dandasana*
- Continue to the second side

Challenge

1. Torso shortens in *IV f-h* transition
2. Chest collapse
3. Difficulty binding

Response

1. Increase sitting height. Transition more slowly from *IV f* to *IV h*, maintaining torso length at each degree. Spend more time in *IV g*. Do not sweep all the way around until length can be retained.
2. *See Response 1.* Lengthen chest forward in *IV f* before sweeping torso toward mid line. Resist hands backward against floor to lift and lengthen from pubis to sternum, *IV m.*
3. Do not attempt wrap until armpit passes tibia. *See Responses 1 + 2* and bring right armpit past right tibia. Resist arm back against tibia before binding. Increase shoulder mobility with *Bharadvajasana A, Explore + Synthesize.*

ॐ *For additional ways to work, see Marichyasana C and Bharadvajasana A*

...can be difficult to Twist along the spine's entire length when seated upright. In this variation of Marichyasana A, the pose is entered from the side, accessing the Twist from lower in the spine. This entry also tends to have a more profound effect on the abdominal organs.

Contact Points

Sitting bones, bent leg foot, extended leg, hands and outer leg and hip (transitional)

External Supports

Bolster or blanket

Essence of Form

Leg extension, leg flexion, hip flexion, lateral torso extension and rotation, spinal twist; legs in slight internal rotation, arms external, internal when binding

IV a
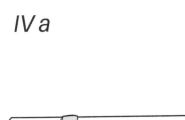

IV b
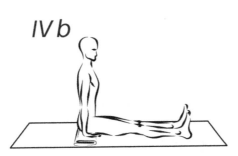

IV c
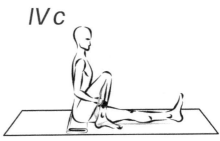

IV d
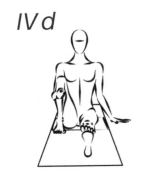

IV e
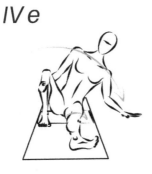

IV f
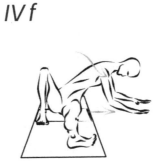

IV g
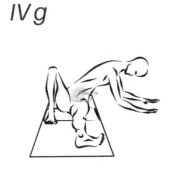

IV h
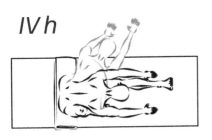

IV i
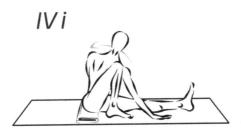

IV j
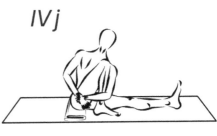

IV k
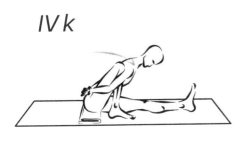

IV l
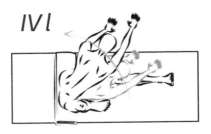

IV m
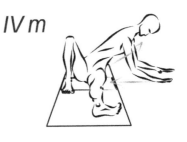

Uttitha Marichyasana C
Sage Marichy's Third Pose, Standing

Simplify

Learn + Practice

Before seated Twists + revolved Standing Poses, After Marichyasana A

Linked Poses

Parivritta Parsvakonasana, Anjaneyasana, Marichyasana A, Uttitha Hasta Padangusthasana

Safety Factors

Lower back strain, groin injury; if pregnant, practice Uttitha Marichyasana A, twisting, I d

Prepare

- Mat's long edge against wall
- Place chair on mat, chair's left side toward wall, block on chair seat
- Set one block on the floor, 6"-1' away from chair and 1-1.5' from wall

Enter

- Stand in *Tadasana* facing chair, right side toward wall
- Step left heel on floor block, block's edge at back of arch, ball of foot to floor, *I a*
- Stack pelvis vertically above left heel
- Without shifting weight forward, step right foot up on chair seat block, *I b*
- Keep the right femur parallel to wall, knee at or above hip crest, tibia vertical
- Pressing down through left heel, lift and lengthen torso from hips to armpits
- Keeping torso length, turn toward wall, placing hands on wall at chest height, *I c*

☸ *If pregnant, Enter with the wall to the left, I d*

Sustain

- Press left heel away from back pelvis
- Gather front iliums and soften pubis inward
- Lengthen right femur and equalize pressure through 4 corners of right foot, particularly the big toe mound
- Keep right femur parallel to wall
- Descend elbows, releasing trapezium and lifting chest
- Without losing spinal length, soften abdomen
- Push right hand into wall, moving right ribs back, away from wall, *I e*
- Without changing left hand position, drag isometrically downward and lift left torso away from left heel, *I f*
- Keeping chest lift, carry left back ribs up and around toward wall

Exit

- Pushing through left heel, inhale and turn torso back to neutral
- Exhaling, lower right foot to floor, then step left foot off block
- *Prepare + Enter* to the left side

☸ *As twist develops, increase bent leg height, I g-h*

Challenge

1. Heel pain, weight shifts forward, *I*
2. Left hip compression
3. Right groin binds
4. Right leg releases laterally

Response

1. Chair is too far away from floor block — decrease distance in *Prepare*. Ensure the block's edge is just in front of heel, not in the arch. Stack pelvis directly above left heel and push more deeply away from back pelvis. If heel sensation is too intense, raise ball of foot on slant board or use rolled mat under heel, *I j-k*
2. Without narrowing groin space, hug femurs inward, creating pelvic lift. Pushing through left heel, move upper left femur backward.
3. Strap from right groin to left sole, *I l*. Bend left leg and tighten strap, then extend leg, dragging right femur and groin downward.
4. Wedge a block between wall and right lower femur, *I m*. Anchor right big toe mound.

Standing upright in Marichyasana C facilitates freer movement in the legs, pelvis, and spine, as well as minimizing some risks associated with combining Forward Bending with Twisting. It is an excellent introduction to seated and standing closed Twists.

Contact Points

Feet, hands

External Supports

Mat, chair, 2 blocks
Strap, rolled mat, slant board, additional blocks

Essence of Form

Leg and groin extension, leg and hip flexion, spinal twist; legs in neutral rotation, arms slightly external

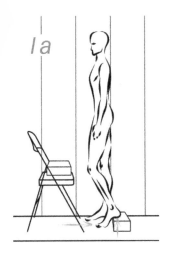

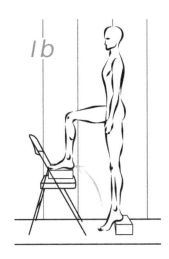

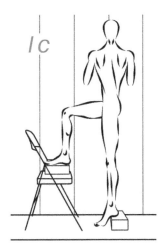

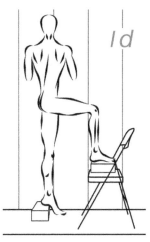

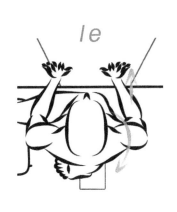

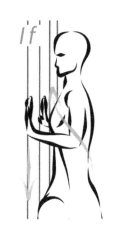

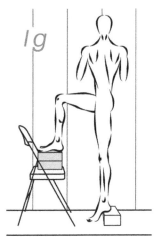

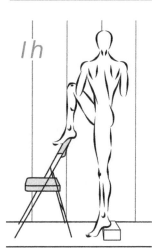

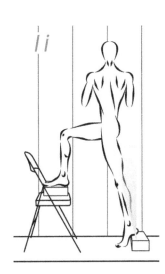

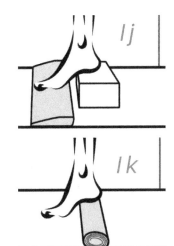

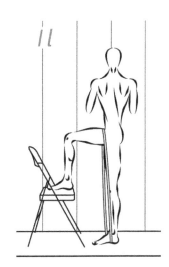

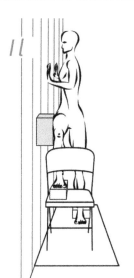

Marichyasana C
Sage Marichy's Third Pose

Explore

Learn + Practice

Once torso twists with ease in Simplify with minimal groin tension

Linked Poses

Marichyasana A, Matsyendrasana, Pashasana, Parivritta Parsvakonasana

Safety Factors

Lower back strain, SI joint injury; turn leftward (Marichyasana A) if pregnant

Prepare

- Place chair on mat facing wall, 2-3' from wall
- Set a block on chair seat

Enter

- Sit in *Dandasana* on the block on chair seat
- Push balls of feet into wall away from back pelvis, heels pressing downward, *ll a*
- Press back femurs into chair lip
- Keep left foot pressing into wall and without lifting left inner femur, bend right leg, bringing right foot to chair seat in front of block, *ll b*
- Exhaling, lean back slightly, moving L4 + L5 inward
- Hold right tibia head with left hand, *ll c*
- Inhaling, lift and lengthen side torso, then bring right hand to backrest, elbow bent, *ll d*
- Without losing torso length, exhale and soften spinal and abdominal muscles
- Keeping length and softness, turn the torso rightward
- If left ribcage passes right thigh, hook left outer elbow on right outer thigh, forearm vertical, *ll e*
- With gaze level, turn head to the right, *ll f*

Sustain

- Extend left leg, pushing through heel and big toe mound
- Contact back of left femur into chair lip
- Gathering front iliums, resist heels laterally
- Press inner right heel into chair seat and spread toes
- Draw right lower femur toward medially, without crossing mid line
- Descending sitting bones equally, soften and deepen inner groins
- Hug left torso toward right thigh if holding tibia, or resist outer left arm against outer right leg
- Pressing right hand into top of backrest, draw elbow down and backward, lifting torso
- Keeping torso extension, continue softening abdomen and turn from that softness

Exit

- Stabilizing left leg, lean back on right hand
- Inhaling, untwist and bring torso upright
- Exhaling, extend right leg to *Dandasana*
- Repeat to the second side

Challenge

1. Block slides on chair seat
2. Pelvis tilts backward
3. Chair lip pressure causes left leg to bend
4. Right groin binds
5. Shoulder restriction

Response

1. Fold mat end through chair back or use mat remnant between chair and block.
2. Increase sitting height, either adding a folded blanket on block or a second block, *ll g-h*.
3. *See Response 2*, or raise left heel on block(s) provided pelvis does not tilt backward, *ll i*.
4. Strap right thigh to chair frame, pulling inner right femur laterally, *ll j*. Strap both thighs for added stability, *ll k*.
5. *Prepare + Enter* with back to wall, 1.5-2' away from it. Extend right arm and push right hand into wall, *ll l*. Begin with fingertips pointing upward and externally rotate arm as capacity increases, *ll m*. *See also Bharadvajasana A, Nourish*.

210 Marichyasana C — *Explore*

Yoga: Point + Process | *Volume 1*

Marichyasana C increases mobility along the spine and between the ribs, balancing strength and flexibility in the intercostals and paraspinal muscles. Often, twisting capacity is restricted by hamstring or groin tightness. Sitting on the chair reduces both of these common restrictions.

Contact Points

Feet, sitting bones, back femur, back hand

External Supports

Mat, chair, block
Blanket, blocks, mat remnant, strap

Essence of Form

Leg and groin extension, leg and hip flexion, spinal twist; legs neutrally rotated, arms external

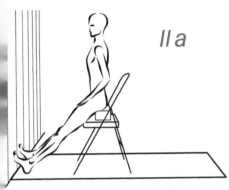
II a

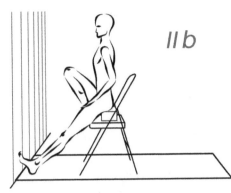
II b

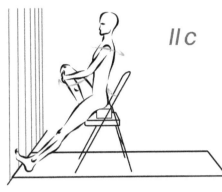
II c

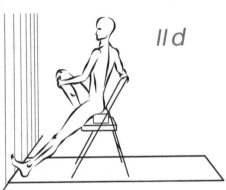
II d

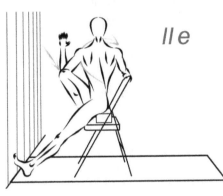
II e

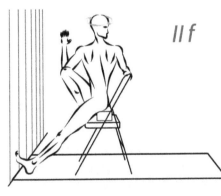
II f

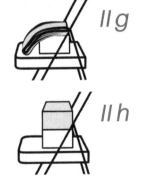
II g

II h

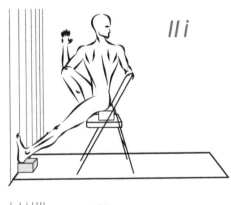
II i

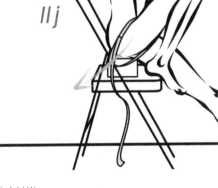
II j

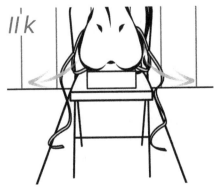
II k

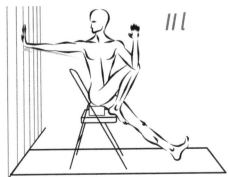
II l

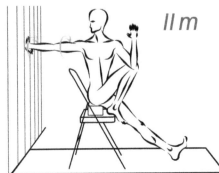
II m

Learn + Practice

After Urdhva Hastasana, once basic shoulder mobility is not challenging

Linked Poses

All Twists, Lateral Standing Poses, Salabhasana

Safety Factors

Shoulder and rib cage injuries, SI joint problems, do not practice if pregnant

Prepare

- Mat's short end to wall
- Set bolster lengthwise to left side of mat
- Have sandbag within reach
- Place folded blanket at mat's head end, *III a*

Enter

- Lie down on left side and extend left leg, pressing left foot into wall
- Bend right leg and place sole of foot on left upper inner thigh, above the knee, *III b*
- Support right leg on bolster and place sandbag on outer right thigh, *III c*
- Facing leftward, extend both arms in front of torso at shoulder level, *III d*
- Without lifting right knee or hand, move right arm through a semicircle along the floor, extending arm first overhead then opening arm and torso to the right, *III e*
- If right hand lifts off floor, wait at that stage, do not continue semicircle
- Keeping right thigh against bolster, turn head and torso naturally as arm passes through overhead range, *III f*

Sustain

- Push left foot to wall, away from back pelvis
- Release right thigh into bolster
- Widen and deepen both inner groins
- Soften abdomen, and lengthen side torso
- Further extend arm before moving to next degree in semicircle
- Keep right palm flat on floor, turning palm upward only once necessary
- Move through range very slowly, possibly not even going through full range

Exit

- From wherever arm is in semicircle with relative ease, gradually reverse arm movement and return to lying on the left side, *III g*
- Repeat movement to capacity 3-5 times
- Push weight off of right thigh and move bolster out from under leg
- Bend left leg and press hands into floor, coming to seated
- *Prepare* and repeat to the second side

Challenge

1. Right thigh lifts, or sandbag is unavailable
2. Right groin binds
3. Right arm bends or lifts
4. Numbness or tingling in right arm or hand

Response

1. Increase thigh support. Press left hand against outer right thigh. Go through movement much more slowly, at least 10 breaths per degree so that right thigh does not lift.
2. Support inner upper right thigh with block, pressing femur away from mid line. Loop strap across inner groin and have a partner gently press foot against outer thigh while pulling upward on strap, *III h.*
3. Move more slowly through semicircle. Support hand on block. Do not complete full range; return to starting position once limit is reached.
4. *See Response 3.* Widen inner humerus away from mid line. Make movement a little quicker (5-10 breaths per degree) and return to difficult ranges once shoulder releases.

This variation of Marichyasana C is also known as Alexander Twist from the Alexander movement technique. It is excellent for increasing shoulder mobility and freeing lateral and cross-lateral fascial chains, especially when practiced slowly for the connective tissue layers to release.

Contact Points

Outer left leg and hip, right inner thigh, back of left arm, shoulder girdle, head

External Supports

Wall, bolster, sandbag
Blanket, additional blocks, strap, assistant

Essence of Form

Leg extension, leg flexion, arm extension, spinal twist; leg rotated slightly internally, arms neutral to slightly external

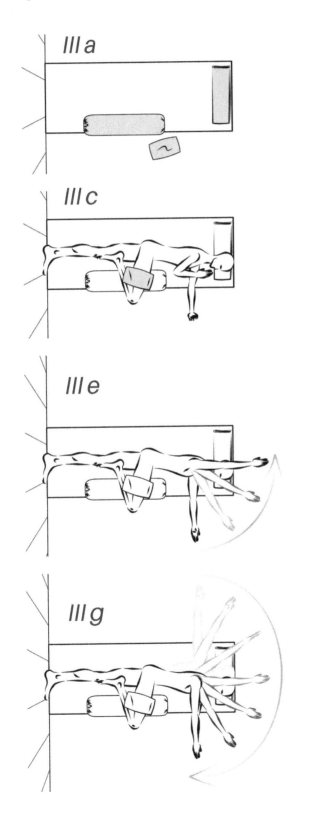

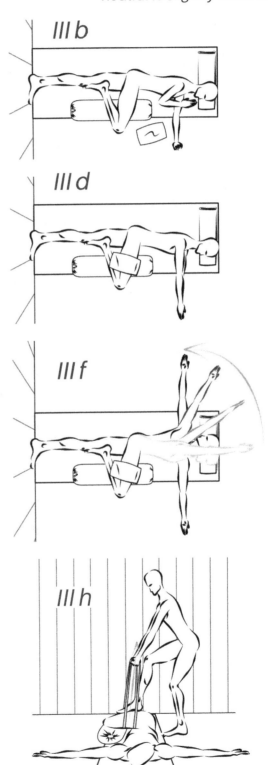

Sage Marichy's Third Pose — Nourish 213

Marichyasana C
Sage Marichy's Third Pose

Synthesize

Learn + Practice

*Once Simplify, Explore +
Nourish are not problematic,
before intermediate Twists*

Linked Poses

Paschima Namaskara,
Paschima Baddhanguliyasana,
Salamba Sarvangasana

Safety Factors

*Collarbone, shoulder, or elbow
injury; lower back or SI joint pain*

Prepare

· Place bolster lengthwise on mat

Enter

· Sit on bolster's end in *Dandasana*
· Descending left femur, bend
right leg and place right foot on
floor, thumbs at knee pit, *IV a*
· Sliding thumbs downward,
bifurcate right calf and
completely fold right leg,
bringing right heel as close to
sitting bone as possible, *IV b*
· Holding right leg with left hand,
place right hand on bolster
12-18" behind pelvis, *IV c*
· Lean back on right hand,
drawing L4 + L5 inward
· Inhaling, lift left arm to *Urdhva
Hastasana*, lengthening
from hips to armpits, *IV d*
· Exhaling, soften spinal and
abdominal muscles
· With abdomen soft, lift and
turn left side torso past mid
line toward right leg, *IV e*
· Keeping left torso length, brace
outer left elbow against outer
right thigh, forearm vertical, *IV f*
· Maintaining twist, lift from
lower lumbars and gradually
bring torso upright, *IV g*

Sustain

· All actions similar to *Explore*,
but without chair
· Resist left arm against right
thigh, broadening chest and
drawing left side ribs to the right
· Repeat *Enter* cycle: lean
back, lengthen, soften, twist,
maintain twist, lift torso upright
· Soften abdominal contents and
unfold from interior layers to
surface layers, without force
· If left armpit passes right thigh,
swiftly internally rotate left arm,
wrapping around right leg, *IV h*
· Bring right arm behind back,
catching right wrist with left
hand and press right hand
into upper left femur, *IV i*

Exit

· If wrapping, release right
hand to bolster
· Lean torso back with
weight on right hand
· Inhaling, untwist and then
bring torso upright
· Exhaling, extend right
leg to *Dandasana*
· Repeat to the second side
· Gradually reduce sitting
height as capacity to maintain
neutral lumbar increases

Challenge

1. Left leg hyperextends
2. SI joint discomfort
3. Groins bind, restricted
   lower abdominal breath
4. Limited twist capacity

Response

1. Support left calf and resist tibia
   upward, *IV j*. If neutral lumbar
   is maintained, reduce height.
2. Reduce overall twist and
   turn from thoracic spine,
   keeping lumbar spine neutral.
   Keeping left leg stable, allow
   pelvis to turn with twist
3. Open left leg 45° from mid
   line, widening groins and
   lower abdomen, *IV k*.
4. Within twist, resist in a counter-
   twisting action. Emphasize
   counter-twist where twist is
   easier, and initiate twist from
   where restriction is felt. *Prepare +
   Enter* with chair to the right, chair
   lip against right outer thigh. Hold
   chair seat's back with left hand
   and push chair lip with right hand,
   IV l. See also Explore, Response 5.

🕉 *For additional ways to work,
see also Marichyasana A
and Bharadvajasana A*

Marichyasana C compresses the abdomen asymmetrically and shifts abdominal contents laterally, which may massage the abdominal organs and increase circulation to them. When wrapping, use care that the spine is twisting to full capacity and the thigh does not force the shoulder forward.

Contact Points

Sitting bones, back of left leg, right foot, back hand
Outer arm, outer thigh, wrists

External Supports

Mat, bolster
Blankets, blocks, chair

Essence of Form

As for Explore; elbows flexed, arms posteriorly extended and internally rotated in wrap

IVa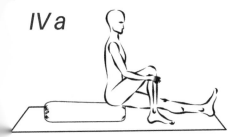

IVb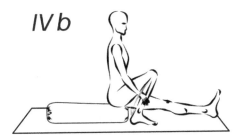

IVc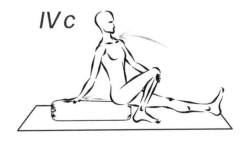

IVd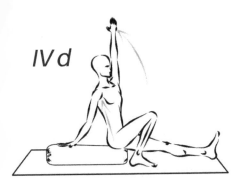

IVe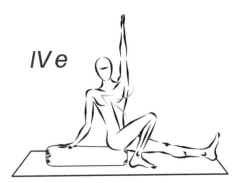

IVf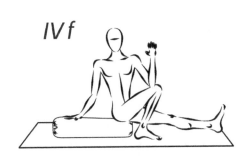

IVg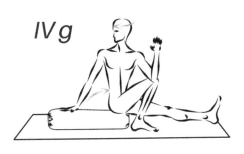

IVh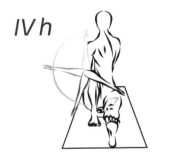

IVi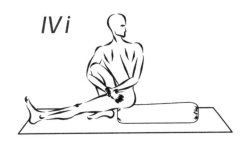

IVj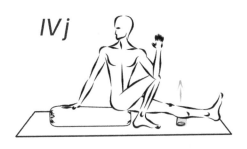

IVk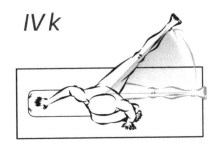

IVl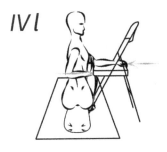

Prepare

- Set chair on mat, away from wall
- Have a block within reach

Enter

- Sit on chair, right side facing chair back, *I a*
- Bend legs, feet hip-width apart, tibias vertical
- If knees are above pelvis, raise pelvis on folded blankets, bringing knees to or below hip joints
- Place block between lower femurs and hold symmetrically, resisting heels laterally, *I b*
- Gather front iliums and soften pubis in and up
- Inhaling, lengthen torso from hips to armpits
- Keeping torso length, exhale, softening spinal and abdominal muscles
- With torso long and spinal muscles soft, turn torso toward chair back, also on exhalation, *I c*
- Hold chair back with left hand, palm facing inward
- Press right hand into chair back, palm facing outward, *I d*
- Keep head neutral, chin in line with sternum

Sustain

- Pressing into big toe mounds, equalize pressure against block
- Continue *Enter* instruction sequence: inhaling, lengthen torso; exhaling, soften spinal and abdominal muscles
- From this length and softness, exhale to twist
- Initiate twist from as low in the pelvis as possible, progressively moving twist up spine
- While twisting, push right hand into chair back and turn right side torso backward, *I e*
- Pull slightly with left hand lifting left side torso forward, around central axis, *I f*
- Descend both elbows, releasing trapezius
- Drawing thoracic spine inward, lift and broaden chest

Exit

- Stabilize feet, legs, and pelvis
- Keeping spinal length, release arm actions
- Inhaling, untwist and return torso to neutral
- Remove block and turn around in chair, left side pelvis toward chair back
- Repeat, twisting to the left

Challenge

1. Legs and pelvis turn with torso
2. Lumbar and SI joint instability
3. Front ribs protrude
4. Upper back rounds and chest collapses

Response

1. Do not let legs collapse toward the right, *I g*, but allow some front-to-back shift, *I h*. Holding block symmetrically, increase right big toe mound and left outer foot pressure.
2. *See Response 1.* If chair seat slopes down from front to back, raise right sitting bone on folded blanket to level pelvis, *I i*. Hug greater trochanters medially, generating pelvic lift. Draw right side of sacrum forward and inward.
3. Soften front ribs inward and ascend back ribs both before and during twist.
4. Draw elbows in, toward side torso and resist them slightly backward. Move bottom shoulder blades forward, lifting chest. *See also Explore, Response 3*— sitting sideways or through chair.

The early variations of Bharadvajasana are among the first spinal Twists learned. Sitting in a chair helps ensure the sacrum does not tip backward as the torso twists. In this variation, thoracic mobility is emphasized as the pelvis and lumbar spine remain relatively stable.

Contact Points

Feet, sitting bones, hands

External Supports

Mat, chair, block
Blanket

Essence of Form

Leg and hip flexion, spinal twist, push/pull arm action; legs in neutral rotation, arms slightly external

Ia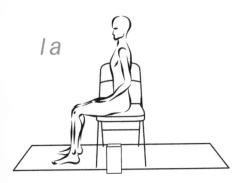

Ib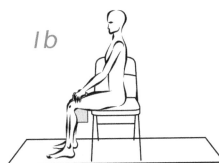

Ic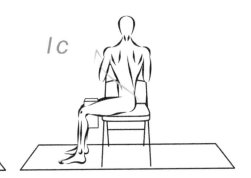

Id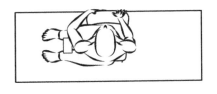

Ie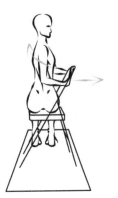

If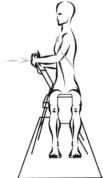

Ig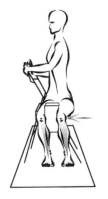

Ih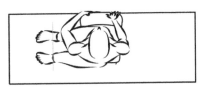

Ii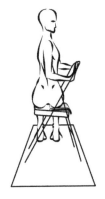

Bharadvajasana A
Twist of Nourishment and Strength

Explore

Learn + Practice

Once twisting capacity is established in Simplify; before introducing binds in any Twist

Linked Poses

Marichyasana C, Utkatasana, Pashasana, Binding Twists, Paschima Namaskara

Safety Factors

Lower back strain, neck and shoulder injury; practice Response 2 if pregnant

Prepare

- As for *Simplify*, use backless chair and elevate seat with blankets if necessary

Enter

- Step legs through chair and sit facing chair back
- Place feet and legs as for *Simplify*, holding block between knees, *ll a*
- Engage leg, pelvis, and torso actions from *Simplify*
- Lift upper sacrum, L4 + L5 in toward front body
- With the abdomen soft, turn belly rightward
- Reach left hand around chair back and place right hand on chair seat behind pelvis, *ll b*
- Pushing right hand into chair seat, further lift right side torso
- Holding length, draw left hand leftward, carrying left side torso to the right, *ll c*
- As twist deepens, walk right hand along chair seat to left back corner, *ll d*
- Keeping head level, turn head rightward, *ll e*
- Once torso twists beyond 90°, reach right hand behind torso to catch chair frame, *ll f*

Sustain

- Equalize foot pressure and hold block symmetrically
- Balance both sitting bones on chair seat
- Without untwisting pelvis, lengthen right inner femur away from right groin, *ll g*
- As right femur lengthens forward, draw left inner groin back, away from block, *ll h*
- Draw head of right humerus backward while broadening shoulder blades
- Soften right front ribs inward and ascend left back ribs
- Let twist develop gradually from softness and without force

Exit

- Stabilizing feet, exhale to release arm actions
- Inhaling, return torso to neutral
- Rest for a few breaths in neutral
- Repeat, turning to the left with left hand to chair seat and right hand holding chair back

🕉 *Can also be done with short hold repetitions, swinging arms to catch chair as torso twists around axis on exhalations*

Challenge

1. Pelvic instability
2. Pelvic space narrows
3. Neck pain, thoracic and shoulder restriction

Response

1. Wedge blanket and/or block between pelvis and chair frame, stabilizing greater trochanters, *ll i*.
2. Straddle chair, shifting pelvis slightly leftward. Brace left inner femur against chair frame, with right femur perpendicular to left leg, *ll j*. While twisting, widen groin space, articulating left hip over left femur, *ll k*.
3. Practice with shoulder jacket, have a partner pull downward while twisting, *ll l-m*. Prepare + Enter with chair sideways, an arm's distance from wall. Extend arm laterally, pressing palm into wall, fingertips upward, *ll n*. Turn chair at 45° increments as capacity increases until back pelvis faces the wall and torso turns 90° or more, *ll o-p*. Gradually externally rotate upper arm until fingertips point backward, *ll q*.

haradvajasana through the chair emphasizes symmetrical torso length while twisting and creates
pinal suppleness by releasing unnecessary tension, increases hip and shoulder mobility, and
ones the abdominal organs. This variation is also a great back release after deep Back Bends.

Contact Points

eet, knees, sitting bones, hands

External Supports

Backless chair, block
Blanket, block, strap, wall

Essence of Form

As for Simplify + posterior
shoulder extension; legs neutral,
arms external (internal in II f)

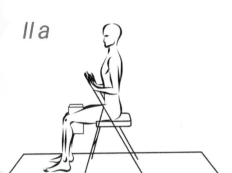
II a

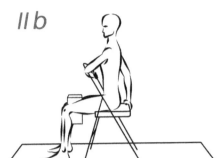
II b

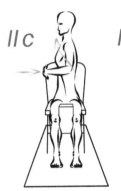
II c

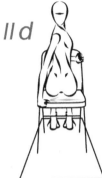
II d

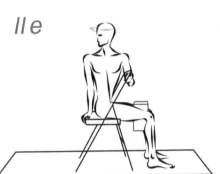
II e

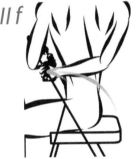
II f

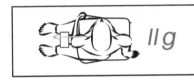
II g

II h

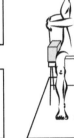
II i

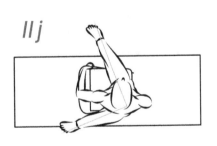
II j

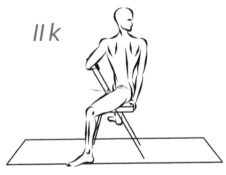
II k

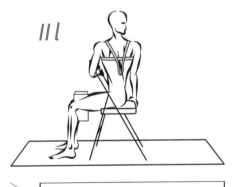
II l

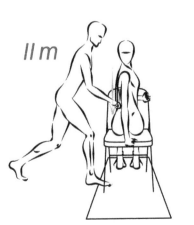
II m

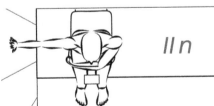
II n

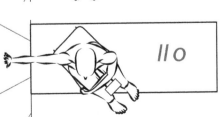
II o

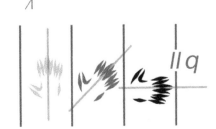
II p

II q

Learn + Practice

Once torso twists with ease in Explore; after Standing Poses and active practice phase

Linked Poses

Bharadvajasana B, Uttana Balasana, Matsyendrasana, Pashasana, Supta Virasana

Safety Factors

As for Simplify + Explore, use care with neck injury; do not practice with abdominal cysts

Prepare

- Mat's short end to wall
- Set bolster lengthwise on mat, 1.5-2' from wall
- Place blocks against wall on their sides, about 1' apart, *III a*
- Set blocks higher for wider pelvis, lower for narrower pelvis

Enter

- Sit between bolster and blocks, left side torso toward wall, *III b*
- Lean to the right and bend both legs, toward the wall, *III c*
- Pressing into hands, lift and shift right outer hip toward wall, underneath torso
- Place right heel against block
- Rest left foot and tibia across blocks, top of foot and tibia against wall, *III d*
- Place hands on either side of bolster, *III e*
- Lifting torso, soften spinal and abdominal muscles
- Extending left femur, turn torso away from wall toward bolster
- Lengthening front body, exhale and lower torso over bolster, resting hands and elbows, *III f*

☸ *As necessary, lift torso, lengthen further, and lower over bolster*

Sustain

- Press right heel gently into block
- Extending left femur, lightly contact left tibia against wall
- Widen greater trochanters, resisting right outer femur into floor, left outer femur toward ceiling
- Gather front iliums, soften pubis skin inward
- Roll left ilium gently toward floor
- Soften abdomen and receive bolster into abdomen and front torso
- Draw right front ribs gently away from bolster
- Roll left side torso toward bolster
- Once shoulder girdle is parallel to floor, turn head toward right shoulder, *III g*
- To deepen further, angle torso and bolster rightward, extending left groin, *III h*

Exit

- Keeping torso position, draw left leg forward, stacking it above right leg, *III i*
- Place hands under shoulders
- Pressing into hands, inhale to lift torso to seated, *III j*
- Repeat to the left, resetting bolster if angled in *III h*

Challenge

1. Knee pain
2. Groin compression, pelvic floor narrows
3. Lumbar discomfort
4. Shoulder tension, neck pain

Response

1. Pad left knee with blanket or mat remnant. Avoid turning foot upward, which torques the knee. Do not let femurs collapse inward, *see Response 2.*
2. Blocks at wall help keep pelvic floor broad — raise block height. Support inner left femur with additional block and resist right femur into floor. Have an assistant loop a strap at left inner groin and pull upward while bracing greater trochanter with foot as for *Marichyasana C, Nourish.*
3. Increase right heel pressure and tuck outer right buttock toward wall. Gather front iliums. Reduce overall twist and turn from throacic spine.
4. Ensure bolster fully supports torso. Raise chest and/or forehead on folded blanket. Keep head neutral. Rest arms forward and to the sides.

A Restorative variation of Bharadvajasana, lying forward over a bolster helps the abdomen and spinal muscles release. Pressure from the bolster also shifts the breath toward the back body and may facilitate a deeper relaxation response. Sequence after the active phase of practice.

Contact Points

Feet, inner tibia, outer leg and hip, front torso, forearms

External Supports

Wall, 2 blocks, bolster Blanket, mat remnant, extra blocks, strap, assistant

Essence of Form

Knee flexion, hip flexion (bottom leg), hip extension (top leg), torso extension and rotation; arms and legs neutrally rotated

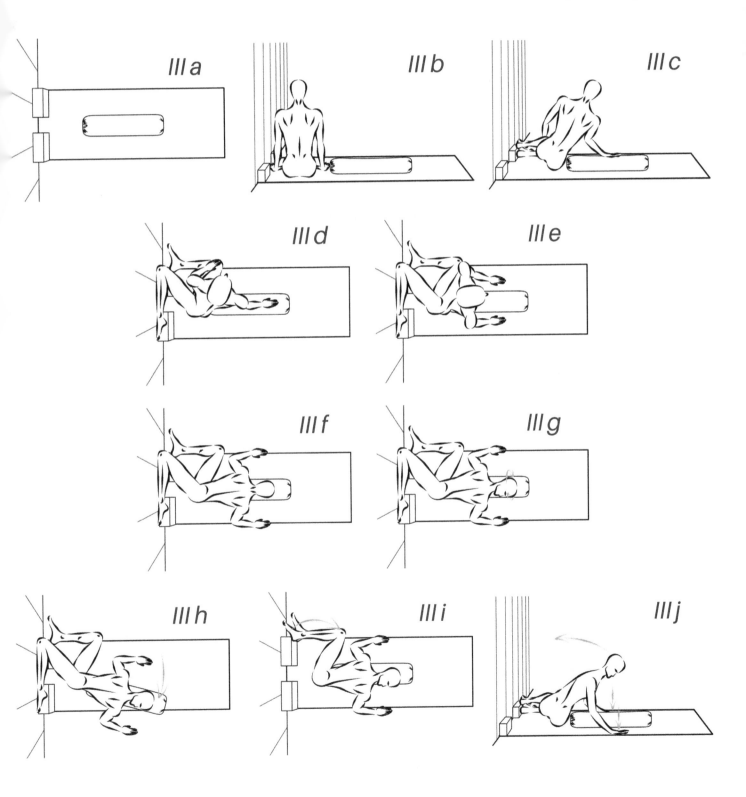

Bharadvajasana A
Twist of Nourishment and Strength

Synthesize

Learn + Practice

After Nourish + Virasana; once bent leg thigh descends fully in Janu Sirsasana

Linked Poses

Virasana, Janu Sirsasana, Bharadvajasana B, Matsyendrasana, Pashasana

Safety Factors

As for Simplify + Explore; use caution with knee or ankle injury, eye strain, and loose stools

Prepare

- Place bolster lengthwise on mat

Enter

- Sit in *Dandasana* on bolster's end, *IV a*
- Bend right leg, bifurcating calf, and bring right foot under left thigh beside left hip, *IV b-c*
- Lean rightward and fold left leg as well, *IV d*
- With left leg completely folded, bring foot beside left hip, top of foot across right arch, *IV e*
- Keep femurs parallel to mid line
- Descend left sitting bone, bringing torso upright
- Place right hand behind pelvis on bolster and lean torso backward, inhaling to lift and lengthen spine, *IV f*
- Keeping torso length, soften abdomen and bring back of left hand against outer right leg, *IV g*
- Initiating from base of pelvis, resist left hand into right thigh and turn torso to the right, *IV h*
- Without untwisting, draw L4 + L5 inward to bring torso upright, sliding left outer hand toward lower right femur, *IV i*
- Keeping head neutral, turn head to the right

Sustain

- Spread toes and draw outer ankles inward
- Gathering front iliums soften pubis skin inward
- Without narrowing inner groins, draw greater trochanters toward each other, lifting pelvis
- Keeping pelvic height, soften left buttock and descend left sitting bone
- Lengthen left side torso from hip to armpit, *IV j*
- Draw left shoulder blade forward as left hand resists backward into right thigh
- As left back ribs lift and broaden, recede right front ribs inward
- Initiating from lower lumbars, and without pushing ribs out, draw thoracic spine in, lifting chest
- Broaden bottom back ribs
- To deepen twist, repeat *Enter* steps: lean backward on right hand, lengthen, soften, turn, and come upright
- Once shoulder girdle turns beyond 90°, reach right hand behind back, catching left forearm if possible, *IV k*
- Continually soften abdominal muscles and release tension behind abdominal wall

🕉 *Can also be practiced beside wall, turning toward it with hands pressing into wall, IV l*

Exit

- Leaning back on right hand, inhale to untwist
- Place left hand behind pelvis on bolster and lean back equally on both hands
- Keeping left leg folded completely, lift left leg through mid line and extend to *Dandasana*
- Extending left leg, bring right leg to *Dandasana* also
- Repeat to the second side
- Reduce pelvic support as capacity to keep pelvis level increases, using blocks if necessary

Challenge

1. Torso shifts rightward and ribs protrude

Response

1. Increase pelvic support. Descend left sitting bone. Avoid leaning to the right, especially before and during transitions. Ascending left bottom back ribs, soften right ribs inward

This classical variation of Bharadvajasana introduces asymmetrical rotations in the legs, which directs the Twist lower down into the pelvis. This variation may have a stimulative effect on the digestive organs, so use caution if digestion is already overactive.

Contact Points

Feet, outer thigh and leg, top of foot, hands

External Supports

Mat, bolster
Blanket, blocks, wall

Essence of Form

Knee and hip flexion, torso extension and rotation; bottom leg externally rotated, top leg internal, arms external, back arm internal in IV k

IV a
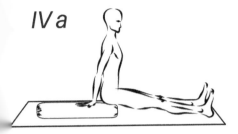

IV b
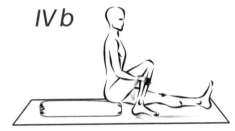

IV c
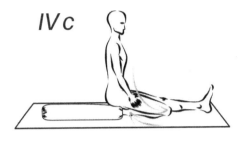

IV d
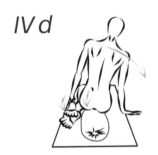

IV e
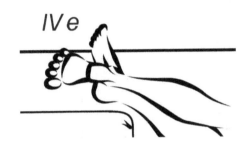

IV f
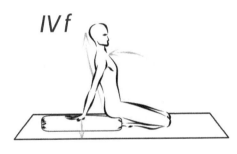

IV g
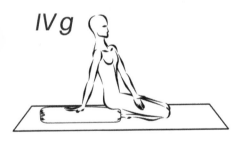

IV h
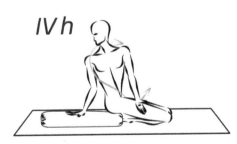

IV i
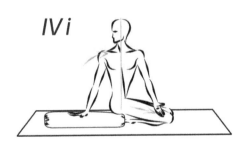

IV j
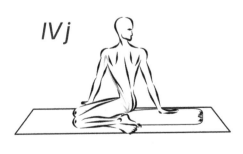

IV k
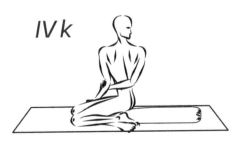

IV l
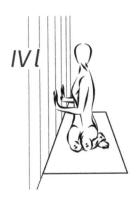

Salabhasana
Locust Pose

Simplify

Learn + Practice

Learn as an introduction to Back Bends; whenever lumbar stability is required

Linked Poses

Urdhva Mukha Svanasana, Chaturanga Dandasana

Safety Factors

Lower back strain; do not practice during pregnancy, or with pelvic/abdominal cysts

Prepare

· Set mat away from obstructions

Enter

· Lie down prone, feet hip-width apart or with big toes touching
· Rest head on backs of hands, elbows to the sides, *I a*, or rest forehead on a blanket
· Spreading toes, press tops of feet to the floor
· Lengthening the legs, internally rotate from the top thighs, rolling outer thighs downward
· Keeping internal rotation, make equal floor contact with pubis and front iliums
· Gather front iliums and resist heels laterally
· Anchoring right foot, lengthen through left leg and lift 2-3″ from floor, *I b*
· Contact front iliums as equally as possible as left leg lifts
· Hold leg lift for 5-10 breaths
· Continuing to lengthen, exhale and lower left leg, toes landing beyond right foot, *I c*
· Repeat, anchoring left foot and lifting right leg
· Once legs lift with minimal pelvic twist, lift both legs, keeping length and internal rotation, *I d*

Sustain

· Soften front ribs inward, away from floor
· Continually gather front iliums, resist heels laterally, and soften pubis inward
· Draw front groins in, away from floor
· Release upper buttocks away from top pelvis, *I e*
· Firm lower buttocks, *I f*
· Engaging upper hamstrings, lift legs from upper femurs without bending at the knees
· Spreading toes, continuously lengthen legs away from back pelvis
· Raise inner thighs higher than outer thighs
· Without tucking, extend sacrum toward heels

Exit

· Do 3-5 repetitions each side
· Place hands under shoulders
· Exhaling, press hands into floor, lifting torso, *I g*
· On the following exhalation, lift thighs back to *Adho Mukha Svanasana*, *I h* or stand up and do *Wall Push*, *I i*
· If finished back bending, rest in *Uttana Balasana*

Challenge

1. Legs bend while lifting
2. Legs externally rotate
3. Lumbar pain

Response

1. Fully engage quadriceps, lifting knees away from floor before leg lifts. Maintain front thigh engagement throughout. Reduce leg lift and increase lengthening action.
2. Widen inner back thighs before lifting legs, *I j*. Decrease overall lift, but lift from upper hamstrings and lower buttocks, rather than squeezing external rotators.
3. *Prepare + Enter* with torso raised on folded blankets, reducing back bend, *I k*. Observe throaco-lumbar asymmetry when lifting both legs: spinal musculature is less voluminous on less active side. To engage muscles on less active side, lift opposite leg until more activated. When lifting both legs, increase length and lift through that leg. Gradually reduce asymmetrical lift as spinal muscles become more equally balanced.

Salabhasana strengthens the lumbar spine and SI joints in preparation for deeper Back Bends, and is a stabilizer for Forward Bends and Twists. Its toning effects may help minimize lower back pain due to weakness. Lifting the legs in isolation and one at a time helps balance the spinal muscles.

Contact Points

Pubis, front iliums, sternum, hands, forearms, forehead

External Supports

Mat
Wall, blankets

Essence of Form

Leg extension, hip extension, torso extension; legs internally rotated, arms neutral

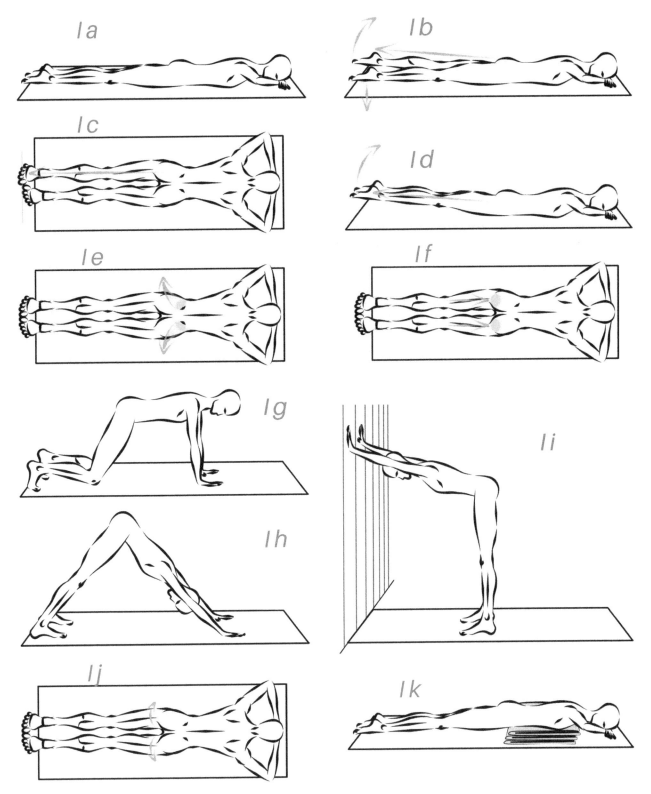

Learn + Practice

After Simplify and Urdhva Hastasana, before Back Bends with overhead arm extension

Linked Poses

Virabhadrasana A + C, Tadasana Urdhva Hastasana, Viparita Dandasana, Urdhva Dhanurasana

Safety Factors

As for Simplify; neck and shoulder strain, hypertension

Prepare

- As for *Simplify*, with 2 blocks within reach

Enter

- Lie down prone as for *Simplify*
- Without lifting legs, engage leg and pelvis actions from *Simplify*
- Rest forehead on floor, not turning head
- Extend arms laterally at shoulder-level, *II a*
- Lengthening from bottom shoulder blades to little fingers, externally rotate upper arms, *II b*
- Without lifting head, further lengthen arms and lift them 2-3" away from floor, *II c*
- Progressively increase external arm rotation before lifting until palms face upward, *II d*
- Once arms lift with ease, set blocks under outer wrists, *II e-f*
- Keep feet and legs anchored, lift arms further by lifting head and torso, *II g*
- Practice also with arms in Y position, *II h*, and extended directly forward, *II i* — first without blocks, then with blocks
- Begin with arms in a reasonable external rotation, and gradually increase

Sustain

- Without lifting legs, maintain leg and pelvis actions from *Simplify*
- Spreading toes, press toenails into floor, drawing outer ankles inward
- Extend and lift arms from as low in the back body as possible
- Maximize length from armpits to little fingers
- Descend outer armpits and draw humerus heads upward
- Lengthen inner shoulder blades toward back pelvis, and gather bottom shoulder blades
- Extend occiput away from mid-upper back, lengthening neck

Exit

- Keeping arm length, lower arms and torso on exhalation
- Rest prone for a few breaths and repeat 3-5 times in each arm position
- Place hands under shoulders and exhaling, press to *Adho Mukha Svanasana*

- ॐ *Once arms and torso lift without pain and legs are well anchored, lift legs, arms, and torso simultaneously, II j*

Challenge

1. Elbows bend or hyperextend
2. Shoulder restriction
3. Neck pain
4. Lumbar pain

Response

1. Fully extend arms before lifting. Lift as a result of length rather than shortening arms to lift. When arms are extended forward, strap upper arms above elbows and hold block between wrists, *II k*. For hyperextension, resist elbows outward into strap, *II l*.
2. Increase external rotation before lifting. Develop shoulder mobility by elevating wrists on blocks before lifting actively
3. See *Response 2*. Keep head in line with torso. Lengthen base of skull away from mid-upper back, tucking chin slightly
4. Strap front iliums. Have an assistant anchor legs while lifting torso, *II m. See also Simplify, Response 3.*

- ॐ *See Tadasana Urdhva Hastasana for additional ways to work*

In addition to stabilizing the lower back and pelvis Salabhasana can help mitigate forward-head posture and rounding in the upper back, which often lead to neck, shoulder, and back pain. This variation utilizes various arm angles to activate different muscle chains.

Contact Points

Tops of feet, pubis, front iliums, wrists, sternum, forehead

External Supports

Mat, 2 blocks, Strap, assistant

Essence of Form

Leg + torso extension, arm extension with abduction; legs internally rotated, arms external

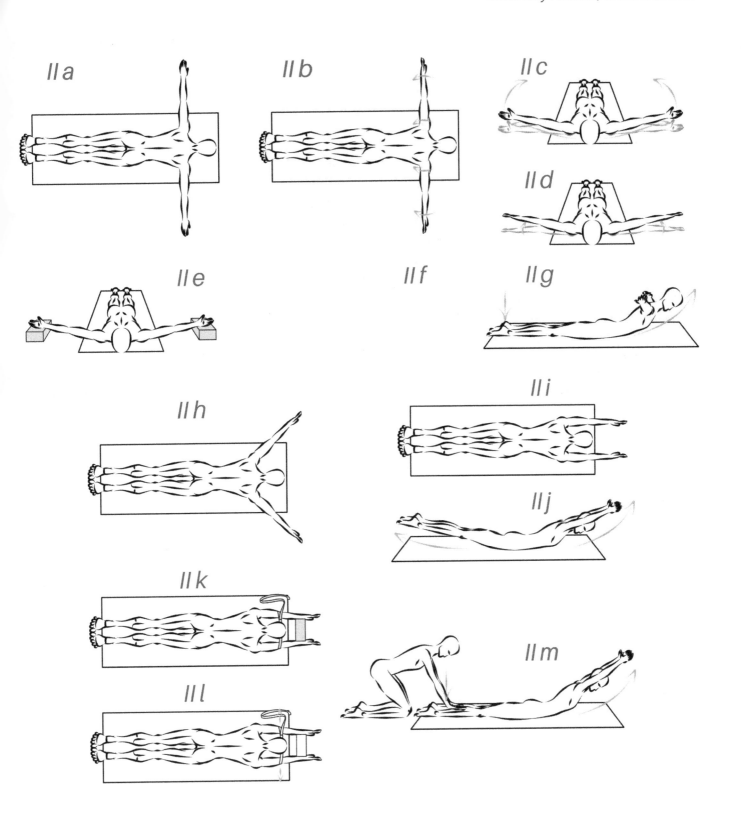

II a

II b

II c

II d

II e

II f

II g

II h

II i

II j

II k

II l

II m

Learn + Practice

After Simplify once there is some shoulder ease in Explore

Linked Poses

Bhujangasana, Urdhva Mukha Svanasana, Virabhadrasana A, Viparita Dandasana

Safety Factors

As for Simplify, neck and shoulder strain, hypertension

Prepare

- Set mat's short end to wall
- Place chair on mat, chair's back against wall

Enter

- Lie down prone in front of chair, an arm's distance from chair
- Place legs and feet as for *Simplify*, engaging leg and pelvis actions, *III a*
- Extend arms, catching chair's front legs, *III b*
- Pushing into chair legs with hands, lengthen and lift legs one at a time as for *Simplify*, *III c*
- Observe hand/arm asymmetry: one hand pushes forward, the other pulls on the chair as leg lifts, usually opposite arm to leg, *III d*
- Lower legs and balance arm action
- Repeat leg lifts, pushing both hands forward symmetrically regardless of which leg lifts, *III e*
- Once arm action is equal, maintain symmetry and lift both legs, *III f*
- Progressively walk hands up chair legs until hands rest on chair seat, *III g*

Sustain

- Continue leg and pelvis actions from *Simplify*
- Without hardening abdomen, draw front ribs in and lift back ribs away from back pelvis
- Pushing hands forward, lengthen from bottom front ribs through armpits to hands
- Lift shoulder girdle and broaden between upper shoulder blades
- Keeping space between shoulder blades, descend outer armpits toward floor, *III h*

Exit

- If lifting legs, lengthen further out of back pelvis and lower tops of feet to floor
- Pressing tops of feet down, activate spinal muscles to stabilize torso position
- With torso lifted and stable, bring hands symmetrically to floor, *III i*
- Gently lower torso, resting head on hands
- Place hands under shoulders and press back to *Adho Mukha Svanasana* on exhalation

☸ *Can also be done with hands to wall, III j*

Challenge

1. Lumbar pain
2. Shoulder restriction
3. Neck pain

Response

1. *See Responses in Simplify + Explore.* When not lifting legs or when lifting both legs, hold a block between thighs and/or strap above ankles and resist outward, *III k.* Strap upper thighs and resist outward, especially when lifting legs.
2. Within arm extension, roll outer arms and armpits downward, widening inner upper arms away from each other. Practice with hands pressing into wall, hands wider than shoulder-width and fingertips pointing outward, *III l.* Bring hands closer toward each other as restriction decreases. Once hands are shoulder-width, set hands progressively higher on wall.
3. *See Response 2. Prepare + Enter* with head supported on a block. Resist hands downward and lift upper thoracic spine. Lengthen occiput away from mid-thoracic spine. Keep ears in line with upper arm bones.

Integrating arm extension with the leg lifts can reveal imbalances in full-body muscle chains. By actively pushing the hands into a resistance such as the chair or a wall in Salabhasana, dynamic traction is created, which may help balance asymmetries with less risk.

Contact Points

Tops of feet, pubis, front iliums, palms

External Supports

Mat, chair, wall
Block, strap

Essence of Form

Leg + torso extension, arm extension; legs internally rotated, arms external

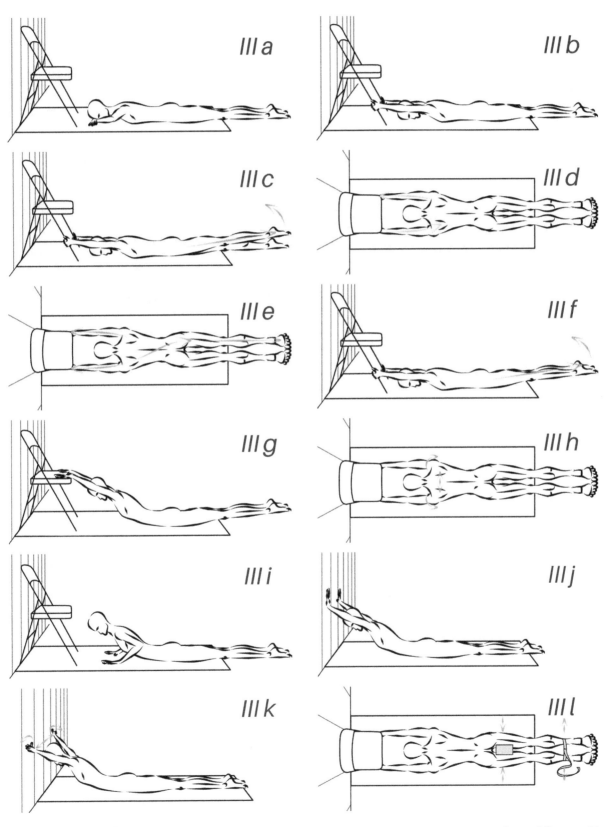

III a

III b

III c

III d

III e

III f

III g

III h

III i

III j

III k

III l

Salabhasana
Locust Pose

Learn + Practice

After Anjaneyasana; before deep Back Bends

Linked Poses

Anjaneyasana, Urdhva Mukha Svanasana, Chaturanga Dandasana

Safety Factors

As for Simplify, neck and shoulder strain, hypertension

Prepare

· Set mat's short end to wall
· Have a block within reach

Enter

· Kneel facing away from wall, with heels to wall, balls of feet against wall/floor juncture, *IV a*
· Place block between thighs
· Holding block between thighs and keeping heel contact against wall, lie down prone, resting thighs on floor with legs bent, *IV b*
· Ensure foot mid lines are parallel
· Rest forehead on crossed hands, elbows to sides
· Squeezing block between thighs, fully extend legs and press heels into wall, *IV c*
· Keeping heel pressure, lift block maximally
· Without losing heel pressure, hold block height and bend legs, lengthening groins further to lower knees to floor, *IV d*

ॐ *Once heel pressure can be maintained throughout, keep legs extended and add arm and torso variations from Explore*

Sustain

· Engage leg and pelvis actions from *Simplify*
· Sharpen inner heel pressure against wall
· Pressing big toe mounds to wall/floor juncture, broaden soles of feet
· Without externally rotating thighs, draw outer ankles inward, *IV e*
· Lift femurs away from front thighs
· Extend backs of femurs away from back pelvis, even when legs are bent
· Lift block by rolling front groins inward and extending inner groins toward heels
· Without tucking pelvis, descend sacrum further in, toward front body

Exit

· Bend legs and lower knees to floor
· Bring hands under shoulders
· Pushing into hands, lift torso
· Exhaling, roll block further backward and press to *Adho Mukha Svanasana*
· Repeat up to 5 times

Challenge

1. Heels lose wall contact
2. Outer ankle fatigue
3. Lumbar discomfort

Response

1. *Prepare + Enter* slightly closer to wall. Anchor pelvis and push heels away from back pelvis rather than pushing pelvis away from wall. Resist urge to generate push with hands. Practice leg action in *Supta Tadasana* first.
2. Extend legs from inner groins to inner heels and big toe mounds, instead of using foot and ankle action exclusively. Rest tops of feet on wall between repetitions, *IV f.*
3. Lift upper femurs before lower femurs, and lengthen groins to extend legs. Draw front iliums forward, away from upper thighs and sink sacrum more deeply into body, *IV g.* Practice *Anjaneyasana* first to lengthen inner groins. Without externally rotating legs, resist thighs laterally and minimally gather back iliums, *IV h.*

230   Salabhasana — *Synthesize*

Yoga: Point + Process | *Volume 1*

In most Back Bends, one of the more difficult actions to learn is extending the groins and keeping the back body long. Pressing the heels into a resistance provides helpful feedback in developing this action. Lifting the block both stabilizes the pelvis and activates the internal rotators.

Contact Points

Soles of feet, inner thighs, pubis, front iliums, sternum, forehead

External Supports

Mat, wall, block

Essence of Form

Groin extension, arm extension; legs internally rotated, arms external

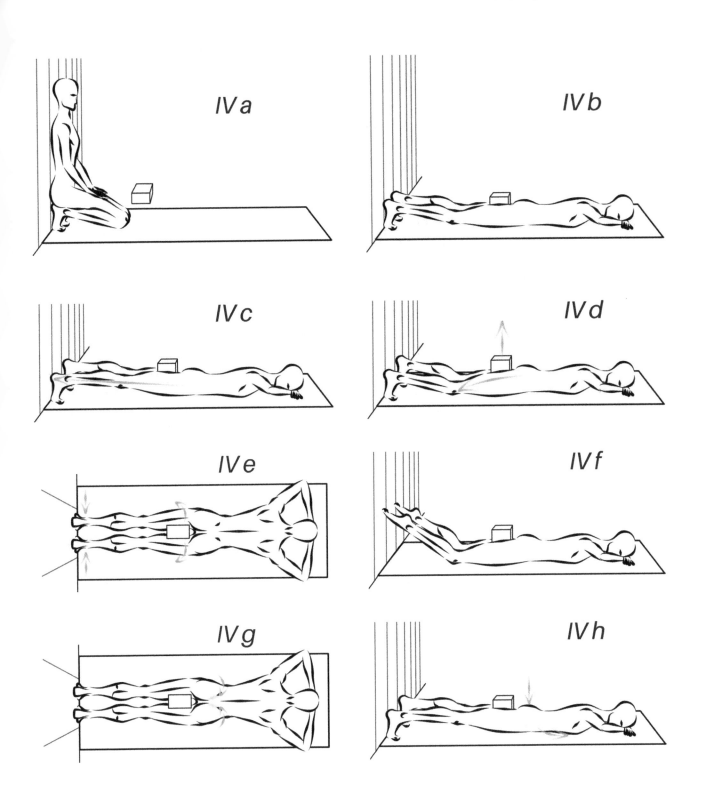

IVa

IVb

IVc

IVd

IVe

IVf

IVg

IVh

Learn + Practice

Once leg actions are learned well in Tadasana and Anjaneyasana

Linked Poses

Salabhasana, Anjaneyasana, Bhujangasana, Chaturanga Dandasana, Purvottanasana

Safety Factors

Some lower back problems; for neck injury, keep head neutral

Prepare

- Mat's short edge to wall

Enter

- Stand facing the wall in *Tadasana*, feet 3-6" from wall and hip-width apart, *l a*
- Ensure foot mid lines are parallel
- Place hands on wall at chest height, *l b*
- Push heels away from back pelvis and resist them laterally
- Press upper femurs backward
- Gather front iliums and lift them upward
- Without lifting heels and keeping femurs pressing backward, bring pelvis to wall, *l c*
- Contact the wall equally with both iliums and pubis
- Keeping wall contact, soften pubis inward and upward
- Drawing sternum gently inward, lengthen from lower sternum to upper sternum
- Without moving hands, push hands into wall and resist downward, lifting chest 3-6" away from wall, *l d*
- Draw chin down and extend back of skull upward

Sustain

- Continue *Enter* actions while increasing chest lift
- Resisting heels laterally, draw lower inner femurs medially
- Balance pressure through both heels
- Equally push upper femurs backward, observing tendency for one femur to collapse forward
- Keep length from coccyx to crown
- Draw upper thoracic spine inward and extend occipital bone upward, then slowly tilt head backward provided there is no dizziness, nausea, or neck compression

Exit

- Deepen heel pressure, extending heels away from back pelvis
- Gather front iliums
- Inhaling, lift torso upright and rest chest on wall
- Pressing hands into wall, step feet back to *Ardha Uttanasana*, *l e*
- Repeat, stepping feet slightly further away from wall as capacity increases

Challenge

1. Lumbar compression
2. Inner knee pain
3. Legs externally rotate
4. Chest collapses backward

Response

1. Strap front iliums toward each other, compressed side toward more stable ilium, *l f*. Without moving, think of drawing the back iliums toward each other. *See Responses 3 and 4.*
2. Internally rotate from the top thighs, not the knees. Without lifting big toe mounds, descend outer heels, lifting inner ankles and arches.
3. Bend legs slightly. Bring hands to posterior thighs and manually draw inner back thighs outward, *l g*. Keeping back femur width, re-straighten legs. Continue only as far as rotation is retained.
4. With pubis resting on wall, interlock fingers behind back. Extend arms downward, *l h*. Lift upper thoracic spine up and forward. Visualize a shelf across bottom shoulder blades and tilt chest up and over this imaginary shelf.

One of the first Back Bends learned in early classes, Urdhva Mukha Svanasana strengthens the spine, wrists, and arms. The classical pose may be too demanding, however, if these areas are vulnerable. Standing with the support of a wall is an accessible introduction.

Contact Points

Feet, pelvis, hands

External Supports

Mat, wall
Strap

Essence of Form

Leg and torso extension, elbow flexion; legs internally rotated, arms slightly external

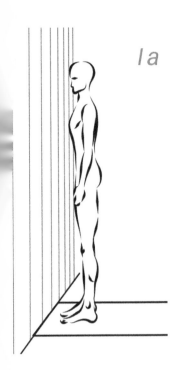
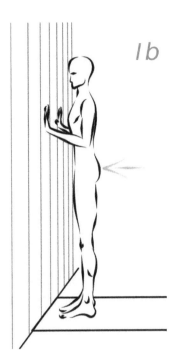
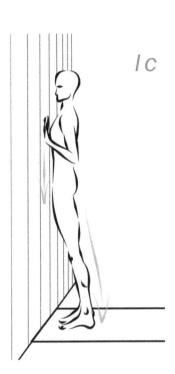
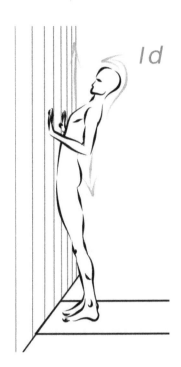

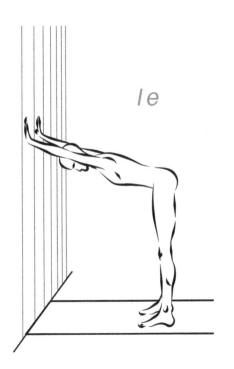
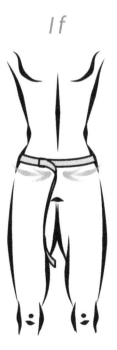
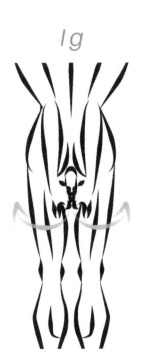
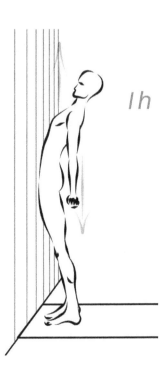

Urdhva Mukha Svanasana
Upward-Facing Dog Pose

Learn + Practice

Once stability is learned in
Phalakasana; after chest
and groin opening

Linked Poses

Anjaneyasana, Phalakasana,
Purvottanasana, Viparita
Dandasana

Safety Factors

Lumbar instability, wrist
injury, shoulder injury

Prepare

· Mat's short edge against wall
· Set chair on mat, slightly less
  than one leg's length from
  wall, seat facing outward

Enter

· Stand in front of chair
· Place hands on floor, *II a*
· Step feet back through
  chair back, *II b*
· Slide backward, bringing
  heels to wall and pubis to
  back of chair seat, *II c*
· Rest torso on chair seat
· Bring hands to sides of chair lip,
  fingers to sides, thumbs forward
· With elbows bent, hug
  elbows inward and lift torso
  slightly off chair seat, *II d*
· Extend legs, pushing heels into
  wall and away from back pelvis
· Resist heels laterally
· Draw front iliums
  toward each other
· Soften pubis inward and
  lift it away from wall
· Without tucking, extend
  back pelvis toward heels
· Pressing hands into chair
  seat, lengthen torso forward
  and lift chest, straightening
  arms on inhalation, *II e*

Sustain

· Keep stabilizing actions
  from *Enter*
· Press outer heels firmly into wall
· Keeping outer heel pressure,
  increase and balance
  inner heel pressure
· Without rotating knees inward,
  widen upper inner back femurs
· Use chair back to guide
  back pelvis toward wall,
  softening sacrum inward
· Keeping heel contact,
  pull hands back to move
  thoracic spine forward
· Pressing into inner hands,
  externally rotate upper
  arms, broadening distance
  between armpits
· Descend inner shoulder blades
  and ascend upper chest

Exit

· Exhaling, lower torso
  to chair seat, *II f*
· Bring hands to floor and walk
  them forward, sliding forward until
  thighs clear the chair seat, *II g*
· Step feet to floor one at a time, *II h*
· Pressing hands to thighs,
  inhale to standing, *II i*

Challenge

1. Heels lift from wall
2. Lumbar compression
3. Chair back interferes
   with pelvic action
4. Front groin pain

Response

1. Slide pelvis and/or chair closer
   to wall. Emphasize leg extension
   from back pelvis to heels. Lift
   upper femurs into back thighs
   to increase heel pressure.
2. Draw thoracic spine forward
   before lifting torso. Resist
   hands backward as chest lifts
   up and forward. Extend back
   pelvis toward wall and lift front
   iliums. Soften sacrum inward.
3. If possible, slide pelvis further
   back through chair while
   Entering. Prepare with chair's
   front legs on blocks, tilting chair.
   If necessary, use backless chair.
4. Pad chair seat with blanket. Use
   pubis as fulcrum, not groins.
   Soften groins away from chair
   pressure. Extend the backs of
   legs more fully than the fronts.
   Prepare + Enter with chair closer
   to wall so that support is on
   upper femurs rather than groins.

234   Urdhva Mukha Svanasana — *Explore*

Yoga: Point + Process | *Volume 1*

nce the essential leg, arm, and torso actions are established with the wall, more of the torso's
eight can be shifted into the arms. Supporting the pelvis on a chair while extending the
eels to a wall helps teach the pelvis to descend as the femurs lift while Back Bending.

Contact Points

eet, pelvis, hands

External Supports

Mat, chair, wall

Essence of Form

Leg, hip, and torso extension,
arm extension; legs internally
rotated, arms external

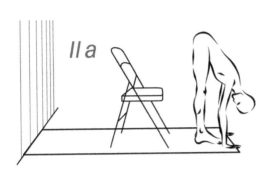

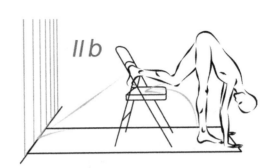

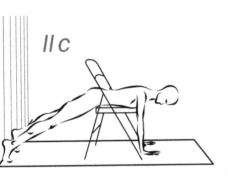

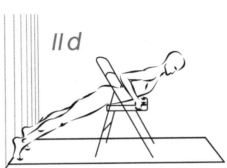

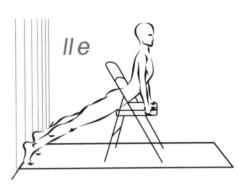

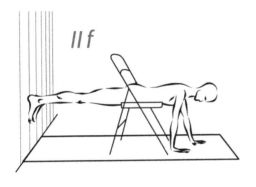

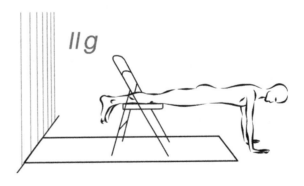

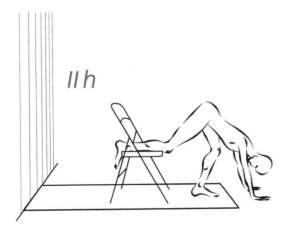

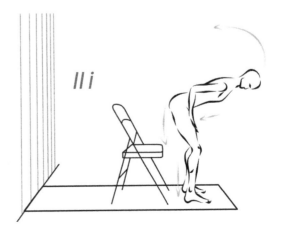

Learn + Practice

After Explore; once leg actions are clear in Phalakasana and Anjaneyasana

Linked Poses

Anjaneyasana, Chaturanga Dandasana, Purvottanasana, Viparita Dandasana

Safety Factors

Groin tear; wrist, shoulder, or lower back injury

Prepare

- Mat's short edge to wall
- Set bolster laterally, $^2/_3$ - $^3/_4$ legs' length from wall to support thighs
- Place blocks 8 - 12" from bolster

Enter

- Kneel between wall and bolster, *III a*
- Walk hands forward onto blocks, *III b*
- Bring balls of feet into wall/floor juncture
- Lifting knees off floor, rest thighs on bolster, elbows bent, *III c*
- Press heels into wall away from back pelvis
- Internally rotate thighs until thigh rotation is neutral
- Gather front iliums and keeping pressure through heels into wall, resist heels laterally
- Soften pubis inward, drawing front iliums forward, away from wall
- Glide sacrum into back pelvis
- Pressing into index finger mounds, lift chest up and forward, straightening arms *III d*
- Stack shoulders vertically above wrists

Sustain

- Maintain leg and pelvis actions from *Simplify + Explore*
- Increase inner heel pressure and draw outer ankles inward
- With continuous heel pressure, alternate resting thighs on bolster and lifting them away from it
- When lifting thighs off bolster, initiate from upper femurs
- Keep thigh and heel actions symmetrical
- Broaden back ribcage
- Move thoracic spine into body
- Descend inner shoulder blades
- Roll armpit chest forward and upward
- Soften sternum inward, lift back of sternum upward

Exit

- Exhaling, lower thighs to bolster and knees to floor, *III e*
- Keeping an upright spine, sit back on the heels
- Press into hands and exhaling, lift thighs up and back to *Adho Mukha Svanasana*, *III f*, before repeating
- Repeat 3-6 times
- Once familiar, lift directly to *Adho Mukha Svanasana* without resting

Challenge

1. Wrist pain
2. Elbow hyperextension
3. Shoulders elevate or roll forward
4. Thighs do no reach bolster

Response

1. Turn hands outward with thumbs pointing forward, *III g*. Distribute weight forward through all bones of the hands and fingers, reducing heel pressure. Broaden palms and narrow forearms, lifting forearms out of wrist joints. Roll up mat's front end and angle blocks downward, *III h*. Move hands (and blocks) slightly forward and engage legs more fully, bringing more weight toward thighs and heels.
2. Without bending elbows, resist forearms laterally outward. Balance internal forearm rotation with external upper arm rotation.
3. Lift front armpits (armpit-chest) more fully. Circularly roll front shoulder skin over top shoulders, drawing back armpits forward, *III i*.
4. Raise bolster height with blocks or blankets, *III j-k*. This also reduces back bend degree.

In addition to its strengthening effects, Urdhva Mukha Svanasana may also build lung capacity, tone abdominal organs, and reduce minor depression as physical resilience develops. In this variation, the thighs remain lightly supported as an additional anchor to extend the torso.

Contact Points

Hands, thighs, feet

External Supports

Mat, 2 blocks, bolster, wall
Blankets, rolled mat,
additional blocks

Essence of Form

Leg, hip, and torso extension,
arm extension; legs internally
rotated, arms external

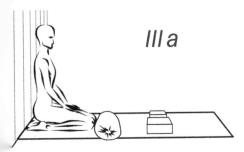
III a

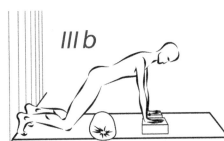
III b

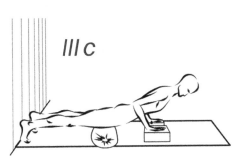
III c

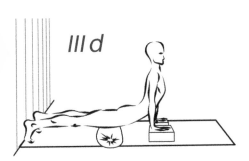
III d

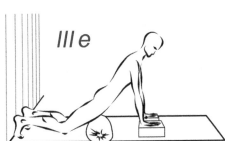
III e

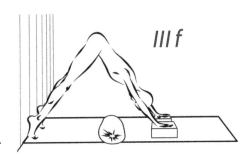
III f

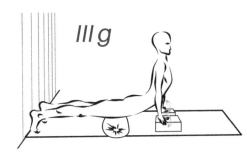
III g

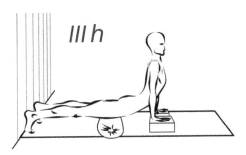
III h

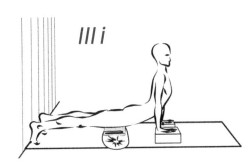
III i

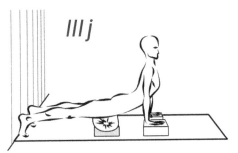
III j

Urdhva Mukha Svanasana
Upward-Facing Dog Pose

Learn + Practice

After Simplify, Explore, + Nourish;
after Chaturanga Dandasana

Linked Poses

Anjaneyasana, Phalakasana,
Chaturanga Dandasana,
Purvottanasana

Safety Factors

Omit Chaturanga Dandasana
for rotator cuff injury, shoulder
tendinitis, elbow injuries

Prepare

· Mat's short edge to wall

Enter

· Lie on belly with legs extended
  and press heels to wall
· Place hands under armpits,
  elbows bent, *IV a*
· Pushing hands into floor and
  heels against wall, exhale
  and lift to *Phalakasana, IV b*
· Ensure pelvis is neutral
· Keeping extension from heels to
  crown and without collapsing
  shoulders, bend elbows 90° to
  Chaturanga Dandasana, IV c
· Reach chest beyond wrists,
  descending no lower
  than elbow height
· Glide tail bone into pelvis and lift
  front iliums away from heels/wall
· Inhaling, press into index
  finger mounds, lifting armpit-
  chest to extend arms, *IV d*
· Without dropping femurs,
  press heels back and
  draw thoracic spine in and
  forward to lift upper chest

🕉 *If Chaturanga Dandasana is
contraindicated, descend pelvis
directly from Phalakasana*

Sustain

· Pressing index finger
  mounds into floor, lift armpit-
  chest away from hands
· Lengthen down from outer
  upper arm to outer heel of hand
· Soften throat and ascend
  occipital bone
· Release jaw muscles
  and soften face
· Broadening collarbones,
  ascend outer collarbones and
  roll front collarbones upward
· Initiating from mid-thoracic
  spine, keep cervical spine
  long and tilt head backward

Exit

· Hold for 5-15 breaths
· Maintain heel/wall contact
· Press into index finger mounds,
  exhale and lift to *Adho
  Mukha Svanasana, IV e*
· From *Adho Mukha Svanasana*:
  inhale *Phalakasana*, exhale
  Chaturanga Dandasana, inhale
  Urdhva Mukha Svanasana, exhale
  again to *Adho Mukha Svanasana*
  and repeat cycle 3-10 times
· When finished, step or
  jump to *Uttanasana*,
  continuing to *Tadasana*

Challenge

1. Heel contact is lost
   during transitions
2. Lumbar pain
3. Shoulders round in
   Chaturanga Dandasana
4. Neck strain

Response

1. Use heel action to initiate
   movements, rather than as
   an afterthought. Practice
   Anjaneyasana variations with
   heels to wall more often.
2. Widen inner back femurs
   and resist heels laterally. Lift
   front iliums more fully before
   transitioning to *Urdhva Mukha
   Svanasana*. Practice away
   from wall with tops of feet on
   floor, descending the tail bone
   to create spinal traction while
   resisting femurs upward, *IV f.*
3. Tie a belt above elbows. Lift
   chest forward, beyond strap
   into *Chaturanga Dandasana,
   IV g*. Or, place blocks in front
   of hands. When lowering,
   stay 1" above blocks, *IV h.*
4. Do not take head back. Draw
   chin in and down. Lengthening
   occiput out of shoulder girdle,
   ascend the crown, *IV i.*

rdhva Mukha Svanasana appears in Surya Namaskara and Vinyasa flow transitions of many
oga styles. Pressing the heels into a wall helps stabilize the pelvis and emphasize the leg
ork when learning this movement pattern before incorporating them into a flow practice.

Contact Points

Hands, feet

External Supports

Wall
Blocks, strap

Essence of Form

Leg, hip, and torso extension, arm extension; legs in mild internal rotation, upper arms external, forearms internal

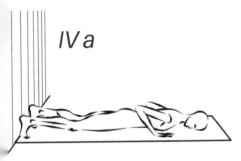

IVa

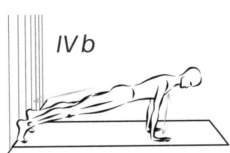

IVb

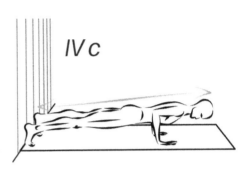

IVc

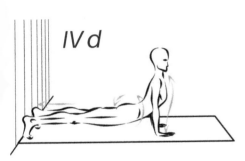

IVd

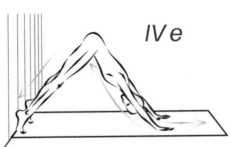

IVe

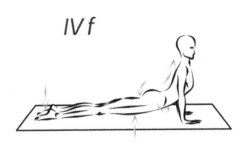

IVf

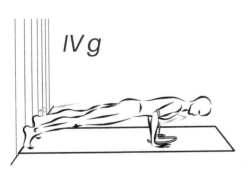

IVg

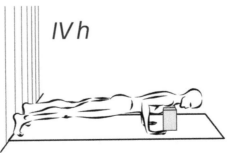

IVh

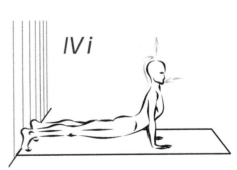

IVi

Phalakasana
Plank Pose

Learn + Practice

Before Back Bends, Inversions + Arm Balances; once legs and pelvis are stable in Tadasana

Linked Poses

Tadasana, Anjaneyasana, Chaturanga Dandasana, Adho Mukha Vrksasana, Sirsasana

Safety Factors

Lower back strain, wrist or shoulder injury

Prepare

- Place mat's short end to wall
- Set block beside mat, within reach

Enter

- Kneel on mat near wall, facing away from it *l a*
- Hold block between upper thighs and walk hands forward to lie down prone
- Bring heels to wall, balls of feet at wall/floor juncture, *l b*
- Place hands directly under shoulders, thumbs at armpit level, *l c*
- Have wrist creases parallel to mat's front edge
- Spread fingertips and press index finger and thumb mounds deeply into floor
- With heels pushing into wall, press down through hands and lift to all fours position on exhalation, *l d*
- Stabilizing hands, squeeze block between thighs
- Push heels into wall and lift knees off floor, *l e*
- Fully extend legs, pushing from heels to crown
- Bring all major joints into a single line, *l f*

Sustain

- Pushing feet away from back pelvis, equalize pressure through all four corners of each foot
- Extending legs, squeeze block and lift inner thighs higher than outer thighs
- Gather front iliums and resist heels laterally
- Softening pubis inward, draw iliums forward
- Without untucking pelvis, lift femurs maximally
- Extend from outer chest to index finger mounds and broaden across palms
- Widen between shoulder blades, lifting back ribs upward
- Draw bottom shoulder blade tips toward front body
- Release unnecessary abdominal tension

Exit

- Pressing heels into wall, bend legs and lower knees to floor
- Lower to prone and rest, press back to kneeling, or press to *Adho Mukha Svanasana, l g*
- Repeat up to 10 times, holding only as long as thighs and pelvis do not collapse

Challenge

1. Thighs and pelvis collapse
2. Pelvis lifts and untucks
3. Shoulder or wrist pain

Response

1. Increase heel pressure and review *Supta Tadasana* leg actions. Support thighs on blocks and bolster (add blanket for additional height if necessary), and lift thighs by extending heels away from back pelvis, *l h*.
2. Without descending thighs, draw front iliums forward and sink sacrum more deeply toward front body. Practice *Anjaneyasana* (which is essentially a one legged plank) to lengthen the groins.
3. Elevate hands on blocks, with a rolled mat under heel end of blocks to decrease wrist flexion, *l i*. Externally rotate arms so that middle fingers point out to the sides, *l j*. Reduce gravitational load by practicing with hands on chair or wall, *l k-l*, first externally rotating arms, then gradually internally rotating forearms. *See also Synthesize, Response 3.*

Phalakasana creates balanced trunk stability in both front and back body, making Back Bends and Inversions safer. It also establishes leg and arm connection, develops shoulder stability, and opens the chest. Also a substitute when Chaturanga Dandasana is contraindicated.

Contact Points

Hands, feet, Heels

External Supports

*Mat, block, wall
Rolled mat, additional blocks, bolster, chair*

Essence of Form

Leg and arm extension, wrist flexion, trunk stability; legs in neutral rotation, arms neutral to slightly external

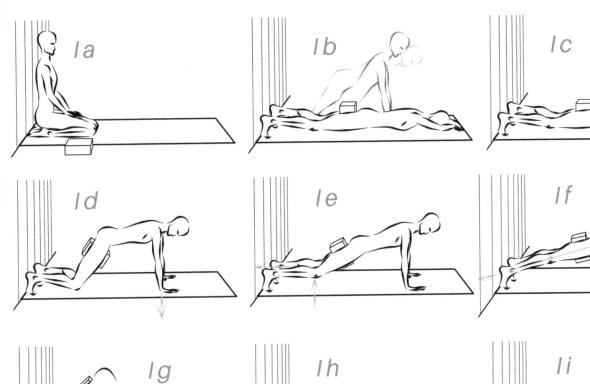

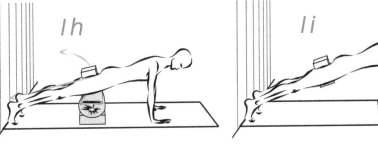

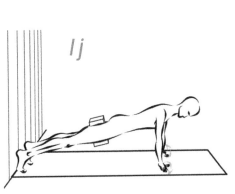

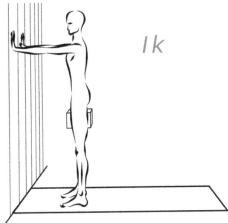

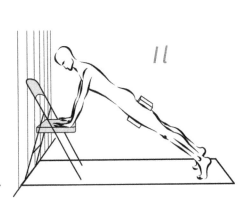

Learn + Practice

Once stability is learned in Simplify; before full Chaturanga Dandasana

Linked Poses

Salamba Sarvangasana, Bakasana, Bhekasana, Pincha Mayurasana, Sirsasana

Safety Factors

Wrist, elbow, or shoulder injury; lumbar instability

Prepare

· Set chair on mat against wall
· Have a strap within reach

Enter

· Stand facing chair, tying strap around upper thighs just below greater trochanters, *ll a*
· Folding forward, place hands on chair and bring shoulders directly above wrists, *ll b*
· Learn first with hands turned out to sides, thumbs on chair seat, *ll c*
· Internally rotate forearms and turn fingertips forward as capacity allows, *ll d*
· Step feet back, fully extending legs and torso in *Phalakasana*, *ll e*
· Gathering front iliums, resist heels laterally and widen greater trochanters into strap
· Reaching back through heels, stabilize legs
· Away from heel extension, lift chest forward
· Further lifting chest and without losing leg action, bend elbows to 90°, hugging them close to side ribs, *ll f*
· Keep heads of humeri drawing back as elbows bend

Sustain

· Engage actions from *Simplify*
· Pushing heels away from back pelvis, press femurs into strap pressure at back thighs
· Lift and broaden bottom back ribs away from back pelvis
· Lengthen side torso from pelvis to armpits
· Extend inner elbows backward, away from armpits and extend collarbones forward
· Draw outer bottom shoulder blades forward
· Soften throat and descend chin slightly
· Keep back of neck long, extending occiput away from mid-upper back

Exit

· Maintain leg and pelvis actions
· Pushing hands into chair seat, straighten arms to *Phalakasana* on inhalation
· Exhaling, press thighs back to *Adho Mukha Svanasana*, *ll g*
· Alternatively, maintain leg and pelvis position, lifting chest to *Urdhva Mukha Svanasana* on inhalation, followed by *Adho Mukha Svanasana* on exhalation, *ll g*

Challenge

1. Wrist compression
2. Elbow pain
3. Shoulders round forward

Response

1. Maintain hand position from *ll c*. Extend legs more fully and utilize leg action to reduce arm and wrist pressure. *See also Synthesize, Response 3.*
2. Externally rotate arms as in *ll c*. Equalize pressure through inner and outer hand. Broaden palms and narrow the forearms.
3. Lift chest before bending elbows. Resist shoulders back and draw upper humeri backward while lowering. Maintain backward action throughout. Tie a strap around the lower humeri, just above the elbows, holding them shoulder-width apart, *ll h*. Lift chest over and beyond strap when lowering. Resist hands backward, lengthening inner arms from elbows to collarbones. Widen the shoulder blades and draw the bottom shoulder blades forward into back ribs.

haturanga Dandasana builds strength in the arms, shoulders, and upper torso. In order to not verload the arms, however, especially when repeating often in Vinyasa-style practices, the legs ust be integrated into the pose. Using a chair emphasizes this, minimizing load on the arms.

Contact Points

eet, hands

External Supports

Mat, chair, strap, wall
Additional strap

Essence of Form

Wrist and elbow flexion, leg and torso extension; legs internally rotated, arms neutral to external

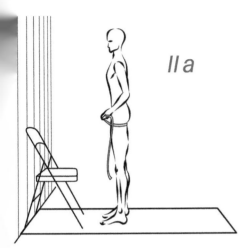
II a

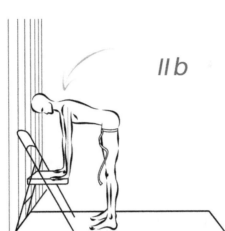
II b

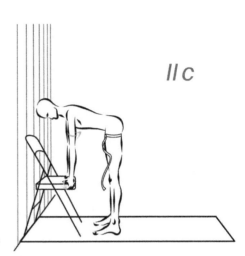
II c

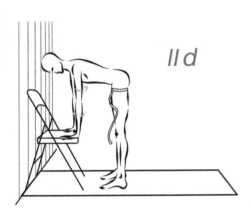
II d

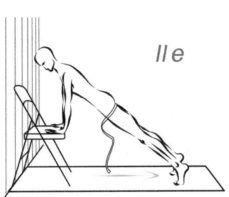
II e

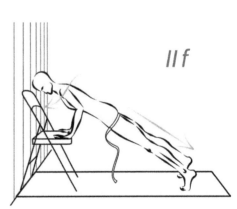
II f

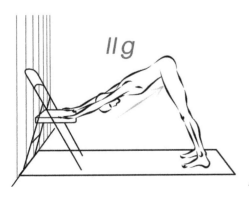
II g

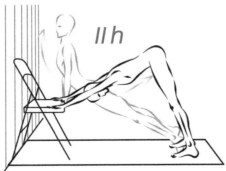
II h

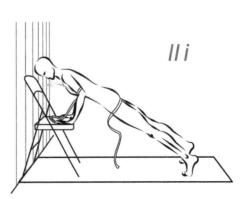
II i

Chaturanga Dandasana
Martial Plank Pose

Learn + Practice

Once leg actions are clear in Simplify + Explore; before full Vinyasa transitions

Linked Poses

Salamba Sarvangasana, Mayurasana, Sirsasana B, Arm Balances

Safety Factors

Do not practice with shoulder, elbow, wrist, or neck injury; some lower back injuries

Prepare

- Mat's short edge to wall
- Set bolster lengthwise, 2/3 - 3/4 legs' length from wall to support torso, *III a*
- Have strap within reach, looped at shoulder-width

Enter

- Kneel between wall and bolster, *III b*
- Place loop around upper humeri, at or just below humeral heads, *III c*
- Tighten strap so that humeral heads are pushed inward with buckle at mid-sternum
- Walk forward on hands to rest chest and pelvis on bolster, throat and head free, *III d*
- Press heels into wall away from back pelvis, balls of feet at wall/floor juncture, *III e*
- Engage leg and pelvis actions from *Simplify + Explore*
- Bring hands below elbows, bending them 90°
- Resist humeri laterally into strap and hug elbows inward
- With heels pushing into wall, increase index finger mound pressure into floor and lift torso slightly off bolster, *III f*

Sustain

- Maintain leg and pelvis *Sustain* actions from *Simplify + Explore*
- Increase inner heel pressure and draw outer ankles inward
- Maximize length from heels to sternum
- Keeping heel pressure, drag hands backward to engage triceps and lift chest, *III g*
- Move thoracic spine into body
- Resisting humeri laterally into strap, extend sternum forward
- Widen upper shoulder blades and extend inner shoulder blades toward pelvis
- Lengthen occiput away from mid-thoracic spine, extending back of neck, *III h*
- Soften throat and release jaw

Exit

- Hold 5-10 breaths and lower torso to bolster
- Repeat up to 10 times
- Lower knees to floor and press to all fours
- Sit back on the heels with spine erect
- When finished, remove strap and press hands to floor, lifting thighs to *Adho Mukha Svanasana*, *III i*

Challenge

1. Wrist pain
2. Shoulders elevate or roll forward
3. Pelvis untucks and buttocks lift

Response

1. Ensure wrists are directly below elbows. Turn hands outward with thumbs pointing forward, *III j*. Distribute weight forward through all bones of the hands and fingers, reducing heel of hand pressure. Decrease wrist flexion by supporting heels of hands with folded strap or rolled mat, *III k*. Using bolster support, press hands down into floor while lifting forearms out of wrists.
2. Lift front armpits (armpit-chest) more fully. Circularly roll front shoulder skin over top shoulders, drawing back armpits forward, *III l*.
3. Review *Tadasana* actions. Keeping heel pressure, resist heels laterally and lift front iliums forward before lifting off bolster. Draw sacrum inward as thighs and torso lift. Initiate lift from pressing humeri laterally into strap. Lift torso as one piece; ribcage and pelvis.

Often, Chaturanga Dandasana is entered by descending from Phalakasana, which can lead to collapse. By supporting the torso from underneath, keeping a feeling of lift away from the floor can be learned before practicing unsupported versions.

Contact Points

Hands, front torso, feet

External Supports

Mat, bolster, strap, wall
Additional straps or rolled mat

Essence of Form

Wrist and elbow flexion, leg and torso extension; legs slightly internally rotated, arms neutral

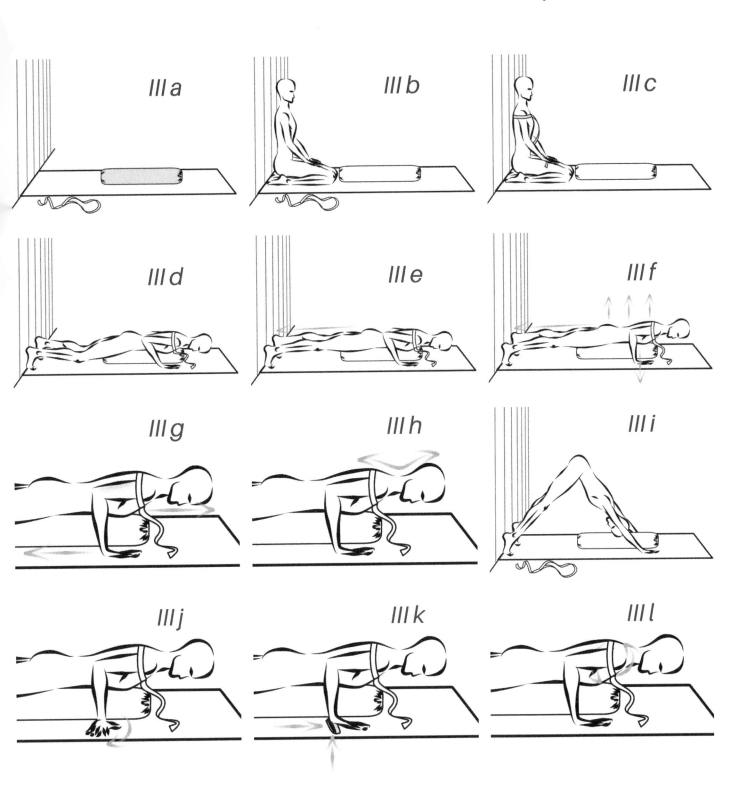

III a
III b
III c
III d
III e
III f
III g
III h
III i
III j
III k
III l

Chaturanga Dandasana
Martial Plank Pose

Synthesize

Learn + Practice

Before full Surya Namaskar and transitions that include Chaturanga Dandasana

Linked Poses

Salamba Sarvangasana, Mayurasana, Sirsasana B, Arm Balances

Safety Factors

Do not practice with shoulder, elbow, wrist, or neck injury; some lower back injuries

Prepare

· Mat's short edge to wall

Enter

· Lie on belly with heels to wall, legs extended
· Place hands under armpits, elbows bent, *IV a*
· Pressing hands to floor and heels to wall, exhale and extend arms fully, pushing to *Phalakasana, IV b*
· Engage leg and pelvis actions as *Simplify, Explore + Nourish*
· Lengthen inner arms form armpit-chest to index finger mounds
· Without losing heel or index finger mound pressure, drag hands backward to lift chest
· Keeping length from heels to crown and without collapsing thighs or shoulders, bend elbows 90° to *Chaturanga Dandasana, IV c*
· Extend chest beyond wrists, descending no lower than elbow height
· Glide tail bone into pelvis and lift front iliums away from heels/wall
· Keep head neutral with back of neck long

Sustain

· Maintain *Sustain* actions from *Simplify, Explore + Nourish*
· Pushing through legs, soften mid and upper abdomen to any degree possible
· Continually deepen index finger mound pressure
· Lengthen inner elbows away from armpits
· Soften lower sternum inward, lengthening back sternum from bottom to top
· Release jaw and soften face

Exit

· Hold for 5-15 breaths
· Maintain heel/wall contact
· Pressing into index finger mounds, inhale and lift chest to *Urdhva Mukha Svanasana, IV d*
· Keeping index finger mound pressure, exhale and press thighs back to *Adho Mukha Svanasana, IV e*
· Repeat entire cycle up to 10 times
· Step or jump to *Uttanasana*, continuing to *Tadasana* or next pose in practice sequence

ॐ *Include this cycle in Vinyasa-style practices*

Challenge

1. Heel contact lost during transitions
2. Shoulders round in *Chaturanga Dandasana*
3. Wrist or elbow pain, index finger mounds lift

Response

1. Initiate heel action before each movement. Set hands slightly further back, not more than 1". Practice lunges with heels to wall
2. *See Explore, Response 3.* Place blocks in front of hands. Lower 1" above blocks *IV f.* Roll front shoulder skin over the top shoulder and draw back armpits toward armpit-chest
3. Turn hands out up to 45° and hug elbows inward. Distribute weight more evenly forward through fingers to take strain off wrists. To strengthen underside of forearms, stand in *Tadasana* 1.5-2' from wall, *IV g.* Lean forward, placing hands to wall at elbow-height, elbows bent 90°, *IV h.* Keeping elbow angle, flick wrists to push away from wall, *IV i.* Repeat 20-30 times

Once Chaturanga Dandasana's structure is clear, keeping the heels against a wall helps maintain leg integration, which is often the first aspect lost when transitioning through the pose. Although this pose strengthens the upper body, it is helpful to think of it as a legs pose.

Contact Points	External Supports	Essence of Form
Hands, feet	Wall Blocks	Elbow and wrist flexion, leg and torso extension; legs in neutral rotation, arms slightly external

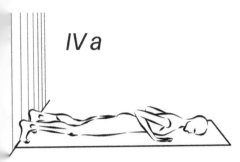

IVa

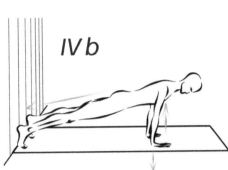

IVb

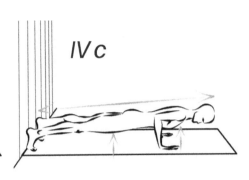

IVc

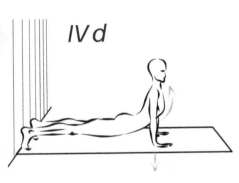

IVd

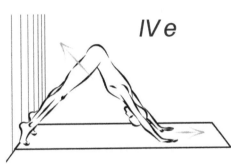

IVe

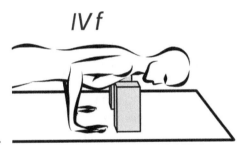

IVf

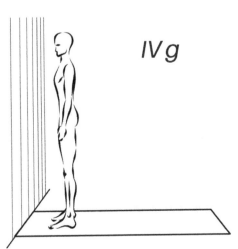

IVg

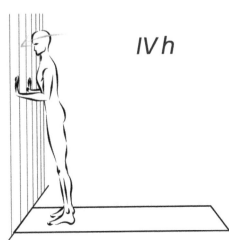

IVh

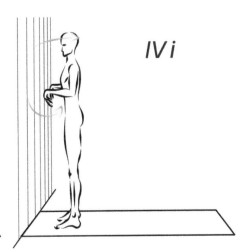

IVi

Purvottanasana
Intense Front-Body Stretch

Simplify

Learn + Practice

Learn before deep Back Bends, use to gradually introduce shoulder openers

Linked Poses

Salamba Sarvangasana, Paschima Namaskara, Paschima Baddhangullyasana

Safety Factors

Shoulder injury, bicep tear, collarbone injury
Use care when rehabilitating

Prepare

- Mat's short end against wall
- Set chair on mat, 8-12"
  from wall, *Ia*

Enter

- Sit at back of chair seat, legs and feet hip width apart, feet flat on floor, *Ib*
- Anchor all four corners of feet into floor
- Without moving legs, resist heels laterally
- Equally settle both sitting bones
- Gathering front iliums, soften pubis inward
- Keeping pelvis neutral, contact bottom back ribs against chair's backrest
- Maintaining back rib contact, extend collarbones up, away from back ribs, *Ic*
- Bring arms behind backrest, arms extended
- Internally rotate arms, palms facing wall, *Id*
- Without collapsing chest or losing back rib contact, raise hands to wall, hands shoulder-width apart, *Ie*
- Keep the head neutral, chin and gaze level to floor

Sustain

- Maintain leg and pelvis actions from *Enter*
- Continue internally rotating upper arms, increasing pressure through index finer mounds, spreading fingertips
- Pressing index finger mounds into wall, lengthen inner arms by lifting armpit-chest away from wall
- With the front armpits lifting broaden armpits away from each other
- Descend inner shoulder blades, widening between bottom shoulder blades
- As capacity increases, press into feet and tilt chair backward, *If*
- Walk hands down wall
- Keeping wall contact through hands and lifting chest, lower chair legs to floor, *Ig*

Exit

- Keeping chest lift, release hands from wall
- Pressing hands to thighs and feet to floor, inhale to standing
- Repeat with chair set further away from wall, as capacity allows, *Ih*

Challenge

1. Hands slide down wall
2. Collarbones roll downward as arms lift
3. Shoulder impingement

Response

1. Bring chair closer to wall and move hands further apart. Move chair further from wall and tip chair as in *If-h*. Change pressure from downward to backward as hands press into wall. Chalk hands to prevent slip.
2. Set chair closer to wall and retain collarbone lift while raising arms. If collarbones still collapse, stand with back against wall. Bring hands alongside upper thighs and press palms into wall, lifting collarbones and broadening chest. Gradually move away from wall, *Ii-k*.
3. In *Tadasana*, hold strap behind legs, hands wider than shoulder-width, *Il*. Resist laterally and raise strap symmetrically to capacity and lower back down, *Im*. Repeat 10-30 times. Gradually reduce hand distance, *In*.

In preparation for the posterior shoulder extension of Purvottanasana, Ustrasana, Sarvangasana, and many other poses, this variation increases that range of motion while also teaching the arms to push actively. It is excellent for minimizing upper back fatigue and neck strain.

Contact Points	External Supports	Essence of Form
Feet, sitting bones, hands	Mat, chair, wall Blocks, strap	Posterior arm extension; legs neutrally rotated, arms internal

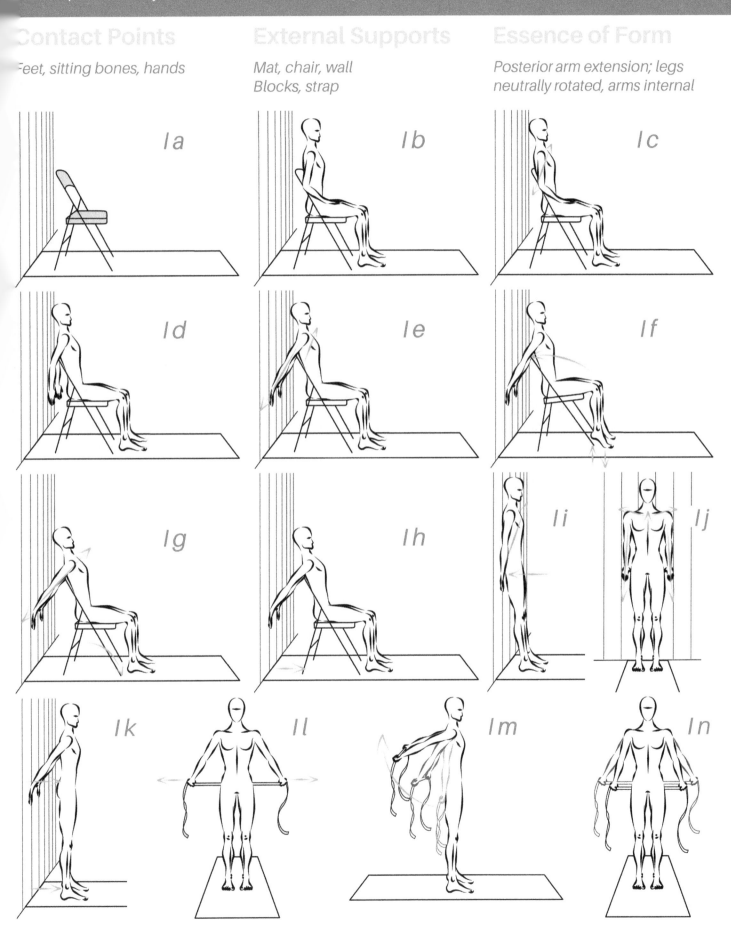

Purvottanasana
Intense Front-Body Stretch

Explore

Learn + Practice

Before unsupported variations of Purvottanasana; as a preparation for Sarvangasana

Linked Poses

Salamba Sarvangasana, Paschima Namaskara, Ustrasana

Safety Factors

Lumbar instability; wrist, elbow, shoulder, or neck injury

Prepare

- Mat's short end against wall
- Set chair against wall, seat facing outward

Enter

- Sit on front edge of chair seat, *ll a*
- Place feet 6-8" forward of knees
- Have thighs and foot mid lines parallel
- Bring hands to chair seat sides, *ll b*
- Pressing hands into chair seat, lift pelvis forward off chair, *ll c*
- Fully extend arms if they are bent
- Walk feet forward until legs extend fully, *ll d*
- Roll big toe mounds downward and press them into floor, then resist heels laterally
- Gather front iliums and soften pubis inward
- Pressing into big toe mounds, press hands downward and backward against chair, lifting chest and pelvis, *ll e*
- Bring shoulders atop wrists, arms vertical, *ll f*
- Keep head neutral, in line with torso, or tuck chin toward chest

Sustain

- Continuously extend legs from back pelvis to big toe mounds
- Deepening big toe mound pressure, internally rotate thighs from upper femurs
- Maintain *Enter* actions in legs and pelvis
- Keeping pelvic height, descend femurs away from front thighs, *ll g*
- Soften and deepen inner groins
- Descending femurs, soften front ribs inward and extend sternum from bottom to top, *ll h*
- Widen across chest, away from sternum, *ll i*
- Slide jaw inward and backward, lengthening occiput away from mid-thoracic spine
- Keeping neck length, draw mid-and upper thoracic spine inward, then carefully tilt head backward if capacity allows, *ll j*

Exit

- Hold for 10-15 breaths
- Exhaling, lower pelvis and sit back on chair
- Repeat up to 5 times

Challenge

1. Legs externally rotate
2. Legs bend or femurs lift
3. Hamstring cramp

Response

1. Keeping leg length, roll front thighs toward each other and back thighs away from each other. Place feet wider apart. Use 2 straps, tying one strap around each thigh, buckles at outer thighs and passing strap end over front thighs through legs. Hold strap ends between hands and chair seat when lifting, *ll k-l*.
2. *See Response 1.* Extend legs more clearly before lifting chest and pelvis. De-emphasize pelvic lift and emphasize chest lift.
3. Hamstring activation is necessary, but legs may overwork when arms/shoulders are under working. Press hands more deeply downward and backward, activating triceps. Elevate balls of feet with block and push feet more deeply away from back pelvis.

...urvottanasana encourages the spine to move anteriorly, which is useful following Forward Bends ...d may help to reduce kyphosis. It also strengthens the triceps, increases shoulder mobility, and ...roadens the chest. In this variation, strain on the arms and wrists is minimized by using a chair.

Contact Points

Feet, hands

External Supports

Mat, chair, wall

Essence of Form

Posterior arm extension, leg, hip, and torso extension; legs and arms internally rotated

II a

II b

II c

II d

II e

II f

II g

II h

II i

II j

II k

II l

Purvottanasana
Intense Front-Body Stretch

Nourish

Learn + Practice

Once basic chest and shoulder opening is established, before Viparita Dandasana

Linked Poses

Viparita Dandasana, Savasana B, Bishmasana, Supta Virasana, Setu Bandha Sarvangasana

Safety Factors

Use care during pregnancy and when deep front body stretch is contraindicated; lower back injury

Prepare

- Mat's short edge to wall
- Set chairs facing each other on mat, about a leg's length from wall
- Place bolster lengthwise on chair seats
- Use folded blanket at bolster's head end
- Have block and two straps within reach

Enter

- Step into chair closest to wall
- Sit near chair back, feet flat on floor, *III a*
- Bring bolster against back pelvis
- Place block lengthwise between thighs
- Strap upper thighs at greater trochanters and lower thighs at least 2" above knees, *III b*
- Extend legs, pressing balls of feet to wall, *III c*
- Gather front iliums and soften pubis inward
- Holding chair back, inhale and lift chest
- Pushing feet away from back pelvis, and keeping chest lift, slide back pelvis toward wall to lie back on bolster, *III d*
- Hold chair back or chair legs with hands

Sustain

- Equalize right and left thigh contact against block and straps
- Pushing feet away from back pelvis, descend thighs away from front strap pressure, toward pressure at back of thighs
- Rest back torso symmetrically into bolster
- Gently and continuously lift and open chest
- Soften abdomen and breathe naturally
- Release throat, neck, jaw, tongue, face, eyes

Exit

- Bring hands to chair back
- Bend legs and place feet flat on floor, *III e*
- Pressing into feet, pull symmetrically with both hands to lift chest and sit upright, *III f*
- Rest a few breaths, then remove block and straps and step out of chair

ॐ *Alternately, keep legs extended and place hands on chair seat, behind pelvis. Push hands into chair seat and symmetrically press to seated, III g*

Challenge

1. Lumbar pain
2. Shoulder and/or neck discomfor
3. Difficulty getting in and out of chair

Response

1. Elevate heels on block(s) to reduce back bend degree, *III h.* Strap front iliums toward each other. Can also be done over 2 bolsters, use blocks and blankets as necessary, *III i.* Review leg, pelvis, and transverse abdominal actions from *Tadasana.*
2. Support arms on chairs, raise arms to shoulder level with folded blankets or bolsters, *III j.* Practice lying over a table (mats under table legs to prevent slide). Raise feet and arms as required, *III k.* Increase head support.
3. Use backless chairs, or replace first with two facing each other to support pelvis and bolster's lower end, *III l.* Or, set chair backs to one side. Alternate which side chair backs face for each practice.

Contact Points

Feet and legs, back body

External Supports

2 chairs, block, 2 straps, bolster, blankets
Additional blankets, chairs, mats, wall, table

Essence of Form

Leg, hip, and torso extension; legs neutral toward internal rotation, arms neutral toward external

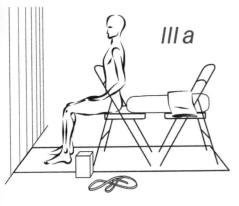

III a

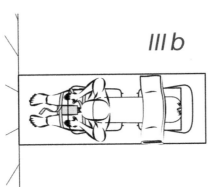

III b

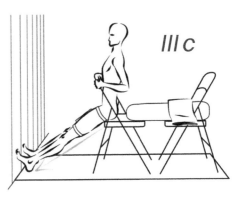

III c

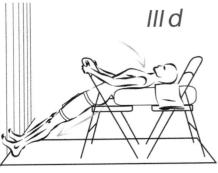

III d

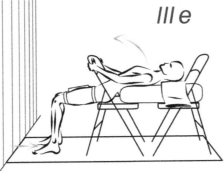

III e

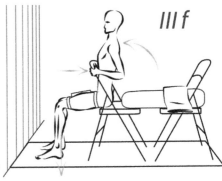

III f

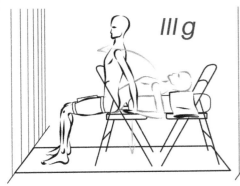

III g

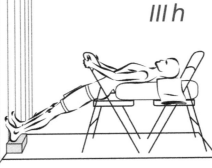

III h

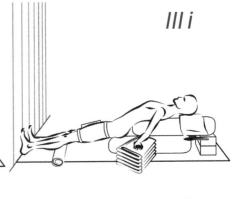

III i

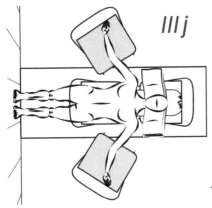

III j

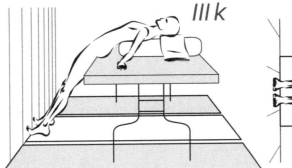

III k

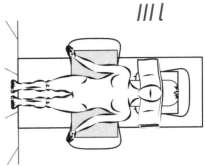

III l

Purvottanasana
Intense Front-Body Stretch

Synthesize

Learn + Practice

*After Explore;
Before Salamba Sarvangasana*

Linked Poses

*Ustrasana, Urdhva Mukha
Svanasana, Setu Bandha
Sarvangasana*

Safety Factors

*Rotator cuff injury, shoulder
tendinitis; wrist or elbow injuries*

Prepare

· Mat can be away from wall

Enter

· Sit on mat in *Dandasana*
· Engage leg and pelvis
 actions from *Explore*
· Leaning back, place hands
 12-16" away from back pelvis,
 fingertips pointing outward, *IV a*
· Pressing hands into floor,
 anchor index finger and
 thumb mounds heavily
· Without protruding bottom
 ribs, lift chest away from
 hands and pelvis, *IV b*
· With chest lifted, bend legs and
 bring feet flat to floor, foot and
 thigh mid lines parallel, *IV c*
· Internally rotate thighs and
 deepen big toe mound pressure
· Glide sacrum away from back ribs
· Pressing into hands and feet,
 draw mid-thoracic spine
 inward, lifting pelvis to shoulder
 height on inhalation, *IV d*
· Initiating from mid-thoracic
 spine, lengthen cervical spine
 and tilt head backward, *IV e*

Sustain

· Maintain leg and pelvis
 actions from *Explore*
· Extend femurs away from back
 pelvis, descending upper
 femurs and lifting front iliums
· Soften sternum inward,
 lengthening upper sternum
 away from lower sternum
· Roll collarbones away from
 upper chest, articulating
 ribs and collarbones
· Draw mid-thoracic spine inward
· Broaden between shoulder
 blades, moving bottom
 shoulder blades into back ribs
· Release jaw and soften face

Exit

· Hold for 5-15 breaths
· Exhaling, tuck chin toward chest
 and slowly lower pelvis, *IV f*
· Extend legs, sitting upright
 in *Dandasana, IV g*
· Repeat up to 5 times, gradually
 internally rotating arms to
 point fingertips forward

❦ *Once familiar, keep legs
 extended when lifting pelvis, IV h*

Challenge

1. Wrist strain
2. Inability to lift pelvis
3. Lumbar pain
4. Shoulders round
5. Neck strain, chest and
 shoulder restriction

Response

1. Externally rotate arms or
 elevate heels of hands on
 slant board or rolled mat, *IV i.*
2. Drag heels backward to engage
 buttocks and hamstrings, *IV j.*
 Ensure shoulder opening is
 adequate in *Simplify + Explore.*
3. Do not splay feet and knees
 outward. Hold block between
 knees or between upper
 thighs, *IV k.* Strap front iliums
 toward each other, and lift front
 iliums away from femurs
4. Roll collarbones up and back
 before lifting pelvis, *IV l.* Practice
 Simplify + Explore until humeri
 extend posteriorly without
 collarbones rolling forward.
5. Draw chin toward chest until
 shoulder mobility increases in
 Simplify, Explore + Nourish.

An invigorating pose, Purvottanasana increases lung capacity, shoulder mobility, broadens the chest, and is an excellent preparation for Sarvangasana, Ustrasana, and Pranayama. This variation using minimal props is common in Vinyasa-style flow classes.

Contact Points	External Supports	Essence of Form
Hands and feet	Mat Block, strap	Hip and torso extension, leg extension (IV h); legs slightly internally rotated, arms internal

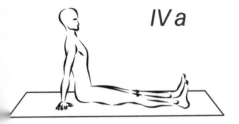

IVa

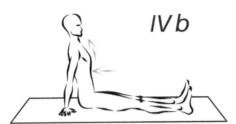

IVb

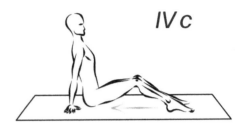

IVc

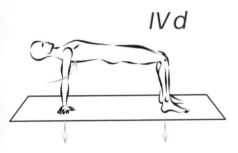

IVd

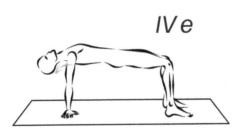

IVe

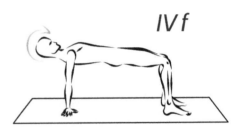

IVf

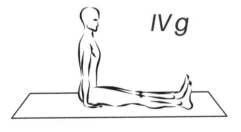

IVg

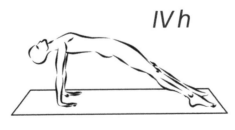

IVh

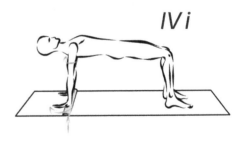

IVi

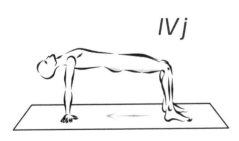

IVj

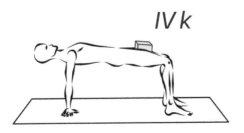

IVk

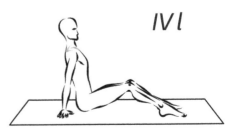

IVl

Intense Front-Body Stretch — *Synthesize*

Viparita Dandasana
Inverted Staff Pose

Simplify

Learn + Practice

After full extension in Urdhva Hastasana, before unsupported Back Bends and Inversions

Linked Poses

Urdhva Hastasana, Upashrayi Dandasana, Pincha Mayurasana, Sirsasana

Safety Factors

Lower back pain, neck injury, eye strain, migraine, insomnia, digestive problems

Prepare

- Place chair on mat, away from wall

Enter

- Sit on chair, legs bent and feet on floor, *l a*
- Set feet 6-8" further forward than knees and hip-width apart
- Press hands to chair seat, beside pelvis
- Lift pelvis and shift forward to clear chair lip
- Bend elbows and descend pelvis and torso, lowering back ribcage to chair seat, *l b*
- Walk feet forward if necessary, *l c*
- Hold chair back with hands, and using chair seat as a fulcrum, press into feet to lift pelvis
- Slide ribs away from backrest until head rests on chair seat, 4-5" away from backrest, *l d*
- One at a time, thread arms through space between chair seat and back rest
- Bend elbows and catch back chair rung, with the palms facing toward the feet, *l e*
- Holding chair rung, slowly descend pelvis away from back ribs to capacity, *l f*

Sustain

- Keep feet firmly anchored, with tibias vertical
- Gather front iliums and soften pubis inward
- Walk hands away from each other and roll elbows inward
- Lengthen inner elbows away from armpits
- Descend upper arm bones
- Broaden between shoulder blades
- Lengthen pack pelvis away from back ribcage

Exit

- Pressing into feet, lift pelvis to chair height
- Exhale, stabilize upper back against chair
- With upper back stable, release grip on chair, then inhale and extend arms, *l g*
- Rest on exhalation
- One at a time, unthread arms from chair
- Holding top of chair back, pull with hands to stabilize ribcage against chair lip, *l h*
- Exhaling, lower pelvis to floor, and lift head simultaneously, then extend legs, *l i-j*
- Pressing hands into floor, sit upright, *l k*

Challenge

1. Arms do not fit through chair space
2. Neck discomfort
3. Back discomfort
4. Numbness in arms or hands

Response

1. Head is often too close to back of chair. Slide away from backrest until shoulder blades are on chair lip. Head should be well supported. If necessary, use a backless chair.
2. Adjust so that chair contacts upper thoracics slightly higher or lower. Widen and descend upper arm bones. Lower pelvis less. Catch top of chair back rather than bringing arms through.
3. *Prepare* with blocks beyond chair seat to rest pelvis on when lowering, *l l*. Lengthen back pelvis forward away from back rib cage while descending, rather than pulling pelvis back toward chair.
4. Pad chair with folded mat. Descend upper humeri. Walk hands toward each other and let elbows release outward into chair frame.

One of the challenges in deep Back Bends is mobility in the shoulders, thoracic spine, and ribcage. This upper back opener is useful in developing this mobility after basic Back Bends, especially before continuing on to Viparita Dandasana in the chair.

Contact Points

Feet, back ribs, shoulder blades, hands
Back pelvis

External Supports

Mat, chair
Blocks, folded mat

Essence of Form

Shoulder and torso extension, elbow flexion, hip and knee flexion; legs neutrally rotated, arms slightly internal

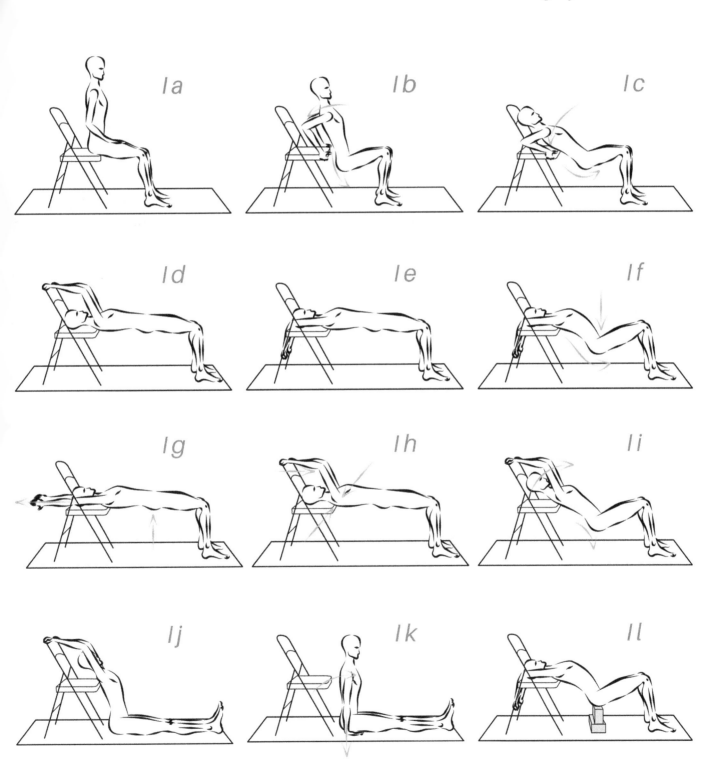

Ia   Ib   Ic

Id   Ie   If

Ig   Ih   Ii

Ij   Ik   Il

Learn + Practice

After Salabhasana and basic Back Bends, before deep Back Bends

Linked Poses

Purvottanasana, Ustrasana, Dhanurasana, Bhekasana

Safety Factors

Lower back pain, anterior disc herniation, neck injury, eye strain, insomnia, spondylosis

Prepare

- Set chair on mat
- Place lengthwise bolster under chair lip, *ll a*
- Have a block near chair, within reach

Enter

- Step legs one at a time through space between backrest and chair seat
- Sit as close to backrest as possible, feet flat on floor and slightly beyond knees, *ll b*
- Place block between inner knees, *ll c*
- Laterally resist heels and gather front iliums
- Holding backrest with hands, inhale to lift chest
- Keeping feet anchored, exhale and lean back on chair seat, sliding pelvis forward, *ll d*
- Lie back symmetrically, controlling descent with arms, resting back ribs on chair seat
- Bring chair lip between shoulder blades
- Rest head on bolster, with the back of neck long, *ll e*
- Keep hands on backrest for first minute, then move hands to back rung, palms up, *ll f*

Sustain

- Stabilize feet with foot mid lines parallel
- Lengthening femurs away from back pelvis, draw upper tibias backward, *ll g*
- Descend upper inner thighs in internal rotation
- Continuously gather front iliums and resist heels laterally
- Soften pubis skin in and up
- Use hands to pull chair seat into upper back, creating chest lift, *ll h*
- Emphasize mobility in upper thoracic spine, drawing lower front ribs gently inward and extending upper ribs away from lower ribs
- Broaden across collarbones
- Release head and neck

Exit

- Stabilize feet, legs, and pelvis
- Bring hands from lower rung to backrest, *ll i*
- Leading with chest, inhale and pull with hands lifting torso symmetrically to seated, *ll j*
- Sit upright for a few breaths
- Step legs out of chair, either sliding pelvis backward or tipping chair forward and standing up, *ll k*

Challenge

1. Lower back pain
2. Neck tension, head does not reach support
3. Chair pressure causes upper back pain
4. Legs do not fit into chair, difficulty stepping in

Response

1. Practice *Anjaneyasana* and *Supta Virasana* first to open groins and quadriceps. Support lumbar curve with rolled mat or blanket. Hold block between thighs and strap around upper thighs. Keep buttocks toned.
2. *Prepare* with more height for under head. Or, slide backward in chair contacting lower on shoulder blades until chest opens more, *ll l.*
3. Skin may be pinched together between bones and chair. Adjust skin away from spine and pelvis. Pad chair seat with folded mat. If the spinous processes protrude, roll mat or mat remnant to support spine lengthwise.
4. Use backless chair. Tip chair backward to step in, then lower chair while sitting.

This deep, but accessible Back Bend prepares the chest, spine, and legs for more advanced work. Supporting the head in this pose simulates the head contact found in unsupported variations of Viparita Dandasana. Though the legs are bent, keep them active to stabilize the spine and pelvis.

Contact Points

Feet, back pelvis, back ribs, crown

External Supports

Mat, chair, block, bolster
Strap, mat or mat remnant, blanket

Essence of Form

Torso and hip extension, knee flexion, shoulder extension; legs slightly internally rotated, arms neutral to external

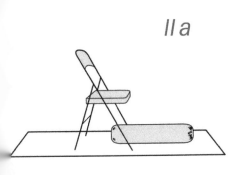

II a

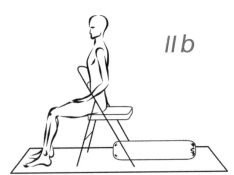

II b

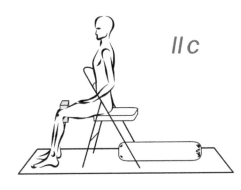

II c

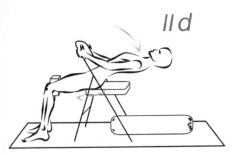

II d

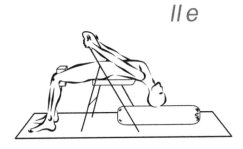

II e

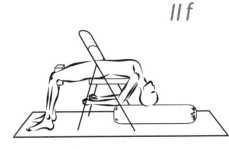

II f

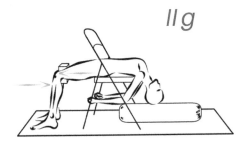

II g

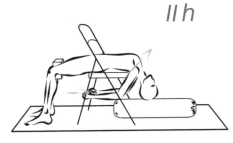

II h

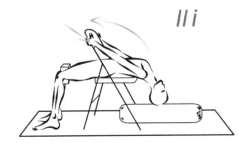

II i

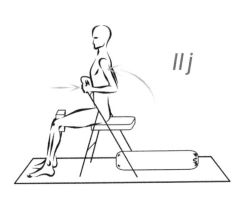

II j

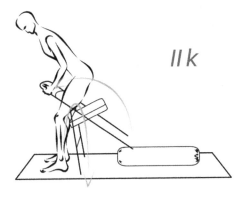

II k

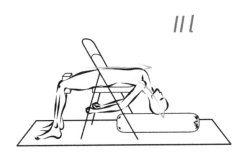

II l

Learn + Practice

Once Explore is stable both Entering and Exiting; before deep unsupported Back Bends

Linked Poses

Purvottanasana, Bhujangasana, Sirsasana, Urdhva Dhanurasana

Safety Factors

As for Explore, extra care for lumbar injury, eye strain, and insomnia

Prepare

- Set chair just less than a leg's length from wall
- Place lengthwise bolster as for *Explore* (optional)
- Have a block and 2 straps nearby

Enter

- Step into chair, sitting at chair seat back, *III a*
- Place block between thighs
- Strap thighs at greater trochanters and lower femurs
- Extend legs in *Dandasana*, pressing balls of feet into wall, away from back pelvis, *III b*
- Adjust chair distance if balls of feet do not reach wall, or if legs do not fully extend
- Press heels to floor, away from back pelvis; heels do not have to touch wall
- Pushing feet deeply away from back pelvis, hold chair back and slide pelvis forward as torso leans back onto chair seat, *III c*
- Pulling chair seat into upper back, lift chest over chair lip and rest head on support, *III d*
- After 10-25 breaths, reach under chair and catch crossbar, palms up, *III e*

Sustain

- Continuously push feet away from back pelvis
- Resist heels and upper femurs laterally
- Squeeze block with inner thighs, lengthening from inner groins to big toe mounds
- Descend upper femurs pressing back into strap
- Rest mid-thoracic region against chair lip, broadening between shoulder blades
- Draw bottom shoulder blades forward
- Gently and continuously pull chair lip into upper back, lifting chest over chair seat

Exit

- Bring hands to chair back if holding crossbar
- Bend the legs and bring feet flat to floor
- Pressing into feet, inhale and pull with hands to bring torso symmetrically upright
- Alternately, keep legs extended and push feet into wall while coming up to seated, *III f*
- Unstrap legs and remove block
- Sit upright, resisting urge to fold forward

Challenge

1. Lumbar pain when *Exiting*
2. Feet lose wall contact
3. Pelvis slides back
4. Neck compression

Response

1. Bring hands to chair seat and push down into chair seat rather than pulling. Descend femurs before and during *Exit*. Once upright, practice *Bharadvajasana* for a few breaths each side before stepping out of chair, *III g*. Do *Adho Mukha Svanasana* with hands on chair after stepping out, *III h*.
2. Move chair slightly closer to wall when *Entering*. Lengthen back body rather than pushing from front thighs. Release back femurs down and away from back pelvis, increasing vertical groin space.
3. Make leg actions clearer. Use mat remnant on chair seat for extra grip. *See Response 2.*
4. Extend occipital bone away from upper back to avoid compression. If using head support, remove or decrease as chest opens.

Viparita Dandasana can be both soothing and energizing. With support directly behind the heart, it may help strengthen the cardiovascular system, boost immune function, and improve circulation. This pose may also be useful in aiding nutrient absorption and digestion.

Contact Points

Feet, back pelvis, back ribs, crown (if using support)

External Supports

Wall, chair, block, 2 straps
Bolster or blankets, mat remnant

Essence of Form

Leg, hip, and torso extension, shoulder extension; legs internally rotated, arms external

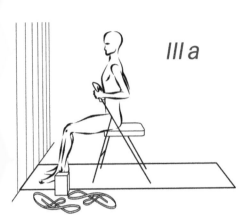

III a

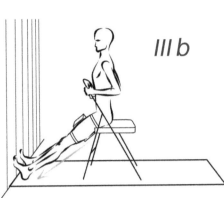

III b

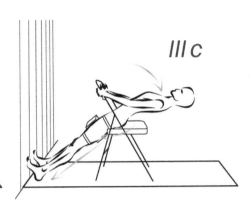

III c

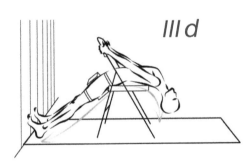

III d

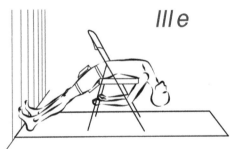

III e

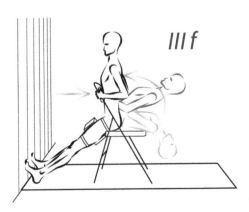

III f

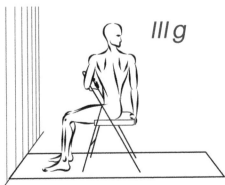

III g

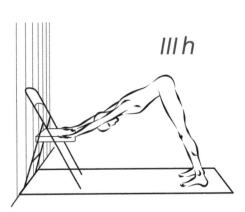

III h

Learn + Practice

*After Simplify + Nourish;
before deep Back Bends*

Linked Poses

*Upashrayi Dandasana, Urdhva
Dhanurasana, Sirsasana,
Kapotasana, Vrschikasana*

Safety Factors

*As for Nourish; if hypertense,
use Nourish arm variations, not
clasping hands behind head*

Prepare

· As for *Nourish*, closer
  to wall if necessary

Enter

· Follow *Enter* instructions
  for *Nourish*
· Hold chair back for 10-25 breath
  cycles, then catch crossbar for
  an additional 10-25 breaths
· Pushing feet and legs deeply
  out of back pelvis, stabilize
  feet, legs, and pelvis
· Maintain internal leg
  rotation, tone buttocks
· Keeping foot/wall contact
  and without sliding pelvis
  away from wall, release
  hands from chair rung
· Anchor mid-thoracic
  spine against chair
· Clasp hands behind head and
  draw elbows toward each other
· Lengthening from mid-thoracic
  spine, extend elbows toward
  floor, away from armpits, *IV a*
· Using chair lip as a fulcrum,
  extend chest over and
  below chair seat, *IV b*
· Reduce or remove head
  support if used
· Catch chair legs if reasonable, *IV c*

Sustain

· Engage leg and pelvis actions
  from *Nourish* and *Tadasana*
· Keeping leg extension,
  descend upper femurs and
  resist tibia heads upward, *IV d*
· Deeply internally rotate
  femurs from hip joint
· With internal thigh rotation,
  tone the buttocks
· Broaden back pelvis and
  lengthen tail bone
· Glide sacrum into back body
· Broaden upper back, rolling outer
  armpits toward front body, *IV e*
· Gather elbows toward each
  other and extend them
  away from armpits, *IV f-g*

Exit

· Keeping leg extension,
  exhale and lift head with
  hands to chair height, *IV h*
· Holding head at chair
  height, release hands and
  hold chair's back, *IV i*
· Pushing feet out of back pelvis,
  pull chair and lead with chest
  to bring torso upright, *IV j*
· Sit upright and resist the
  urge to fold forward

Challenge

1. Lumbar pain
2. Sliding out of chair
3. Shoulder pain
4. Eye/head pressure

Response

1. Raise feet on blocks to reduce
   back bend degree, *IV k*. Descend
   femurs and internally rotate
   thighs. Resist inner femurs
   laterally. *See Response 2.*
2. Hang a strap from backless chair,
   supporting pelvis in loop, *IV l-m*.
   Lengthen back body rather than
   extending from front body, *IV n*.
3. Practice *Simplify* and *Upashrayi
   Dandasana* (*Dandasana*,
   Nourish) to develop more
   shoulder mobility. Broaden
   between shoulder blades
   and roll outer armpits forward.
   Draw humeral heads back
   and into shoulder girdle, *IV o*.
4. Support head, with pressure
   on the crown, *IV p*. Tuck chin,
   extending occiput out of mid-
   thoracic spine to decompress
   cervical arteries, *IV q*.

Though supported in a chair, transitioning from holding the chair to bringing the arms overhead [i]s quite demanding. Viparita Dandasana teaches the deep relationship between leg stability [an]d spinal freedom, integrating action through the entire body from heels to hands.

Contact Points

[F]eet, back pelvis, back ribs, [c]rown (if using support)

External Supports

Wall, chair, block, 2 straps, bolster
Backless chair, blocks, strap

Essence of Form

Leg, hip, and torso extension, shoulder and elbow flexion; legs internally rotated, arms external

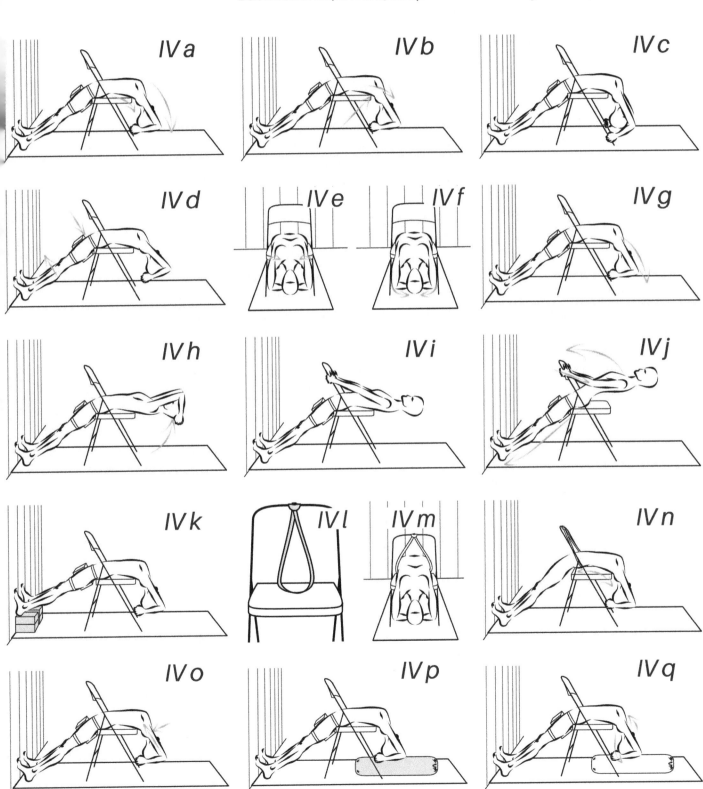

IVa IVb IVc
IVd IVe IVf IVg
IVh IVi IVj
IVk IVl IVm IVn
IVo IVp IVq

Ustrasana
Camel Pose

Learn + Practice

After Anjaneyasana, Purvottanasana, Supta Virasana; learn well before intermediate Back Bends

Linked Poses

Anjaneyasana, Supta Virasana, Urdhva Mukha Svanasana, Purvottanasana, Viparita Dandasana

Safety Factors

Lower back strain, knee pressure; practice with chair against wall if pregnant, I o-p

Prepare

- Short end of mat to wall
- Place blocks on end 1.5-2' from wall, shoulder-width apart, *I a*

Enter

- Kneel in *Virasana*, knees touching wall, blocks lateral to feet and upper thighs, *I b*
- Gather front iliums and resist heels laterally
- Spreading toes, press tops of feet to floor
- With feet pressing down, exhale to lift pelvis, bringing front thighs and iliums to wall, *I c*
- Soften pubis skin away from wall
- Lengthening thighs, internally rotate top thighs
- Descend back pelvis heavily
- Place hands on wall at chest height, elbows bent and descending toward floor, *I d*
- Without moving hands, press hands into wall and drag downward, lifting back rib cage, *I e*
- Keeping back rib height, lift chest up and back
- Exhaling, symmetrically lower hands to blocks
- Pushing hands to blocks, further lift chest, *I f*

Sustain

- Keeping front iliums against wall, draw upper femurs backward, *I g*
- Without tucking pelvis, descend sacrum away from bottom ribs, lifting bottom ribs off pelvis
- Pressing into hands, roll elbows toward each other, externally rotating arms, *I h*
- Broaden across collarbones and roll front shoulder skin over the shoulders toward back body, *I i*
- Slide shoulder blades down as back ribs lift
- Soften throat and extend occiput away from thoracic spine, *I j*

Exit

- Pressing feet and tibias down into floor, bring hands to back pelvis, *I k*
- Descending back pelvis and pressing into hands, inhale to lift torso upright, *I l*
- Exhaling, sit back in *Virasana*
- Stand up and do *Ardha Uttanasana* (*Adho Mukha Svanasana*, *Simplify*), or extend arms up, placing hands at wall, *I m*
- Repeat 3-5 times

Challenge

1. Knee pressure
2. Inability to reach blocks, or hands lower asymmetrically
3. Lumbar discomfort
4. Neck strain

Response

1. Use folded blanket or mat for padding under knees, *I n*.
2. *Prepare* with chair against wall, *I o*. Press hands into chair seat and lift chest upward, *I p*. Also appropriate if pregnant.
3. Drag back pelvis down with hands as torso lifts up and back, *I q*. Manually internally rotate thighs, *I r*. Keep gaze forward and reduce degree. Practice *Anjaneyasana* and *Supta Virasana* to open groins and thighs more. *See Response 2.*
4. Draw thoracic spine more deeply into body, and open upper chest more fully. Keep gaze forward toward wall, *I s*. When bringing arms backward, externally rotate arms with fingertips pointing away from wall, thumbs out, *I t*. Practice *Trikonasana* more frequently to strengthen neck musculature. *See also Explore + Nourish.*

Resembling the high arch of a camel's hump, Ustrasana lengthens the anterior chain, opening the thighs, groins, and chest. Practicing it with the thighs against a wall prevents them from sinking back, which reduces the pose's efficacy. This variation also helps retain torso lift.

Contact Points

Tops of feet, tibias, front iliums, hands

External Supports

Mat, wall, 2 blocks
Additional blocks, blanket, chair, strap

Essence of Form

Hip and spine extension, knee and shoulder flexion; legs slightly internal, arms internal (external in I t)

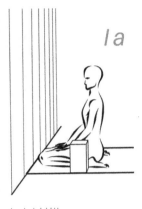

I a

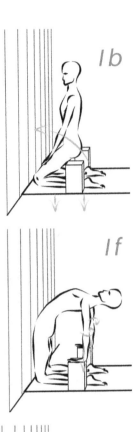

I b

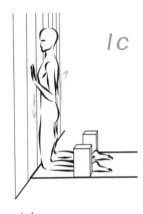

I c

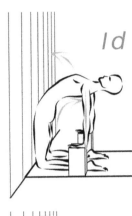

I d

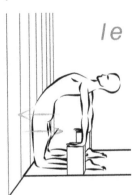

I e

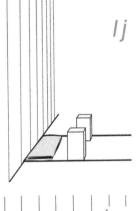

I f

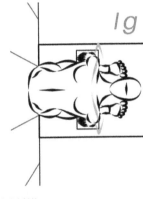

I g

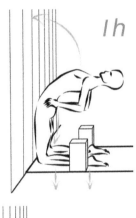

I h

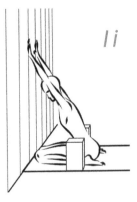

I i

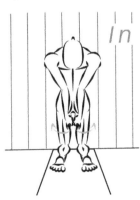

I j

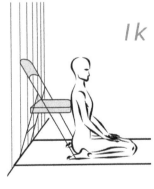

I k

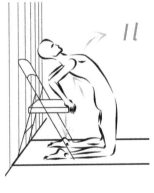

I l

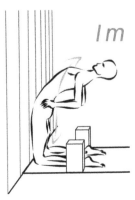

I m

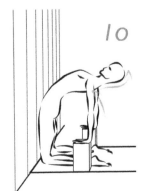

I n

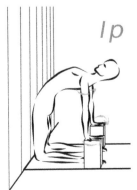

I o

I p

Ustrasana
Camel Pose

Explore

Learn + Practice

Learn after Simplify and after
Viparita Dandasana; before
deep thoracic Back Bends

Linked Poses

Anjaneyasana, Supta Virasana,
Viparita Dandasana, Kapotasana

Safety Factors

Lumbar instability, wrist injury,
shoulder injury; use care with
neck injury or discomfort

Prepare

· Short end of mat to wall
· Rest folded chair against
  wall, chair seat toward wall
· Place folded blanket 1.5-2
  feet from wall or fold mat for
  padding if necessary, *ll a*

Enter

· Sit in *Virasana* facing
  away from wall
· Gather front iliums and
  resist heels laterally
· Soften pubis skin inward
  and upward
· Catch chair with both hands, *ll b*
· Pressing tops of feet to floor,
  exhale and lift pelvis, to
  bring thighs vertical while
  tipping chair forward, *ll c*
· Bring chair to bottom shoulder
  blade tips and brace chair
  legs in wall/floor juncture, *ll d*
· Lengthening down through
  femurs, lift chest
· Keeping pelvis atop thighs,
  arch upper torso over chair
  back toward wall, *ll e*
· Gaze forward or, if appropriate,
  lengthen back of neck and
  tilt head backward, *ll f*

Sustain

· Continue actions from *Simplify*
· Lengthen through femurs and
  press upper femurs backward,
  internally rotating thighs
· Symmetrically walk hands
  down chair legs, pulling chair
  into thoracic spine, *ll g*
· Using chair, lift back ribs
  away from pelvis

Exit

· If tiling head backward,
  release hands from chair and
  manually lift head to upright
· Gathering front iliums, and
  pressing tops of feet to floor,
  inhale to bring torso upright, *ll h*
· Catch chair with hands and
  lean chair against wall while
  bringing chair legs forward 2-3"
· Exhaling, sit back in *Virasana*, *ll i*
· Once proficient, leaning chair
  to wall and sitting in *Virasana*
  can be done simultaneously
· Sit upright in *Virasana* or walk
  hands forward and exhale to
  Adho Mukha Svanasana, *ll j*
· Repeat, moving chair back
  either higher or lower on upper
  back for a different opening

Challenge

1. Chair sits too high or
   low on upper back
2. Chair unfolds
3. Neck pain
4. Knee pain

Response

1. Chair back too high: move
   further from wall; too low: move
   closer to wall or elevate chair
   legs on blocks, *ll k*. Keep pelvis
   well forward, with femurs vertical
   to ensure correct chair angle.
2. Hold folded chair legs
   together before using full
   support. Alternately, strap
   chair legs together.
3. Do not tilt head backward.
   Prepare with vertical bolster
   between wall and chair and rest
   head on bolster's end when
   Entering, *ll l*. Deepen back bend
   from thoracic spine, not the neck.
4. Pad knees. Draw knee skin
   forward from under knees
   before sitting up from *Virasana*.
   Press tops of feet more firmly
   down to reduce direct load.
   Practice *Anjaneyasana* and
   Supta Virasana to release
   thighs and groins, *ll m-o*.

...strasana generally helps reduce kyphosis and rounded shoulders by moving the thoracic spine forward. This feature is emphasized by using a chair to support the rib cage — the chair acts as a fulcrum to lift the chest. Explore placing the chair at different heights for a variety of openings.

Contact Points

Tops of feet, tibias, thoracic spine, hands

External Supports

Mat, chair, wall
2 blocks, strap, bolster

Essence of Form

Hip and spine extension, Knee flexion, shoulder extension; legs slightly internally rotated, arms external

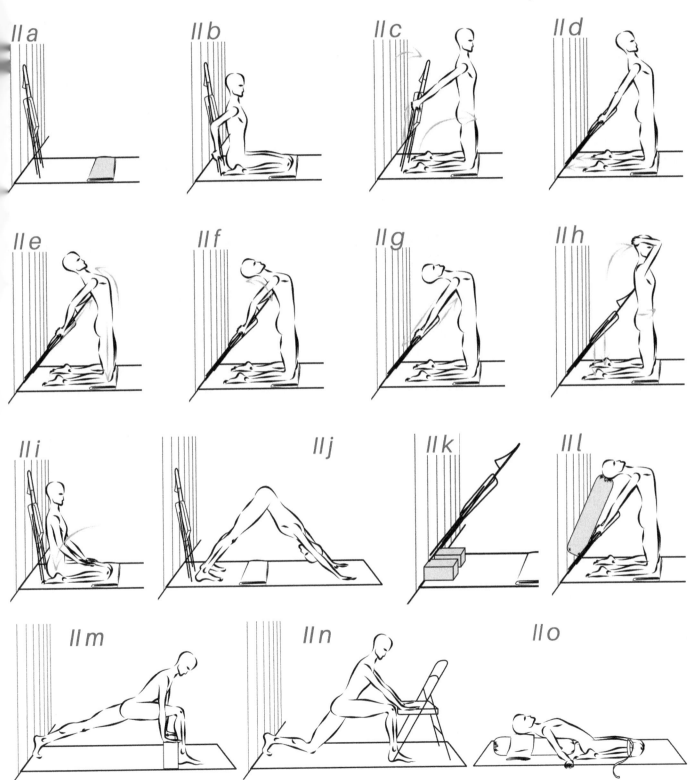

II a

II b

II c

II d

II e

II f

II g

II h

II i

II j

II k

II l

II m

II n

II o

Learn + Practice

After Simplify + Explore, before intermediate Back Bends

Linked Poses

Supta Virasana, Upashrayi Dandasana, Purvottanasana, Viparita Dandasana

Safety Factors

Use care with back and neck injury; avoid for moderate to severe knee discomfort

Prepare

- Chair on mat, block and strap within reach
- Place one folded blanket in front of chair, and set second blanket on chair's backrest
- Stack 2 bolsters lengthwise on chair seat
- Offset top bolster slightly further back, *III a*

Enter

- Kneel in front of chair with thighs vertical and back pelvis against chair lip, *III b*
- Internally rotate upper thighs and place block between thighs, holding by its faces (narrow), *III c*
- Strap upper thighs at greater trochanters, *III d*
- Gather front iliums and soften pubis skin inward
- Pressing hands into bolster, inhale to lift chest and back ribs away from back pelvis, *III e*
- Keeping lift, exhale to rest back on bolsters
- Using hands, manually drag occiput away from thoracic spine
- With back of neck long, rest head on chair back
- Release arms to sides, gently catching chair's front legs, *III f*

Sustain

- Maintain leg and pelvis actions from *Simplify + Explore*
- Spread toes, descending the little toe
- Without externally rotating lower legs, draw outer ankles medially inward
- Resist greater trochanters laterally
- Settling back ribs, widen shoulder blades and firm them against back rib cage
- Circularly roll armpit chest forward and up
- Soften abdomen and breathe freely
- Create vertical space between femurs and pelvis, and between navel and diaphragm, then between ribs from diaphragm to collarbones

Exit

- Stabilizing legs and pelvis, release hands
- Inhaling, manually lift head upright, *III g*
- Press hands into chair seat and inhale to bring torso upright, *III h*
- Walk hands forward and exhale to *Adho Mukha Svanasana*

Challenge

1. Lumbar pain
2. Back body not fully supported
3. Neck discomfort
4. Shoulder discomfort

Response

ॐ *Tailor Preparation with additional props according to body proportions and capacity*

1. Practice *Upashrayi Virasana, III i.* Support torso at a higher angle, reducing back bend degree. *See Response 3.*
2. Fill gaps between bolsters and back body with folded or rolled blankets, *III j.*
3. Use additional height under head and a rolled blanket to support cervical curve. *See also Responses 1 + 4.*
4. *Prepare* with two additional chairs, lateral to the central one and at 45-60° from mid line. Rest arms on chair seats at or just slightly below shoulder-level, *III k.* Adjust height with folded blankets or bolsters as necessary, *III l.*

In this variation of Ustrasana, the back is fully supported, allowing the deeper tissues to release over time. Though supported, this variation is often much more intense than the active versions. Use props generously and reduce as ease is found.

Contact Points

Tops of feet, tibias, knees, back torso

External Supports

Mat, backless chair, 2 bolsters, 2 folded blankets, strap, block
Extra chairs, bolsters and blankets

Essence of Form

Hip and spine extension, knee flexion, shoulder extension; legs slightly internally rotated, arms external

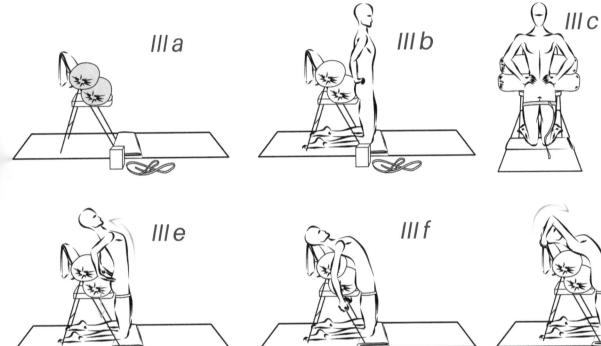

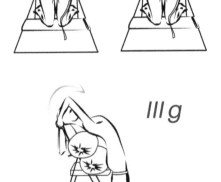

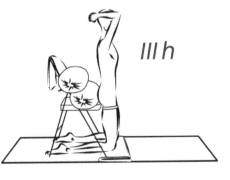

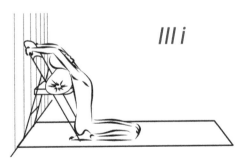

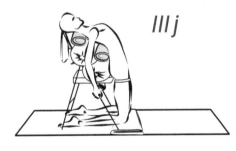

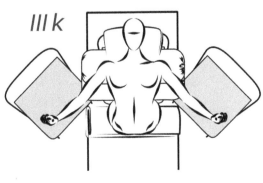

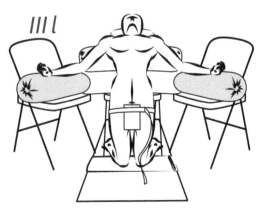

Ustrasana
Camel Pose

Synthesize

Learn + Practice

After Simplify, Explore + Nourish; before intermediate and advanced Back Bends

Linked Poses

Supta Virasana, Upashrayi Dandasana, Purvottanasana, Viparita Dandasana

Safety Factors

As for Simplify, Explore + Nourish; avoid standing knees for longer than 30 seconds before bending back

Prepare

- Place supports (if used) on mat for *Virasana*
- Use folded blanket under knees if necessary

Enter

- Sit in *Virasana* with hands on back pelvis, fingertips pointing downward, *IV a*
- Gathering front iliums, soften pubis inward
- Spreading toes and pressing tops of feet down into floor, exhale and lift pelvis, standing vertically on knees, *IV b*
- Dragging buttock flesh downward with hands, inhale and lift back ribcage away from pelvis
- Drawing thoracic spine inward and forward, arch upper torso backward, *IV c*
- Once sternum is horizontal, release hands from back pelvis and without twisting, exhale to symmetrically place hands on heels or catch ankles, *IV d*

- ॐ *Alternatively, place hands on heels while in Virasana and lift pelvis and torso directly into Ustrasana, IV e*

Sustain

- Maintain actions from *Simplify, Explore + Nourish*
- Pressing hands into feet, further lift torso away from hands, *IV f*
- Keeping pelvis moving forward, press upper femurs backward
- Inhaling, broaden back body and draw spine forward, from sacrum to upper thoracic
- Soften face, jaw, and throat
- Initiating from mid-thoracic spine, extend occiput away from upper thoracic spine and tilt head back

Exit

- Stabilizing feet and legs, symmetrically place hands on back pelvis
- Drag back pelvis down and press pelvis slightly forward with hands, *IV g*
- Pushing firmly down through feet, inhale to lift torso vertical
- Exhaling, sit back in *Virasana*
- Rest a few breaths in *Virasana* and repeat 3-5 times
- Exhale to *Adho Mukha Svanasana*

- ॐ *Alternatively, sit directly back from Ustrasana*

Challenge

1. Lumbar discomfort
2. Shoulder strain, inability to reach feet
3. Chest collapses when reaching feet
4. Neck strain

Response

1. Deepen internal thigh rotation. Lift front iliums and widen inner back femurs while *Entering*. Strap front iliums toward each other. Lumbar pain may be alleviated by tucking chin toward chest, as cervical and lumbar curves reflect each other. *See Responses 2 + 3.*
2. *Prepare* with blocks beside feet in *Virasana*, as for *Simplify*. As capacity increases, lower block height, *IV h*. Practice *Purvottanasana, Simplify*, to increase shoulder mobility.
3. Practice *Simplify + Explore* until thoracic lift is learned more fully. *See also Response 2.*
4. Roll armpit-chest toward ceiling and ensure neck action originates in mid-thoracic spine. Set chair behind torso in *Prepare* and rest head on chair's back. Use blankets if necessary, *IV i*.

270   Ustrasana — *Synthesize*

Yoga: Point + Process | *Volume 1*

This classical variation of Ustrasana incorporates the actions and effects of the earlier variations. Using minimal props, it can be integrated into Vinyasa-style practices. Experiment with short hold repetitions and longer holds for different results.

Contact Points

Tops of feet, tibias, knees, hands, heels

External Supports

Mat, blanket
Strap, blocks

Essence of Form

Hip and spine extension, Knee flexion, shoulder extension; legs slightly internally rotated, arms external

IV a

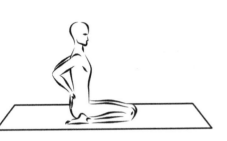

IV b

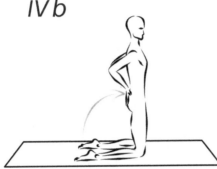

IV c

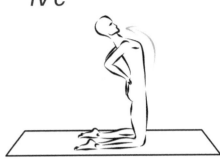

IV d

IV e

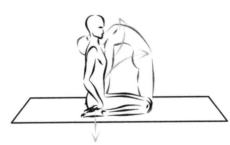

IV f

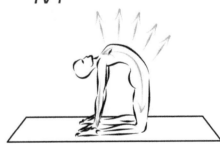

IV g

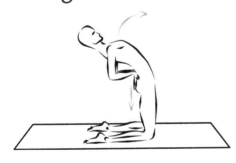

IV h

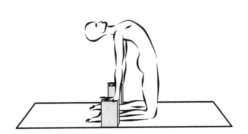

IV i

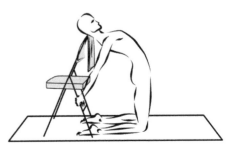

Antaramsasana
Upper Chest Opening Pose

Learn + Practice

Learn before lifting pelvis in Explore; before Salamba Sarvangasana and its relatives

Linked Poses

Paschima Namaskara, Ratniprishthaka Vakrasana, Salamba Sarvangasana

Safety Factors

Use care with rotator cuff injury and shoulder restriction

Prepare

- Measure shoulder-width loop in strap, *I a*
- Set strap beside mat, within easy reach

Enter

- Lie on back, legs bent, feet hip width apart
- Bring one arm through strap loop, placing loop just above elbow, *I b*
- Pressing into feet, exhale to lift pelvis slightly off floor
- Pass looped strap under pelvis, behind torso and thread second arm through loop, *I c*
- Exhaling, lower pelvis to floor
- Descend bottom back ribs into strap
- Establish neutral cervical and lumbar curves
- Bend elbows 90°, bringing forearms vertical, *I d*
- Turn palms to face head, externally rotating forearms, *I e*
- Without lifting bottom ribs, and keeping 90° elbow bend, externally rotate upper arms, moving hands away from each other, *I f*
- Continue externally rotating arms until thumbs touch floor, *I g*

Sustain

- Maintain 90° elbow bend; do not bend or straighten arms to lower hands, *I h*
- Descend back ribs into strap and floor as symmetrically as possible
- Anchor top shoulder blades and extend inner shoulder blades toward pelvis
- Lengthen from armpits to inner elbows
- Equalize rotation in each arm; reducing degree on more extreme side, *I i*
- Broaden across collarbones, lifting them away from upper ribs to open upper chest, *I j*
- Reduce unnecessary effort in the abdomen

Exit

- Hold 10-15 breaths
- Inhaling, return to neutral arm rotation, forearms vertical
- Pressing into feet, lift pelvis and unthread arms from strap
- Descend pelvis and rest arms beside torso
- Roll to the right and press to seated

Challenge

1. Shoulder restriction
2. Ribs protrude
3. Throat restriction, head tilts backward

Response

1. Practice without the strap until there is a little more ease. Do not force rotation, if necessary support wrists/forearms with bolsters or blocks, *I k*. Lengthen humeri and draw shoulder blades against outer back rib cage, so that rotation involves shoulder structure more completely.
2. If strap is too tight it will not allow ribs to descend, so loosen the strap enough to accommodate the torso. Reduce external arm rotation until ribs descend.
3. Support head with folded blanket(s) until forehead slopes down toward nose, *I l*.

❀ *When lifting pelvis in later variations of Setu Bandha Sarvangasana, support shoulders, not head.*

Before lifting the pelvis into Chatush Padasana or Setu Bandha Sarvangasana, some opening through the upper chest and shoulders is helpful. Antaramsa is the space within the chest cavity, which can experienced as infinite though it is finite. In this pose, let consciousness broaden within.

Contact Points

Feet, back pelvis, back ribs, shoulder blades, back of humeri, thumbs, back of skull

External Supports

Mat, strap
Blanket, strap, sandbags

Essence of Form

Knee, hip, and elbow flexion; legs neutrally rotated, arms external

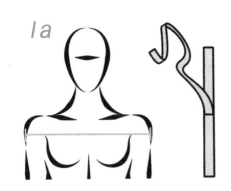
I a

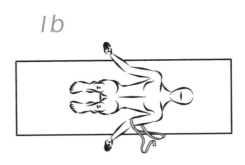
I b

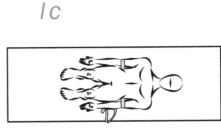
I c

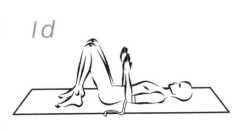
I d

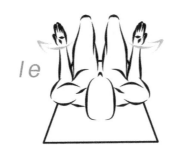
I e

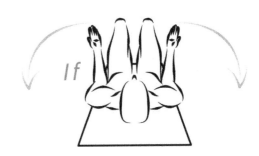
I f

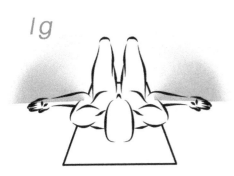
I g

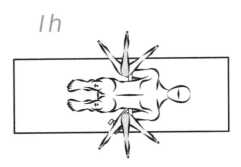
I h

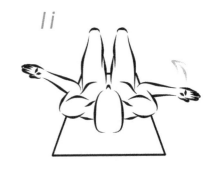
I i

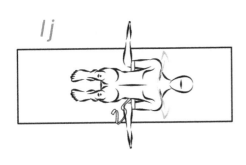
I j

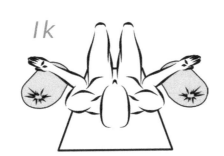
I k

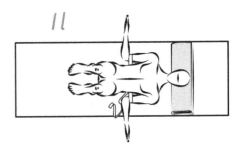
I l

Chatush Padasana
Joining of Four Limbs Pose

Explore

Learn + Practice

Learn before active and deep Back Bends; before supported variations and Inversions

Linked Poses

Setu Bandha Sarvangasana, Ustrasana, Dhanurasana

Safety Factors

Use care with lower back strain, neck and shoulder injury/restriction

Prepare

- Prepare two looped straps, each loop 8"-12"
- Set block beside mat, within easy reach

Enter

- Lie on back with the legs bent
- Feet hip width apart, heels 2-3" from sitting bones
- Bring strap loops around ankles, ensuring buckles do not touch skin, *II a*
- Place block between knees and hold symmetrically, *II b*
- Extend arms beside torso, reaching fingertips toward heels
- Turn palms downward, internally rotating arms to widen between shoulder blades
- Catch loops with fingertips and externally rotate upper arms, turning palms upward, *II c*
- Without losing block contact and holding straps, resist heels and shoulders away from each other in all directions, *II d*
- Keeping expansive action, press big toe mounds and upper shoulders into floor
- Gather front iliums and soften pubis inward
- Exhaling, lift pelvis to capacity, *II e*

Sustain

- Maintain big toe mound pressure into floor and spread toes laterally
- Descend pubis and deepen groins as outer hips lift
- Draw heels toward pelvis, toning hamstrings and buttocks 30-50%, *II f*
- Resist upper tibias backward
- Descending upper femurs, lengthen back femurs away from back pelvis, *II g*
- Extending through arms, lift armpit chest
- Gradually walk hands along straps toward ankles to capacity
- Without turning the head, soften the face, throat, and back of neck

Exit

- Hold for 10-15 breaths
- Keeping block pressure, exhale to lower pelvis, leading with pubis and ascending outer hips
- Rest and repeat 2-5 times
- Remove block and straps
- Once finished, bend legs and roll to the right, pressing hands into floor and come to seated

❁ *Once familiar, remove straps and catch ankles with hands when lifting pelvis in Enter, II h*

Challenge

1. Knee pain
2. Lumbar discomfort
3. Neck strain, cervical curve flattens

Response

1. Elevate heels on folded mat, *II i*. Slightly untuck pelvis. Draw heels toward pelvis to activate hamstrings, but keep tibias vertical — walk shoulders toward feet, not the other way around. Practice *Supta Virasana* and *Anjaneyasana* to release quadriceps.
2. Strap big toes toward each other before placing block. Spread toes away from strap, *II j*. Tie straps around each thigh, with strap ends circling from outer thighs across front thighs to back thighs. Press strap ends down with heels, pulling inner thighs downward as pelvis lifts, *II k. See Response 1.*
3. Support upper arms with folded blankets. Use enough height that once pelvis is lifted, neck flexion does not flatten cervical curve, *II l*. Without lifting chin, gently press occiput directly into floor, drawing cervical curve inward.

hatush Padasana is both a pose of joining and dividing — as the hands and ankles connect, they provide an anchor away from which to expand. This pose creates dynamic tension that develops stability for later, deeper Back Bends.

Contact Points

Feet, back pelvis, back of humeri, shoulders, back of skull

External Supports

Mat, block
Blanket, blocks, straps

Essence of Form

Neck and knee flexion; hip, torso, and arm extension; legs internally rotated, arms external

II a

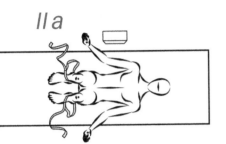

II b

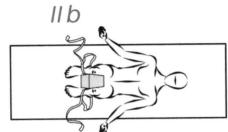

II c

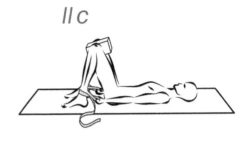

II d

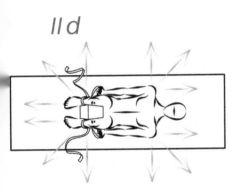

II e

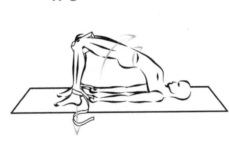

II f

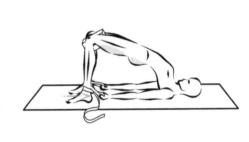

II g

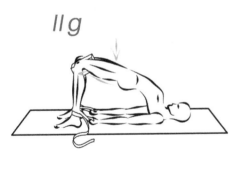

II h

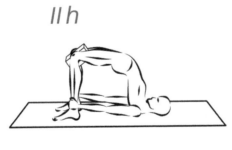

II i

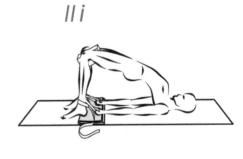

II j

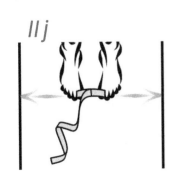

II k

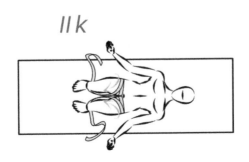

II l

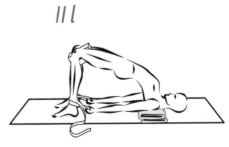

Learn + Practice

Learn early, as capacity allows. Include in most Restorative sequences and as a finishing pose

Linked Poses

Chatush Padasana, Salamba Sarvangasana, Back Bending Poses

Safety Factors

As for Explore; keep feet below pelvis during menstruation, practice moderately in therapeutic applications

Prepare

- Short end of mat to wall
- Place 2 blocks at wall, one on its face and one on its side; both laterally, *III a*
- Have strap and a third block within reach

Enter

- Strap upper thighs 1" below greater trochanters
- Lie on back, sitting bones 2-3' from wall (less than a full leg's length), *III b*
- Legs bent, feet parallel and hip-width apart
- Gathering front iliums, resist heels laterally
- Soften pubis skin in and up
- Bend elbows 90°, hugging elbows into side body
- Pressing elbows and big toe mounds into floor, lift pelvis and roll onto upper shoulders
- Stabilizing upper shoulder blades, place block lengthwise vertically under sacrum, *III c*
- With buttocks toned, rest sacrum on block
- Keeping upper shoulder blades and sacrum stable, extend legs, resting heels on blocks and pressing feet to wall, *III d*

Sustain

- Engage *Tadasana* actions in legs and pelvis
- Continue gathering front iliums, resisting heels laterally, and softening pubis skin
- Descend and widen inner back femurs, internally rotating thighs
- Without externally rotating thighs, keep buttocks toned throughout
- Roll the back armpits forward while softly lifting the chest away from the pubis
- Broaden collarbones away from sternum
- Head neutral, chin neither lifted nor tucked

Exit

- Stabilize sacrum on block
- With sacrum stable, bend legs one at a time and rest feet flat on floor
- Without externally rotating legs, press into feet and lift pelvis off block
- Remove block and slowly lower pelvis to floor
- Rest until pelvis neutralizes, then roll to the right and press into hands to seated

Challenge

1. Lumbar discomfort
2. Chest collapse

Response

1. Use wider and lower pelvic supports, *III e*. Lower height incrementally when *Exiting*, resting at each height, *III f*. Counter pose with forward-bending *Sukhasana*, forehead supported on wall, chair, or blocks, *III g*.
2. *Prepare + Enter* closer to wall. Pin shoulder blades to mat before straightening legs. Do not walk shoulders away from wall; rather, lift chest as legs straighten, *III h*. Place a rolled cloth lengthwise in thoracic spine, *III i*.

ॐ *Can also be practiced with lengthwise bolster, III j. Set bolster 1.5-2' from wall and sit on bolster. Lie back so that bolster's upper end supports mid-thoracic spine, and shoulders descend to floor. Exit by bending legs and resting feet on bolster, then either sliding back off bolster or rolling to the right, III k-l*

Setu Bandha Sarvangasana is an essential Restorative Back Bend that lengthens the anterior chain, rests the heart and abdominal organs, soothes the nervous system, and resets the sacrum. It may help relieve back pain and is an ideal counter pose to Forward Bends and Twists.

Contact Points

Feet, back pelvis, shoulders, back of skull

External Supports

Mat, wall, folded blanket, 3-4 blocks, Straps, rolled mat, bolsters, blankets

Essence of Form

Leg, hip, and torso extension, neck flexion; legs internally rotated, arms neutral

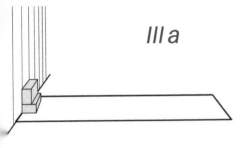

III a

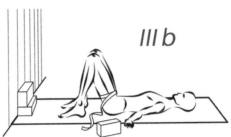

III b

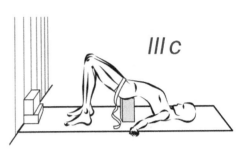

III c

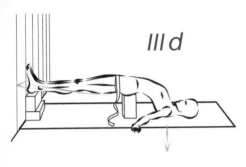

III d

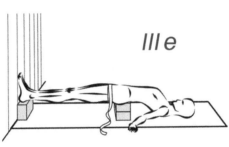

III e

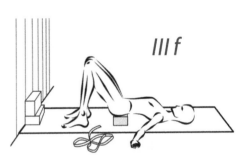

III f

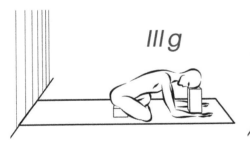

III g

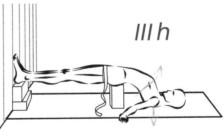

III h

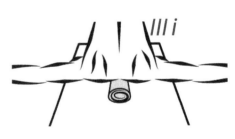

III i

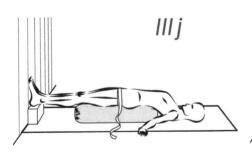

III j

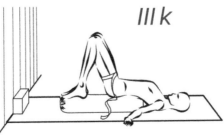

III k

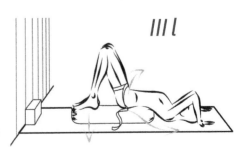

III l

Learn + Practice

Learn before deep Back Bends and Practice after Twists and Forward Bends

Linked Poses

Viparita Dandasana, Viparita Karani, Salamba Sarvangasana, Urdhva Dhanurasana

Safety Factors

Use care with lower back and neck injuries, SI joint instability, and during pregnancy

Prepare

- Short end of mat to wall
- Place a chair on mat, against wall
- Set folded blanket(s) 2-3' from chair lip, *IV a*
- Have a strap and two blocks nearby

Enter

- Lie down on mat, shoulders on blanket
- Place feet on chair lip, *IV b*
- Tie strap around upper thighs, holding legs in internal rotation
- Bend elbows 90° and anchor humeri
- Pressing down through feet and elbows, lift pelvis on exhalation
- Stabilize upper shoulder blades
- With shoulder blades anchored, keep pelvis lifted and place blocks, one block flat and lengthwise, second block vertical, *IV c*
- Exhaling, rest sacrum on block
- Once pelvis is stable, extend legs, resting calves and heels on chair seat, *IV d*

ॐ *Place base block lengthwise to prevent top block from tipping if adjusted, IV e*

Sustain

- Extend inner legs from sacrum through inner groins to big toe mounds, *IV f*
- Gather front iliums and resist heels laterally
- Soften pubis skin inward and upward
- Descend inner femurs and soften groins
- Release shoulders heavily into blanket
- Keep buttocks toned throughout
- Continually soften pelvic/abdominal contents

Exit

- Stabilize sacrum on block
- Bending legs, bring feet to chair lip
- Pressing feet into chair lip, lift pelvis and remove top block
- With pelvis lifted, turn bottom block laterally
- Lower pelvis, resting it on bottom block, *IV g*
- Rest here until pelvis and lower back sensations neutralize
- Lift pelvis again and remove block
- Lower pelvis to floor and rest for 5-10 breaths
- Roll to the right and press to seated

Challenge

1. Unstable block or its edge digs into sacrum
2. Inability to lift pelvis sufficiently
3. Neck flexion too extreme
4. Lumbar instability after *Exiting*

Response

1. Ensure block is not tipped, and that its base is flush. Adjust block so that its edge does not dig directly into upper sacrum. Pad block with mat remnant; which also adds stability. Move block slightly away from top pelvis.
2. *Enter* closer to chair. Leverage is more difficult when too far from the chair. Press feet down toward floor, not toward wall.
3. *Prepare + Enter* with more folded blankets under shoulders to lift shoulder girdle and reduce neck flexion, *IV h*.
4. Pause at *IV g*. Without lifting pelvis, maintain block contact while engaging legs and pelvis as though lifting. Maintain engagement for 5 breaths, then release engagement. Repeat 3-5 times before removing each block. Review transverse abdominus actions from *Supta Tadasana*, *Nourish*.

In this more extreme variation of Setu Bandha Sarvangasana, maximum elevation of the pelvis accentuates the Inversion. Here, a chair is used not only to support the feet in the pose, but also to help create leverage in lifting the pelvis. Its effects are similar to Nourish, but more profound.

Contact Points

Heels, sacrum, top of shoulders, back of skull

External Supports

Mat, wall, Chair, 2 blocks, strap, blankets
Additional blankets, mat remnant

Essence of Form

Leg, hip, and torso extension, neck flexion; legs internally rotated, arms passively external

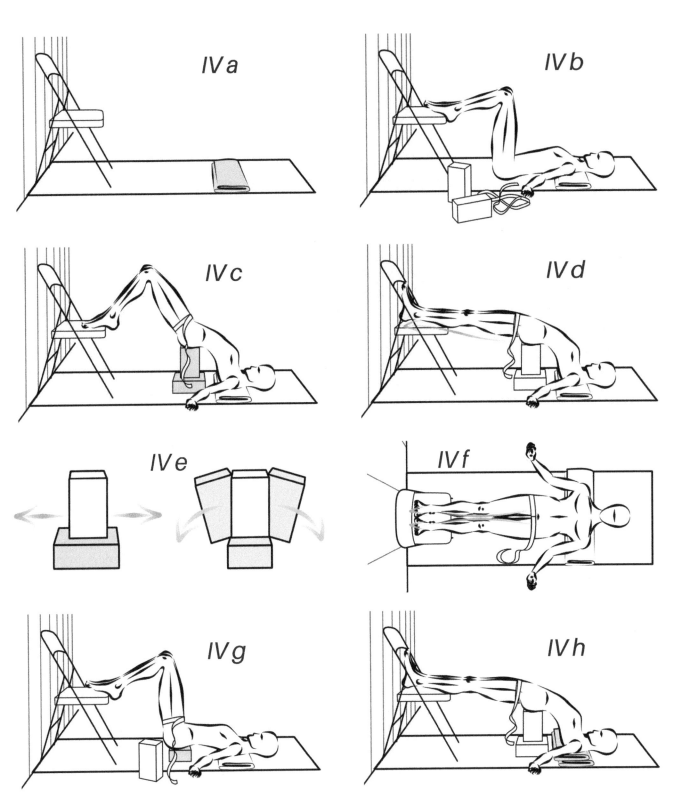

Urdhva Prasarita Padasana
Inverted Leg Extension

Learn + Practice

Learn early, prepares hamstrings at beginning of practice and establishes leg + pelvis actions

Linked Poses

Dandasana, Ardha Uttanasana, Supta Padangusthasana A, Viparita Karani

Safety Factors

Lower back strain, hamstring injury

Prepare

- Place folded blanket at mat's head end
- Keep strap within reach, *Ia*

Enter

- Lie on the back with legs bent, feet hip width apart, *Ib*
- Establish neutral spinal curves
- Rest femurs into pelvis, away from front iliums
- Evenly balance weight across back pelvis
- Gathering front iliums, draw pubis in and up
- Exhaling, lift feet off floor
- With legs bent, loop strap across soles of feet, *Ic*
- Hold strap ends in each hand
- Draw humeri into floor and hug elbows inward
- Pin upper outer shoulder blades to floor
- Keeping legs bent move upper femurs away from torso, until back pelvis descends fully, *Id*
- Pressing back pelvis into floor, lead with upper inner femurs as legs extend on exhalation
- Lengthen legs fully at 90° from torso, not closer, keeping neutral lumbar curve with feet directly above pelvis, *Ie*

Sustain

- Descend sacrum, continually increasing contact against floor through back pelvis
- Draw L4 + L5 away from floor
- Press up equally through 4 corners of each foot, planes of soles parallel to ceiling
- Broaden soles of feet, spreading toes
- Gathering front iliums, resist heels laterally
- Maximize inner thigh length from pubis to big toe mounds
- Soften behind pubis and draw pubis in and up
- Descend forehead skin towards the nose
- Soften the face, throat, and back of neck

Exit

- Hold 10-15 breaths
- Exhaling, bend both legs and lower feet to floor, re-establishing neutral breath and spine
- Set strap aside and rest arms beside torso, palms facing upward
- Rest for a few breaths and observe changes
- Roll to the right press into hands to seated

Challenge

1. Pelvis lifts and lumbar flattens
2. Legs do not fully extend
3. Groins bind
4. Pushing action is not clear

Response

1. Lumbar curve may contact floor, but should be less than back pelvis contact. Move legs away from torso when extending to open angle between legs and torso and relieve hamstring strain, *If*. Support back pelvis with folded blanket or support lumbar curve, *Ig-h*. Practice *Nourish* and/or *Supta Padangusthasana A* first.
2. Place a second, large looped strap around upper femurs. Have a partner pull on both ends of loop while pressing feet into back femurs, providing resistance. Extend legs by pressing femurs into partner's resistance, *Ii-j. See also Response 1 and Nourish*.
3. *See Response 2 and Nourish.*
4. Pull gently on strap, making back pelvis heavier. Press the feet up into this resistance. *See also Response 2.*

Urdhva Prasarita Padasana lengthens the hamstrings and stabilizes the back pelvis, in a dynamic relationship. It can be used as either a warm-up or cool-down pose, helping to reduce leg and ankle swelling and inflammation while increasing pelvic circulation.

Feet, back pelvis, back ribcage, upper arm bones, back of skull

Mat, blanket, strap
Additional strap, assistant

Leg extension, hip and elbow flexion; legs slightly internally rotated, arms neutral

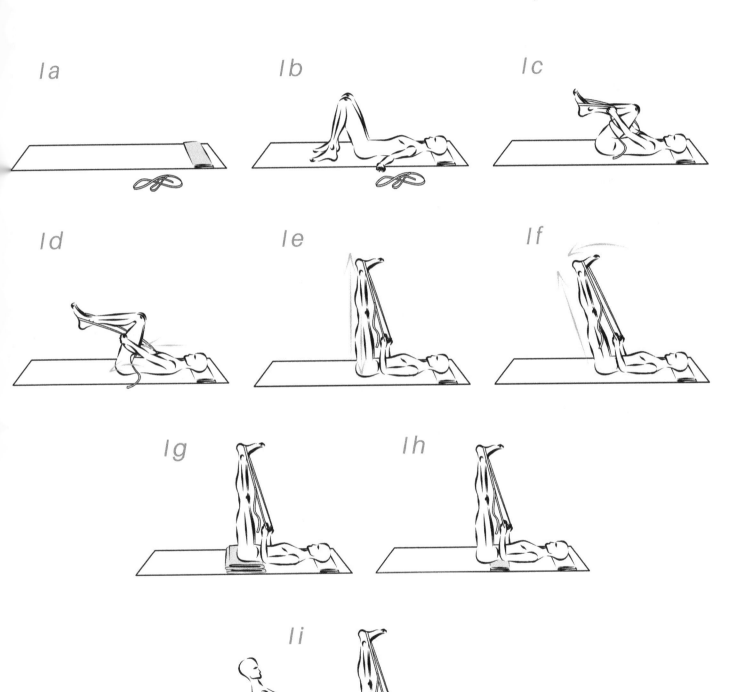

I a

I b

I c

I d

I e

I f

I g

I h

I i

Learn + Practice

*Learn early, can be practiced
near the beginning or
end of sequences*

Linked Poses

*Dandasana, Ardha Uttanasana,
Supta Padangusthasana A,
Viparita Karani*

Safety Factors

*Use care with hamstring
injury; support lumbar curve
for lower back injury*

Prepare

- Place mat's short end to wall
- Set folded blanket a torso's
  length from wall
- Have tightly rolled thin mat
  and 4 straps nearby

Enter

- Sit with left side facing the wall
  in *Dandasana*, buttocks near
  the mat's long edge, *II a*
- Manually internally rotate thighs
- Place tightly rolled mat between
  legs, top end close to perineum
- Strap legs at four levels: 1"
  below greater trochanters, 2"
  above knees, widest part of
  calf, 2" above ankles, *II b*
- Lean rightward onto right
  hand and scoot sitting bones
  toward wall, bringing outer
  side of right pelvis against
  the floor, close to wall, *II c*
- Still leaning to the right, swing legs
  up wall and roll onto back, *II d*
- Adjust torso, bringing spine
  perpendicular to wall and
  ensure legs are vertical, *II e*
- Rest arms beside torso,
  palms facing upward

Sustain

- Balance weight equally
  across back pelvis
- Contact sitting bones
  symmetrically against wall
- Push feet away from back pelvis,
  continually extending legs
- Apply *Tadasana +
  Dandasana* leg actions
- Where strap contact is felt less,
  gently press outward; where
  strap contact is felt more,
  recede away from contact
- Once overall strap pressure is
  equal, move upper thighs away
  from front of straps and more
  deeply into back of straps
- Keeping balanced strap
  pressure, gradually reduce
  effort in extending legs
- Descend forehead skin
  towards the nose
- Soften the face, throat,
  and back of neck

Exit

- Hold 5-15 minutes
- Exhaling, loosen straps
  and remove rolled mat
- Bend both legs and roll to
  the right on exhalation
- Pressing into hands,
  inhale to seated

Challenge

1. Pelvis lifts and lumbar flattens
2. Legs do not fully extend
3. Ankle fatigue
4. Numbness/tingling in feet

Response

1. Move away from wall until back
   pelvis descends fully and lumbar
   spine no longer presses heavily
   into floor. Fill gap between wall
   and sitting bones with blocks, *II f*.
2. Roll stick within mat and use
   additional strap at mid-thigh.
   Set block atop soles of feet
   and place weighted bag on
   block, *II g*. Receive weight into
   legs and pelvis, while pushing
   feet up into weighted block.
3. Use spacer between ankles.
   Strap around outer ankles.
   See Responses 1 + 2.
4. Loosen straps slightly if pressure
   is too great. Place folded
   blanket against wall for under
   pelvis and torso, *II h*. Bring legs
   to *Baddha Konasana* before
   Exiting, II i. See also Response 3.

s a Viparita Karani precursor, Urdhva Prasarita Padasana carries similar circulatory benefits and
a viable alternative when elevating the pelvis above the heart is contraindicated. This variation
ay also help reduce back, hip, and knee pain by correcting minor leg misalignments.

Contact Points

Back pelvis, back ribs,
shoulder blades, humeri,
back of skull, legs

External Supports

2 mats, 4 straps, blanket
Block, sandbag

Essence of Form

*Hip flexion, leg extension;
legs in slight internal rotation,
arms slightly external*

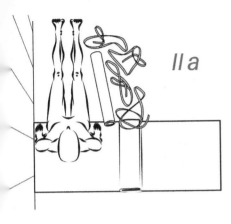

II a

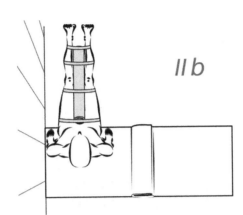

II b

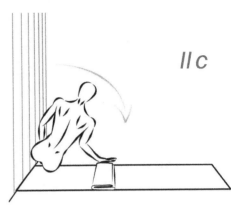

II c

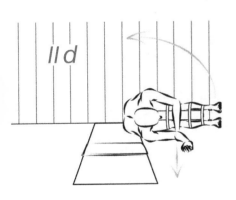

II d

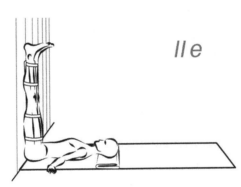

II e

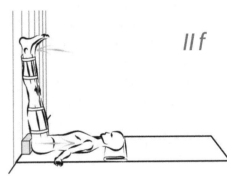

II f

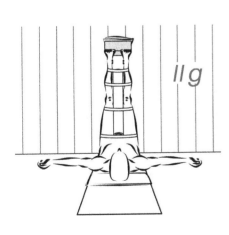

II g

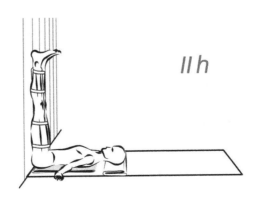

II h

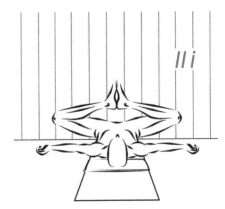

II i

Viparita Karani
Inverted Lake

Nourish

Learn + Practice

Learn after Urdhva Prasarita Padasana, practice at the end of sequences

Linked Poses

Urdhva Prasarita Padasana, Setu Bandha Sarvangasana, Salamba Sarvangasana

Safety Factors

Practice Explore for circulatory conditions; use lengthwise bolster when menstruating

Prepare

- Set bolster laterally, parallel to wall, with a 4-6" gap between wall and bolster, *III a*
- Have a strap nearby

Enter

- Tie strap around upper thighs, 1" below greater trochanters
- Sit on bolster's end, left side of torso toward wall, *III b*
- Lean rightward onto right hand, slide right side hip under torso and onto bolster's end, bringing buttocks against wall, *III c*
- Exhaling, roll onto back and swing legs up on wall
- Bending the legs, press feet into wall
- Lift pelvis to adjust placement, bringing spine perpendicular to wall and legs vertical
- Exhaling, lower pelvis into space between wall and bolster
- Descend pubis and rest buttocks on wall
- Settle shoulders fully, resting arms beside torso with palms facing upward, *III d*

🕉 *Set bolster lengthwise when menstruating, supporting head and torso above pelvis, III e*

Sustain

- Descending pelvis into gap between wall and bolster, extend legs away from back pelvis
- As pelvis descends, softly lift sternum
- Roll outer armpits up and forward, top shoulder skin down and backward
- Bring pubis, anterior pelvic rims, and bottom front ribs in line parallel to floor
- Soften abdominal wall, and release tension in the pelvic/abdominal cavity
- Breathe freely and naturally
- Soften the senses and sense organs
- Ensure skull does not tilt backward and rest brain toward back of skull

Exit

- Rest for 10-20 minutes
- Loosen strap around thighs
- Bring legs to *Baddha Konasana* and rest for up to an additional 5 minutes, *III f*
- Use hands to gather legs toward mid line
- Roll to the right and press into hands to seated
- Use care when rolling off the bolster

Challenge

1. Pelvis slides off bolster in *Enter*
2. Legs bend; ankle discomfort
3. Tingling or numbness in legs or feet
4. Chest collapse; neck strain

Response

1. Set bolster further from wall. Ensure pelvis is beyond bolster before swinging legs up.
2. *See Response 3 and Responses 2 + 3 in Explore.*
3. Bring legs to *Baddha Konasana*, *III f*, until sensation dissipates, then re-extend legs. If problem persists, practice with legs bent:

- Set chair on mat, bolster beside mat, *III g*
- Lie down with buttocks near chair seat
- Press feet into chair seat and elevate pelvis, bringing bolster under pelvis lengthwise, *III h*
- Settle pelvis and rest calves on chair, *III i*

4. Descend pelvis over bolster, into gap between bolster and wall, *III j*. Increase shoulder and/or pelvic height with folded blankets, *III k-l*.

An excellent calming and finishing pose, Viparita Karani introduces a mild Inversion and is Salamba Sarvangasana relative. It settles the nervous system, eases the breath, and helps reduce swelling in the legs by aiding venous return. It may also aid some digestive problems.

Contact Points

Back of skull, upper shoulder blades, back pelvis, back of legs

External Supports

Wall, bolster, strap Blankets, rolled mat, additional straps, chair

Essence of Form

Leg extension with hip flexion, Torso extension, neck flexion; legs in slight internal rotation, arms slightly external

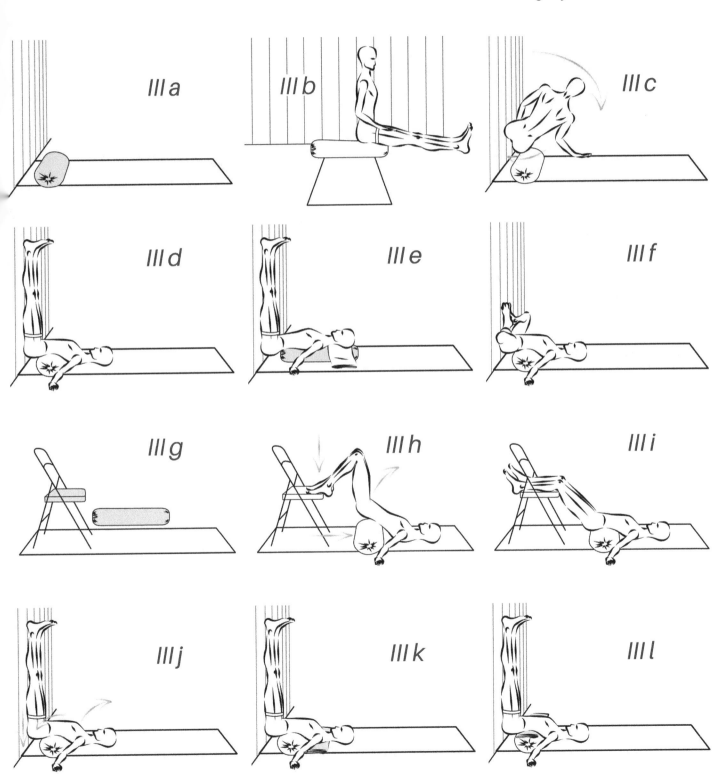

Viparita Karani
Inverted Lake

Learn + Practice

*After Urdhva Prasarita Padasana;
use as a finishing pose*

Linked Poses

*Urdhva Prasarita Padasana,
Setu Bandha Sarvangasana,
Salamba Sarvangasana*

Safety Factors

*Do not practice while
menstruating, use lower block if
neck flexion is contraindicated*

Prepare

· Set block beside mat

Enter

· Lie on back, legs bent, feet
  hip-width apart, *IV a*
· Pressing into feet, exhale
  and lift pelvis, *IV b*
· Stabilizing shoulder blades and
  without turning head, stand block
  on end under upper sacrum
· Exhaling, settle pelvis on block,
  resting on as much of the block's
  surface as possible, *IV c*
· Keeping back pelvis on
  block, and without tucking
  pelvis, raise legs with knees
  bent (hold block with hands
  for added stability, *IV d*)
· Descending pubis and lifting
  chest, extend legs vertically,
  feet hip-width apart
· Once legs are extended and
  block is stable, rest arms beside
  torso, palms facing upward, *IV e*

🕉 *Alternatively, bring hands to the
back pelvis and instead of using
a block, support the pelvis on
the hands and forearms, IV f*

Sustain

· Gather front iliums and
  resist heels laterally
· Soften the space between
  pubis and sacrum
· Broaden back pelvis
  as sacrum settles
· Descending bottom pelvis,
  bring pelvic floor diaphragm
  perpendicular to floor
· Spread toes and widen
  across back thighs
· Soften and deepen groins,
  extending inner legs from
  groins to big toe mounds
· Descend tops of shoulders,
  expanding collarbones
  away from top front ribs

Exit

· Stabilize block with hands
· Keeping legs elevated,
  exhale and bend legs,
  lowering feet to floor
· Pressing into feet, elevate
  pelvis and turn block
  laterally and on its face
· Rest pelvis on lowered block
  for 10-20 breaths, *IV g*
· Lift pelvis again and remove
  block, then lower pelvis to floor
· Let sensations dissipate
  before rolling to the right
  and pressing to seated

Challenge

1. Block tips or is unstable
2. Block digs into upper sacrum
3. Chest collapses
4. Legs shake

Response

1. Block base is too close to
   shoulders, causing instability.
   Move block base away
   from shoulders. Block may
   also tip if pelvis tucks. Using
   block's edge against upper
   sacrum as a fulcrum, descend
   mid and lower sacrum.
2. Rest pelvis on more of block's
   surface by untucking pelvis
   and descending lower pelvis,
   IV h. See Response 1.
3. Chest often collapses when
   pelvis tucks. Once sacrum
   descends into block fully, chest
   will lift. If more lift is required, use
   a rolled cloth between shoulder
   blades, *IV i,* or elevate shoulders
   on a folded blanket, *IV j.*
4. Leg shaking is normal after
   vigorous practice; maintain leg
   extension and reduce overall
   effort. Develop endurance
   over time. If shaking persists,
   strap legs or have an assistant
   apply weight to feet, *IV k-l.*

In this active variation of Viparita Karani, the leg engagement resets the sacrum and is an ideal counter pose to deep Back Bends and vigorous Standing Poses. Use in conjunction with Setu Bandha Sarvangasana and as a Salamba Sarvangasana alternative.

Contact Points

Back of skull, upper shoulder blades, sacrum Hands in IV #

External Supports

Mat, block
Blanket, additional block

Essence of Form

Leg and torso extension, hip and neck flexion; legs slightly internally rotated, arms external

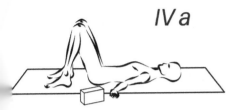
IVa

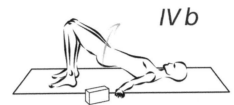
IVb

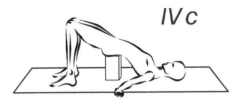
IVc

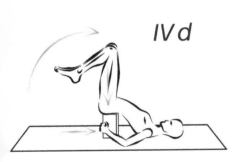
IVd

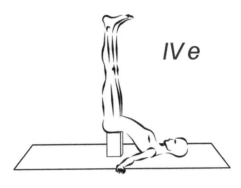
IVe

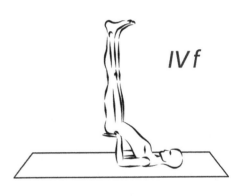
IVf

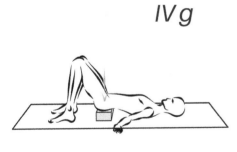
IVg

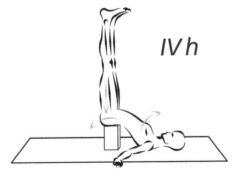
IVh

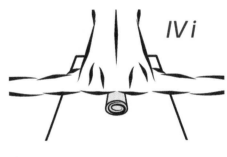
IVi

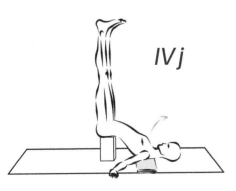
IVj

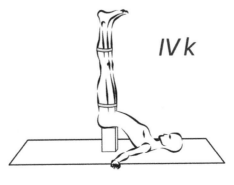
IVk

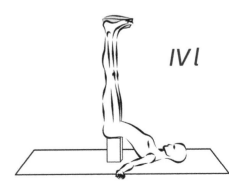
IVl

Ratniprishthaka Vakrasana
Bent-Elbow Shoulder Opener

Simplify

Learn + Practice

Well before considering full Sarvangasana; after Purvottanasana, Simplify

Linked Poses

Paschima Namaskara, Setu Bandha Sarvangasana, Salamba Sarvangasana,

Safety Factors

Use care with shoulder, elbow, or wrist injury

Prepare

- Mat's short end to wall
- Place chair on mat, chair back against wall

Enter

- Sit on edge of chair seat, *l a*
- Place feet forward of knees, 6-8"
- Feet and thighs hip-width apart
- Foot mid lines parallel
- Gather front iliums and soften pubis inward
- Resist heels and greater trochanters laterally
- Place hands to chair seat on either side of pelvis, fingers pointing outward, *l b*
- Pressing into hands, lift pelvis and shift forward just enough to clear the chair, *l c*
- Staying close to chair lip, lift the chest, and bend elbows to descend pelvis on exhalation, *l d*
- Draw elbows toward each other as pelvis descends
- Without collapsing chest lower to capacity
- If the pelvis reaches floor, extend legs to *Dandasana*, *l e*
- Keep the chin and gaze level without turning the head

Sustain

- Gather front iliums and soften pubis inward
- Anchor big toe mounds and spread toes, widening soles of feet
- Resist lower femurs inward while resisting heels and upper femurs outward
- Draw tibia heads back as legs bend
- Deepen and release the inner groins
- Soften sternum inward and lengthen top and bottom sternum away from each other
- Press heads of upper arm bones laterally
- Extend from inner elbows to back armpits
- Widen between shoulder blades
- Roll front shoulder skin over the shoulders toward the back

Exit

- Pressing into hands and feet, extend arms to lift pelvis and sit on chair
- Rest and repeat up to 5 times
- Gradually increase length of holds

Challenge

1. Legs collapse
2. Pelvis moves too far from chair, *l*
3. Elbows fall outward
4. Shoulders protract, or shoulder pain

Response

1. For outward collapse, squeeze block between thighs. For inward collapse, strap lower femurs and resist outward.
2. Walk feet back slightly. Resist pelvis backward to prevent forward movement. Lift chest before and while descending pelvis; do not descend as far.
3. Strap the upper arms, just above elbows. Draw elbows away from the strap until no longer necessary.
4. Practice shoulder jacket. Pass strap across bottom shoulder blades, forward under armpits, over front shoulders, and across the back, *l g-j*. Tie a stick to the strap ends and push downward, *l k*. Strap around humerus heads and resist outward, *l l*. Transfer this action to *Salamba Sarvangasana*.

Salamba Sarvangasana requires deep posterior shoulder extension. This shoulder opener increases shoulder mobility while bearing weight, which develops both range of motion and stability in preparation for Shoulderstand. It may also reduce minor neck and upper back pain.

Contact Points

Feet, hands

External Supports

Chair
Block, strap, stick

Essence of Form

Posterior arm extension, elbow flexion; ams externally rotated, legs neutral

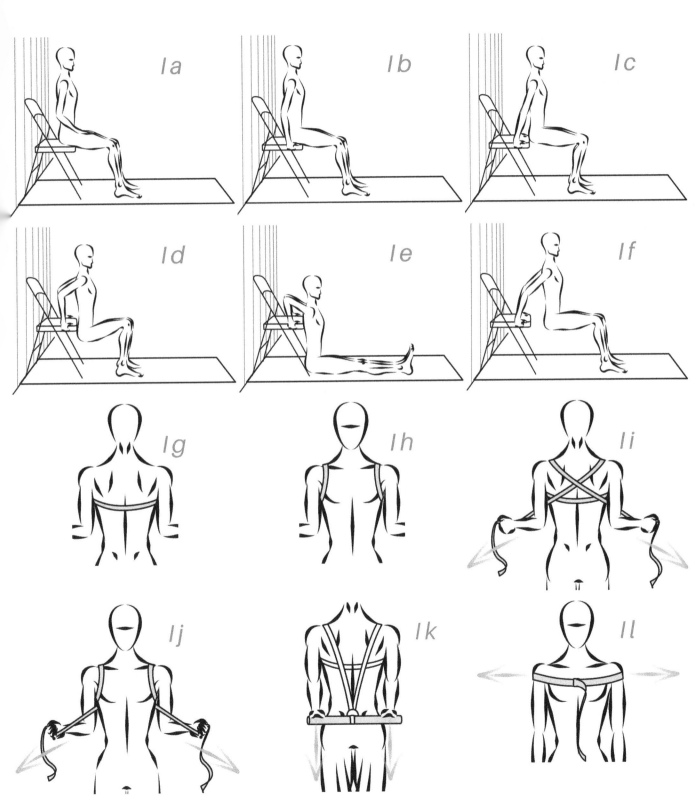

I a

I b

I c

I d

I e

I f

I g

I h

I i

I j

I k

I l

Before considering full Sarvangasana, after learning Viparita Karani

Purvottanasana, Setu Bandha Sarvangasana, Salamba Sarvangasana

Neck or shoulder injury, eye pressure, glaucoma, high or low blood pressure

Prepare

- Place a chair on mat, both against wall
- Stack 2-4 wide-fold blankets 6-8″ from chair
- Ensure blanket's folded edges face away from wall, *II a*
- Measure belt's loop shoulder-width
- Set strap and block beside mat

Enter

- Lie down with shoulders 2″ from blanket edges, head on mat, *II b*
- Step feet on chair, chair lip at back of arch, heels off chair's edge
- Place block between lower thighs, *II c*
- Pressing feet into chair, lift pelvis and thread arms through strap, *II d*
- With strap above elbows, press upper arms down into blankets from shoulders to elbows
- Bend elbows 90°, palms facing each other with fingers extended, *II e*
- Pressing feet and upper arm bones downward, exhale and raise pelvis toward the ceiling, *II f*

Sustain

- Anchor big toe mounds, extending inner femurs away from pubis
- Gather front iliums and resist heels laterally
- Squeeze block to generate pelvic lift, lengthening from pubis to inner knees
- Lengthen inner elbows away from back armpits
- Roll inner elbows downward
- Widen outer shoulders and descend diagonally away from inner elbows
- Lift side rib cage away from floor and arms
- Soften throat and face
- Keep plane of face parallel to floor
- Do not turn the head

Exit

- Keeping elbows stable, lower pelvis on exhalation
- Rest for a few breaths and then lift pelvis just enough to unstrap arms
- Remove block from between thighs
- Roll to the right and press into the hands, coming to seated

Challenge

1. Pelvis lifts minimally
2. Shoulders slide off blankets
3. Shoulder pain
4. Neck strain
5. Lumbar pain

Response

1. Anchor shoulders and elbows more firmly, and push feet directly down into chair, not toward wall. Emphasize rib cage lift more, let pelvis follow.
2. *Enter* with shoulders further away from blanket edges. Use extra mat on top of blankets to prevent slide. *See also Response 1.*
3. Widen shoulder girdle before lifting pelvis (*as in Simplify, Response 4, II*). Extend arms, fully externally rotate, bringing outer shoulders to floor. Keep outer shoulders anchored and bend elbows.
4. Use more blankets. *Also see Response 3.*
5. Internally rotate thighs. Tuck pelvis while lifting. Minimally gather back iliums. *Enter* slightly further from chair.

This variation, which is halfway between Setu Bandha Sarvangasana and Salamba Sarvangasana, teaches pelvic lift and helps develop weight-bearing in the elbows — both of which can be challenging in full Shoulderstand once the shoulders are relatively free.

Contact Points

Back of skull, upper arms, shoulders, feet

External Supports

2-4 blankets, block, chair, strap

Essence of Form

Neck, elbow, and knee flexion, shoulder and hip extension; legs neutrally rotated, arms slightly external

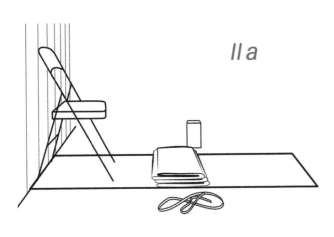

II a

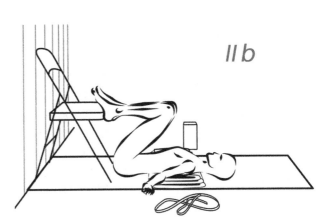

II b

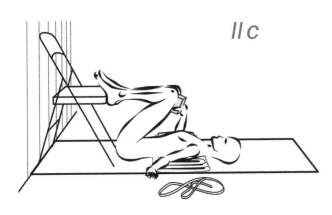

II c

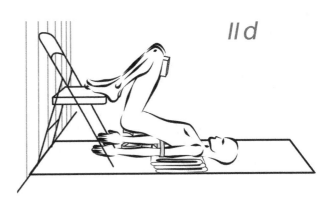

II d

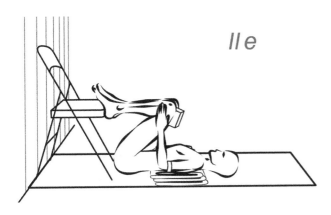

II e

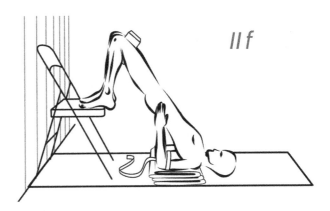

II f

Salamba Sarvangasana
Chair Shoulderstand

Learn + Practice

After learning Viparita Karani, before unsupported Sarvangasana

Linked Poses

Viparita Karani, Setu Bandha Sarvangasana, Salamba Sarvangasana

Safety Factors

Eye pressure, glaucoma, menstruation, excessively high or low blood pressure

Prepare

- Set chair on mat, away from wall
- Place 2-4 long-fold blankets in front of chair legs, folded edges away from chair

Enter

- Sit facing chair back
- Swing legs over top of chair's backrest, *III a*
- Holding chair back with hands, lift chest
- Without twisting torso or tilting head backward, lean back, *III b*
- Controlling descent with hands and calves on chair, lower shoulders to blankets, head to floor beyond blankets, *III c*
- Do not look for blankets/floor
- Once shoulders reach blankets, stabilize shoulders
- With shoulders stable, hold crossbar with palms up, *III d*
- Bring chair lip just below pelvic rims
- Descend back pelvis into chair seat and extend legs vertically atop pelvis, *III e*
- Do not turn the head
- Once familiar, strap upper thighs together before descending torso

Sustain

- Similar to *Explore*
- Broaden between shoulder blades
- Lift back armpits toward ceiling
- Soften neck and without lifting chin, draw cervical spine gently inward
- Soften sternum inward, lengthening top away from bottom sternum
- Bring sacral plate flat into chair seat
- Deepen front groins, softening pubis inward and toward sternum
- Extend inner legs from pubis to big toe mounds
- Widen feet, pulling little toes downward

Exit

- Bend legs, bringing feet to chair seat
- Stabilizing pelvis and shoulders, bring hands beside head, palms down, fingertips back, *III f*
- Pressing into feet and hands, lift pelvis and shoulders slightly, *III g*
- Without scraping pelvis on chair, scoot backward until pelvis rests on blankets
- Roll to the right and press to seated

Challenge

1. Pelvis slides off chair
2. Shoulders do not reach blankets
3. Chair pressure too intense, lumbar pain
4. Legs fall back or forward, groins bind

Response

1. Place sticky mat on chair seat, blanket on mat. Slide pelvis forward and use calves to control descent. *See Response 2.*
2. Use more blankets (or a bolster) and/or move them closer to chair. Slide pelvis slightly further back when descending. Use L5/S1 juncture as fulcrum.
3. Bending legs bring feet to chair back. Stabilizing chair with hands, lift and tuck pelvis, sliding back pelvis flesh toward feet. Re-descend pelvis. Pad chair with folded mat and blanket.
4. Descend sacrum evenly. Settle legs' weight into pelvis, extending legs out of back pelvis. Lengthen pubis toward chair back. Use a bolster behind thighs, *III h*.

Using a chair for support introduces the full Inversion with minimal effort to sustain the pose for a more restorative and rejuvenating effect. Salamba Sarvangasana is believed to balance hormones, increase circulation to the brain, decompress the pelvic organs, and restore vitality.

Contact Points

Back of skull, shoulders, pelvis

External Supports

Chair, 2-4 blankets
or bolster, strap
Mat remnant, additional blankets
Neck and hip flexion, torso

Essence of Form

and leg extension, shoulder
extension; legs neutrally
rotated, arms external

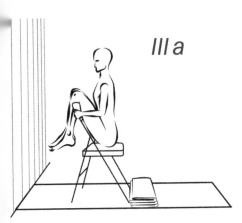

III a

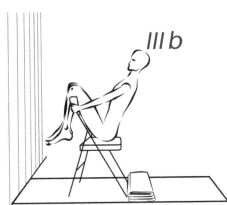

III b

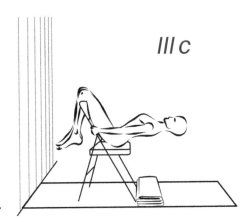

III c

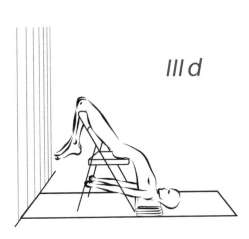

III d

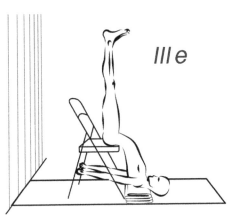

III e

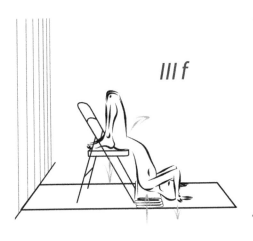

III f

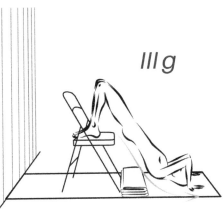

III g

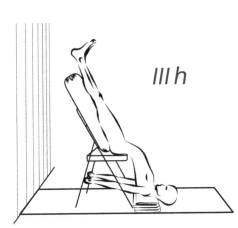

III h

Learn + Practice

After Nourish, before full Inversions; practice near the end of sequences, after Sirsasana

Linked Poses

Setu Bandha Sarvangasana, Paschima Namaskara, Gomukhasana (arms)

Safety Factors

Neck or shoulder injury, eye pressure, glaucoma menstruation, high or low blood pressure

Prepare

- Stack 4-6 blankets mid-mat, folded edges away from wall
- Fold mat's wall end over blankets, *IV a*, sandwiching blankets between mat layers
- Slide mat/blanket bundle near wall, folded edges 18-24" from wall, *IV b*
- Have a shoulder-width looped strap within reach

Enter

- Lie down on blanket/mat bundle, shoulders 2" from blankets' far edges, head off blankets on mat, *IV c*
- Ensure both shoulders are equidistant from blanket edges
- Place feet on wall, parallel and hip-width apart, legs bent
- Take strap around one arm
- Lift pelvis and loop strap around second arm, just above elbows, *IV d*
- Anchoring shoulders and elbows, press feet to wall, lifting torso and pelvis, *IV e*
- Adjust foot height so that tibias are horizontal, femurs vertical, legs bent 90°
- Bring hands to back ribcage, fingertips vertical, *IV f*

Sustain

- Same arm actions as *Simplify* + *Explore*
- Stack thighs, pelvis, and torso vertically
- Descending elbows, lift back ribs with hands
- Draw 7th cervical vertebra inward
- Without turning head, soften face and throat, keeping facial plane horizontal
- Continually lift pelvis away from wall
- Inner femurs long, upper femurs toward wall

🕉 *Once thighs and pelvis lift above shoulders with weight in the hands and elbows, keep pelvis away from wall and extend legs one at a time, IV g-h*

Exit

- Keeping shoulders and elbows stable, remove hands from back ribs
- Extending up through femurs, lower torso and pelvis
- Remove strap from elbows
- Roll to the right, press to seated

🕉 **Do not turn the head at any stage**

Challenge

1. C7 collapses, neck strain
2. Elbows lift
3. Torso is not vertical
4. Pelvis falls toward wall
5. Chest compression on *Exit*

Response

1. *Prepare* blankets in two parallel stacks, with a gap between them, *IV i*. Use more height.
2. Use more blankets to raise shoulders, bringing elbows and shoulders level. Place additional long-fold blanket or slant board under elbows for firm support.
3. *Prepare + Enter* closer to wall. Pelvis will not be on floor before lifting into pose. Anchor elbows more heavily. Pressing into feet and elbows, lift side ribs and bring pelvis as far from wall as possible. Keep femurs behind pelvis. *Enter* with a block between inner knees as for *Explore*.
4. Separate thighs slightly. Tuck tail bone, then return thighs toward each other. *See previous Responses.*
5. Do *Uttanasana* with the head supported until compression dissipates, *IV j*.

This classic pose has similar effects as the Nourish variation, but is more active. Using a wall to support the feet helps the pelvis stack vertically above the shoulders, bringing weight directly into the elbows. It is best to learn this variation under the guidance of an experienced teacher.

Contact Points

Shoulders, elbows, upper arm bones, back of skull, feet

External Supports

4-6 blankets, mat, wall, strap
Additional blankets,
slanted board, block(s)

Essence of Form

Elbow and neck flexion; shoulder, torso, and hip extension; legs slightly internally rotated, arms external

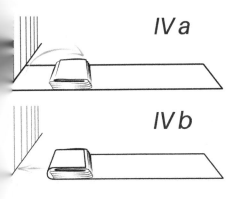
IV a

IV b

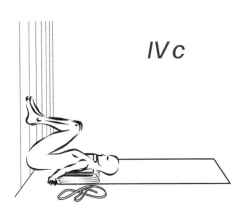
IV c

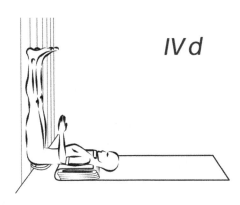
IV d

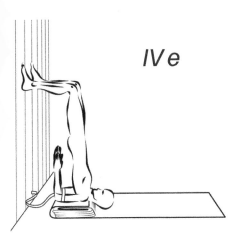
IV e

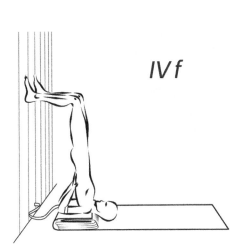
IV f

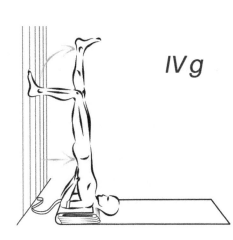
IV g

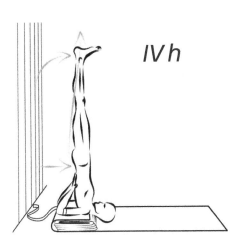
IV h

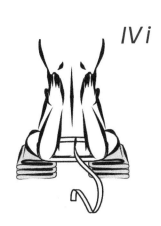
IV i

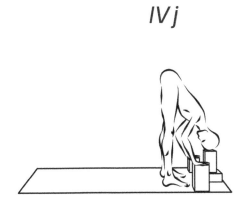
IV j

Learn + Practice

Can be learned at any point, practiced at the beginning or end of sequences, or between poses

Linked Poses

Supta Tadasana, Savasana, All Restorative Poses

Safety Factors

Use a bolster to elevate the torso for vertigo and after the third trimester if pregnant

Prepare

- Set mat away from walls and obstructions
- Place folded blanket on mat to support head
- Have a strap within reach

Enter

- Lie down on mat with head resting on folded blanket
- Lift feet off floor and loosely tie strap around lower thighs, about hip-width, *I a*
- Keep strap buckle away from skin, tail where it is unobtrusive
- Bring feet to floor, with the legs bent, feet and thighs parallel, hip-width apart, *I b*
- Have the feet close enough to pelvis for abdomen and groins to remain soft; but far enough away that the lumbar is neutral
- Without tucking pelvis, slide buttock flesh toward feet and away from mid line, *I c-d*
- Using hands, draw back body skin away from mid line and settle back ribs, *I e*
- Manually lift the head and slide skin at back of skull away from neck, *I f*
- Rest arms beside torso, 30-45°, turning palms upward

Sustain

- Settle feet and feel their weight resting into the floor
- Release feet and ankles away from lower legs
- Rest thighs into strap's support
- Settle pelvis, feeling its weight descend into the floor
- Receive thigh and femur weight into the pelvis
- Soften groins and abdomen
- Settle skull and back rib cage, letting them become heavy while releasing tension in the neck and chest
- Soften the throat, jaw, lips, tongue, eyes, and forehead skin
- Breathe softly, naturally, and consciously

Exit

- Rest for 5-30 minutes
- Gradually deepen the breath over 3-10 cycles, resting consciousness on the breath
- When ready, loosen and remove the strap
- Roll to the right and lie on the right side for 10-20 breaths
- Keeping the head heavy and initiating with the pelvis, press into the hands and inhale to seated

Challenge

1. Sense of anxiety or panic when eyes are closed
2. Discomfort after long holds at points of contact
3. Body temperature drops
4. Groin, thigh, or abdomen tension persists, lumbar flattens

Response

1. Keep the eyes open, but soften gaze. If in a safe environment, try using an eye pillow, but know that it can be removed and the eyes opened at any time.
2. *Prepare* with blankets on mat to pad the pelvis, rib cage, shoulder blades, and skull.
3. Cover torso and/or legs with blankets in *Enter*. Keep the breath moving through the nose.
4. Instead of tying the strap around the lower thighs, pass strap over front thighs, between the outer hips and ankles, around the ankles, and once again over the front thighs before buckling, *I g-h*. Once tied, walk feet away from pelvis to draw upper femurs away from front iliums, opening front groin and abdominal space.

Vishramastha Padartha, or Constructive Rest Pose, re-establishes neutral spinal curves, facilitating natural breath. Some practitioners may find more rest by supporting the legs with a strap. Resting in this stability may also help balance cerebral spinal fluid rhythm.

Contact Points

Feet, back pelvis, back rib cage, shoulder blades, backs of arms and hands, back of skull

External Supports

Blanket, strap
Additional blankets, eye pillow

Essence of Form

Hip and knee flexion; legs in neutral rotation, arms slightly external

Ia
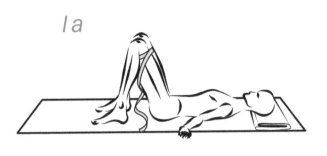

Ib
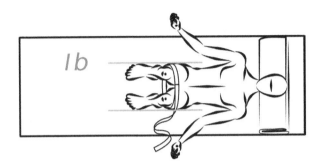

Ic
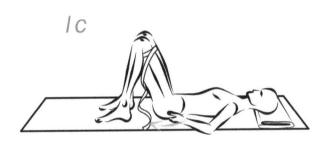

Id
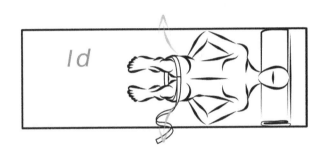

Ie
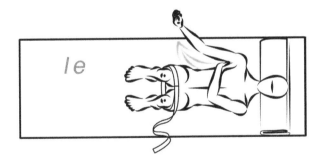

If
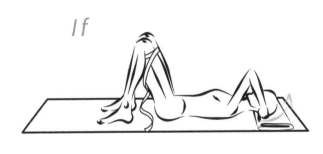

Ig
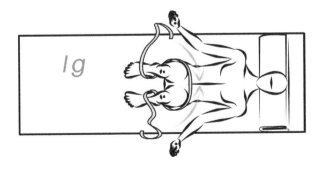

Ih
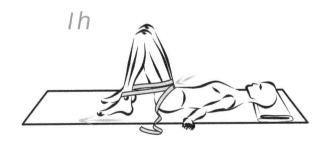

Janvakna Savasana
Bent-Leg Pose of Repose

Learn + Practice

Learn at any time, and practice at the end of sequences to finish

Linked Poses

Vishramastha Padartha, Supta Tadasana, Savasana

Safety Factors

As for Simplify; support torso with bolster if pregnant

Prepare

- Set mat away from walls and obstructions with folded blanket to support head
- Have a bolster and any additional props such as sandbags, eye pillows, extra blankets, etc, within reach

Enter

- Sit at mid-mat with legs bent
- Slide bolster under upper thighs, close to pelvis, *II a*
- Partially extend legs, resting thighs into bolster
- Descend heels to floor, walking them away from the bolster and pelvis
- If using weight on thighs, or covering legs with blanket, apply those props while seated
- Placing hands behind pelvis, use hands to gently lower torso and lie down, head supported by blanket, *II b*
- If desired, apply weight to shoulders, hands, and/ or forehead, or have an assistant do so
- Allow thighs to roll into passive external rotation, *II c*
- Repeat manual adjustments from *Simplify*

Sustain

- Continue all applicable actions from *Simplify*
- Settle the weight of both heels symmetrically
- Release calf muscles away from the backs of knees
- Soften the buttocks and release them away from the back ribs
- Passively descend the back rib cage
- Let go of unnecessary tension in the thighs, groins, and abdomen
- Gently broaden the chest on the first few inhalations, and then rest passively with that opening
- Feel the bones becoming heavy and release their weight into the floor/supports
- Allow the breath to become smooth and subtle
- Follow the breath to draw consciousness deeper into body experience

Exit

- Rest for 5-30 minutes
- *Exit* as for *Simplify*, sliding weights off to the sides and lifting legs off the bolster before rolling to the right and pressing to seated

Challenge

1. Lumbar pain
2. Lying supine contraindicated
3. Heel pain or knee compression
4. Agitation prevents relaxation

Response

1. Slide buttock skin toward bolster. Elevate pelvis and/or lumbar spine with folded blanket, *II d*. Support calves instead of thighs with a chair, 2 bolsters, or stack of 6-10 folded blankets, *II e-g* . Angle femurs away from torso, not vertical, and that lumbar curve is long. *See also Nourish.*
2. Support torso with bolster, *II h*. If support causes sharp lumbar bend or other discomfort, elevate bolster on blocks or chair to raise angle, *II i-j*.
3. Support heels on folded blankets or a second bolster, *II k. See also Response 1.*
4. Apply weight to thighs, hands, and shoulders. If sandbags are too heavy, use stacked, folded blankets on thighs and to cover torso, *II l. See also Synthesize, Response 1.*

☙ *Rolled blanket can be used instead of bolster*

298   Janvakna Savasana — *Explore*

Yoga: Point + Process | *Volume 1*

For some, lying flat on the floor in Savasana can cause some lumbar discomfort, especially when the legs are relaxed. Supporting the legs with the knees bent may alleviate this common problem, which then allows for a more full relaxation and surrender.

Contact Points

Feet, back pelvis, back rib cage, shoulder blades, backs of arms and hands, back of skull

External Supports

Mat, bolster, blanket
Chair, additional bolster and/ or blankets, sandbag

Essence of Form

Mild hip and knee flexion; legs in passive external rotation, arms slightly external

II a
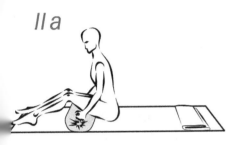

II b
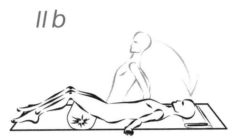

II c
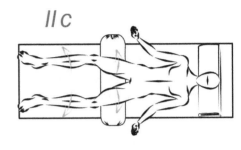

II d
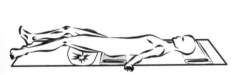

II e
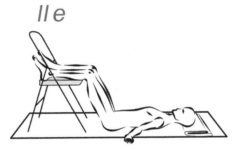

II f
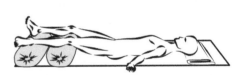

II g

II h
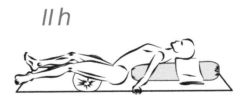

II i
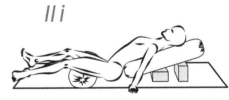

II j
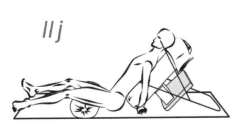

II k
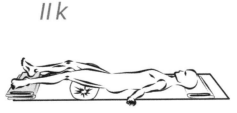

II l
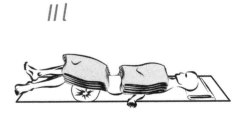

Learn + Practice

Learn early, practice after Back Bends and back body expansion is desired

Linked Poses

Makarasana, Uttana Balasana, Chaturanga Dandasana, Salabhasana, Savasana

Safety Factors

Pregnancy and abdominal cysts; when abdominal compression is contraindicated

Prepare

- Set a bolster lengthwise on mat
- Place a folded blanket on mat beyond bolster for head support

Enter

- Kneel on mat at foot end of bolster, *III a*
- Walking the hands forward, lift the pelvis and bring torso above bolster, *III b*
- Have bolster under sternum, abdomen, and pubis
- Bending the elbows on exhalation, gently lower front torso to bolster support
- Ensure head and throat are not touching bolster; slide forward of necessary
- Rest the forehead on folded blanket or crossed palms, *III c*
- Extend the legs and walk knees away from pelvis
- Exhaling, lower knees to floor and drape thighs over bolster
- Roll backs of thighs and heels away from each other, internally rotating the thighs, *III d*
- Walk elbows out laterally and away from torso, widening between shoulder blades, *III e*
- Ensure weight is supported by bolster, not arms

Sustain

- Receive bolster pressure into front body, softening chest and abdomen
- Release back of skull away from upper back
- Ensure forehead skin slides toward nose, not toward scalp
- Broaden back body skin with each inhalation, release away from spine on exhalations
- Soften buttock flesh away from back ribs
- Allow femurs to hang away from pelvis
- Breathe naturally, observing breath shift from front body to back body

Exit

- Rest for 10-30 minutes
- Exhaling, place hands under the shoulders, *III f*
- Tuck the toes and on exhalation press into hands, lifting torso off bolster
- Walk the hands backward and settle the pelvis toward the heels, sitting upright
- If desired, draw bolster toward pelvis, between thighs, and fold forward into *Uttana Balasana, Nourish, III g*

Challenge

1. Breath restriction
2. Breast tenderness
3. Lumbar compression
4. Neck or shoulder pain
5. Knee or ankle discomfort

Response

1. Support torso with stacked folded blankets instead, *III h*. Use rolled blanket across abdomen or in hip creases, *III i. See also Response 2.*
2. Place folded blanket laterally across lower ribs, below breasts to redistribute weight, *III j*. Manually adjust breasts in *Enter* so that breasts drape on each side of bolster rather than being compressed by it.
3. Apply weight to sacrum, dragging sacrum toward heels. Internally rotate thighs more in *Enter. See Responses 1, 2, + 5.*
4. Increase head support or elevate bolster so that head hangs more freely into support, depending on proportions. Ensure arms are not supporting weight.
5. Place rolled blanket under front ankles or fold lengthwise blankets to support tibias, *III k-l.*

This supported prone position can help mitigate discomfort from lying supine for an extended period. It releases the back body, encouraging a deep, receptive front body release. Adho Mukha Savasana also induces back body expansion for a more complete breathing experience.

Contact Points

Tops of feet, knees, pubis, abdomen, sternum, forehead, elbows, hands

External Supports

Mat, bolster, blanket
Additional blankets, sandbag, block

Essence of Form

Prone position; mild knee, hip, and neck flexion; legs internally rotated, arms neutral

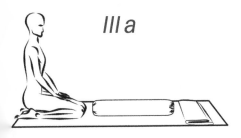

III a

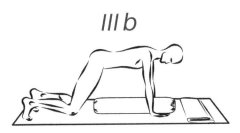

III b

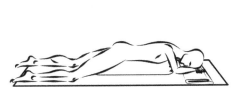

III c

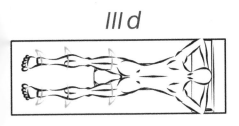

III d

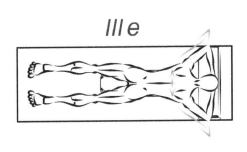

III e

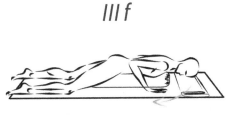

III f

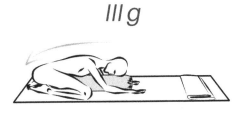

III g

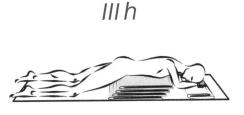

III h

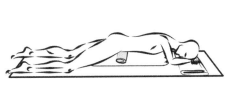

III i

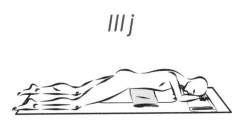

III j

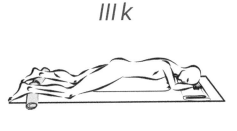

III k

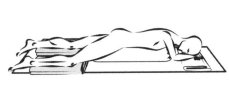

III l

Savasana A
Pose of Repose

Synthesize

Learn + Practice

As for Simplify; once Simplify + Explore are comfortable

Linked Poses

Supta Tadasana, Vishramastha Padartha, All Restorative Poses

Safety Factors

Vertigo, beyond third trimester if pregnant; use care for back pain

Prepare

- Set folded blanket at head end of mat
- Place additional props nearby, clear all unnecessary props well away from mat

Enter

- Sit mid-mat with legs bent, feet flat on floor
- Manually drag buttock flesh toward heels
- Holding back thighs, carefully and symmetrically roll spine to floor, resting head on blanket
- Extend legs along floor in neutral rotation, heels close to each other, *IV a*
- Pinning calves and outer thigh skin to mat, roll thighs outward drawing outer leg skin toward mid line, *IV b*
- Repeat manual adjustments from *Simplify*
- Rest arms beside torso, ensuring armpit skin does not contact side torso, *IV c*
- Roll palms upward and descend index finger knuckles toward floor
- Tuck elbows gently toward torso and roll outer back shoulders toward floor, *IV d*

Sustain

- Settle each heel equally into floor
- Release femurs, tibias, and heels away from pelvis and into floor
- Soften the abdomen and breathe naturally
- Let the skin settle and spread into the floor at all contact points
- Soften the palms and allow fingers to curl naturally toward palms
- Release all skin away from mid line and toward floor
- Let go of tension from the skin inward through the muscles to the organs
- Observe layers of tension release as relaxation deepens
- Soften the sense organs and draw the senses inward
- Visualize the body's elements gradually dissolving

Exit

- Rest for 10-40 minutes
- Using the breath as an anchor, take 3-10 gradually deeper breaths, re-establishing body and spatial awareness
- Continue *Exiting* as described for *Simplify + Explore*

Challenge

1. Head rolls to the right or left
2. Neck tension
3. Lumbar discomfort

Response

1. Fold a rolled blanket into a loop, closing the ends with a strap, *IV e*. Rest head in blanket loop, *IV f*. Set blocks beyond head support in *Prepare*, with a sandbag atop blocks. Slide bottom portion of sandbag onto forehead in *Enter, IV g*.
2. Roll a blanket to support cervical curve and increase head support so that head does not tilt backward, *IV h*. Loop a strap around a chair's crossbar. Bring the loop over the chair seat so that it hangs 1-2" above floor. Rest head in loop, creating traction, , *IV i. See also Response 1.*
3. Support outer thighs with rolled blankets to prevent excessive external rotation, *IV j*. Loosely tie a strap between the big toes or around the mid-calves to hold neutral rotation as legs release, *IV k-l.*

❀ *See also Simplify + Explore*

avasana is a pose of both dissolution and resolution, where the body rests and integrates effects
om the practice while also casting off the actions leading to those effects. It is a pose of time and
melessness, in which to observe passing cycles while experiencing enduring consciousness.

Contact Points

Outer heels, outer calves
nd thighs, back pelvis, back
'b cage, shoulder blades,
outer arms, back of skull

External Supports

Mat, blanket
Additional blankets, sandbags,
6-10 blocks, strap

Essence of Form

Neutral, supine position;
legs and arms passively
externally rotated

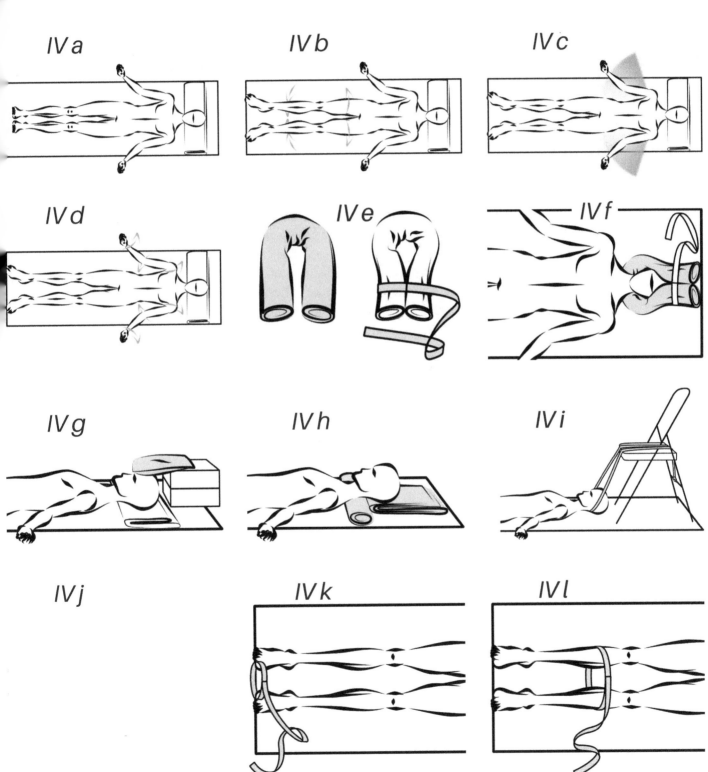

IV a

IV b

IV c

IV d

IV e

IV f

IV g

IV h

IV i

IV j

IV k

IV l

Pose Categories

Back Bends

Back Bends open the shoulders, chest, groins, quadriceps, and the entire front body. They counter the effects of slouching and sitting for long periods of time by activating the posterior postural muscles and extending the spine.

Back Bends tend to be invigorating — elevating mood and boosting energy. This group of poses is also thought to increase immune function, strengthen the heart and improve cardiovascular health, as well as tone and stimulate the nervous system.

Learn these poses after gaining some postural stability and groin length in Standing Poses such as *Tadasana, Urdhva Hastasana, Anjaneyasana, Trikonasana, Parsvakonasana,* and *Virabhadrasana A.*

Practice Back Bends in the morning or early afternoon, before calming and Restorative Poses. Some Restorative Poses are also Back Bends, and can be used to prepare for more active Back Bends or help transition from active practice to more passive phases.

Back Bends in this book are *Upashrayi Dandasana,* *Supta Baddha Konasana, Supta Virasana, Salabhasana, Urdhva Mukha Svanasana, Purvottanasana, Viprarita Dandasana, Ustrasana,* and *Setu Bandha Sarvangasana.*

Forward Bends

Forward Bends release the spine and back body. They are usually done standing or seated, but can be done in nearly any orientation. Most Forward Bends lengthen the hamstrings, and all forward bends increase hip mobility.

Forward Bends are usually calming and facilitate introspection. They can also be depressive, so use them sparingly if you struggle with depression, and finish the practice with a mild, Restorative Back Bend.

This group of poses is thought to stimulate elimination by compressing the abdominal organs while reducing stress and fatigue.

Learn deep Forward Bends after preparing the hips and hamstrings in poses like *Supta Padangusthasana, Ardha Uttanasana,* and *Urdhva Prasarita Padasana.*

Practice Forward Bends in the morning or evening, and after active poses like Standing Poses and vigorous Back Bends.

Forward Bends in this book are *Uttana Balasana, Ardha Uttanasana, Adho Mukha Svanasana, Prasarita Padottanasana, Uttanasana, Parsvottanasana, Adho Mukha Virasana, Paschimottanasana, Janu Sirsasana, Trianga Mukhaikapada Paschimottanasana,* and *Marichyasana A.*

Inversions

Inversions turn the body upside-down, either fully or partially, which reverses some of the cumulative gravitational effects when the body is upright. They are thought to decompress the pelvic and abdominal organs while strengthening the heart.

Inversions increase circulation to the head, and can therefore also increase pressure inside the skull, particularly behind the eyes. Do not practice full Inversions and use care in partial Inversions if you have any eye related issues, such as glaucoma or detached retina. Increased eye pressure can also be a safety consideration for diabetes.

Because of their circulatory effect, Inversions can help reduce swelling and fatigue in the legs, as well as aiding lymphatic drainage.

Partial Inversions are poses that lower the head and/or heart below the pelvis, or elevate the legs or pelvis above the head and heart but not the legs and pelvis at the same time. Most of the Inversions in this book are partial: *Adho Mukha Svanasana, Prasarita Padottanasana, Uttanasana, Viparita Dandasana, Setu Bandha Sarvangasana, Urdhva Prasarita Padasana*, and *Viparita Karani.*

Full Inversions are those where the heart, pelvis, and legs are all above the head. Full Inversions in this book are *Viparita Karani* and *Salamba Sarvangasana.*

Restorative Poses

Restorative Poses are long-held supported poses that are on the range between semi-active and completely passive. Most Restorative Poses are supine, as this is a naturally restful position, but with adequate support can be done in any orientation.

Savasana is a Restorative Pose that is done in nearly every style of yoga, and its value is highly recognized. Many

Restorative Poses are variations of *Savasana*, or are structured in a way to induce a *Savasana*-like sensation and effect.

Inversions are also considered extremely Restorative, due to their effects on the circulatory system and how they reverse some negative gravitational effects. Finishing practice with *Sarvangasana* and poses from the *Sarvangasana* family (*Setu Bandha Sarvangasana, Halasana, Viparita Karani*), is thought to ensure the practice is rejuvenating and not depleting.

Restoratives can be learned at any time, and often a Restorative variation is the entry point for learning deep and/or complex poses.

Practice Restoratives in the afternoon or evening, and use them near the beginning or end of practice, but try not to intersperse them throughout a practice, unless it's a Restorative practice.

Many poses in this book are Restorative or have Restorative variations: *Supta Tadasana, Uttana Balasana, Supta Padangusthasana, Uttanasana, Supta Parsvakonasana, Upashrayi Dandasana, Supta Baddha Konasana, Supta Virasana, Adho Mukha Virasana, Adho Mukha*

Bharadvajasana, Purvottanasana, Viparita Dandasana, Setu Bandha Sarvangasana, Urdhva Prasarita Padasana, Viparita Karani, Salamba Sarvangasana, and *Savasana.*

Seated Poses

All **Seated Poses** are at least partial forward bends, due to hip flexion, but warrant their own category because many maintain an upright, neutral spine, and do not have the same effects as Seated Forward Bends.

Seated Poses develop stability and are usually grounding. They are the foundation of meditation practice, and develop spinal resilience for long periods of sitting upright.

A primary challenge in Seated Poses is keeping the pelvis and lumbar spine erect. Rounding the lumbar spine backward can place excessive load on the lumbar spine and contribute to or aggravate disc problems and other issues further up in the torso.

Tilting the pelvis back in Seated Poses also causes the hip flexors and lower abdomen to hold excess tension, which makes bringing and keeping the pelvis upright even more challenging.

Pose Categories

Seated Poses can be learned at any time, but be sure to sit on adequate height to keep the groins and abdomen soft, the pelvis upright, and the lumbar neutral.

Practice Seated Poses at any time throughout the day, particularly when a calming and grounding effect is desired. Practicing *Supta Padangusthasana* first may help keep the pelvis upright in Seated Poses.

The Seated Poses in this book are *Uttana Balasana, Dandasana, Upavistha Konasana, Baddha Konasana, Virsana, Paschimottanasana, Janu Sirsasana, Trianga Mukhaikapada Paschimottanasana, Marichyasana A, Marichyasana C,* and *Bharadvajasana.*

Side Bends

Side Bends stretch the torso laterally and open the intercostals, side waist, and side groins between the iliums and greater trochanters.

Side Bends are also believed to have an organic effect, releasing and creating space on one side while gently compressing the opposite side, which is thought to "squeeze and soak" organ tissue,

wringing stagnant blood out by squeezing, and then replenishing with fresh, nourishing blood when the compression is released.

Learn mild Side Bends at any point, though the deeper Side Bends may be better learned at the Intermediate stage of practice, after lateral Standing Poses and basic Twists are well integrated.

Practice Side Bends at any time of day, with the possible exception being immediately after eating. It may also be wise to bend to the right first, so that matter in the colon is pushed from the ascending colon toward the descending colon first.

If Side Bends cause digestive or deep abdominal pain, bend only very mildly or avoid them altogether.

Side Bends are best practiced in conjunction with Twists and lateral Standing Poses, but also make an excellent adjunct to Back Bends and Forward Bends. Practice symmetrical poses after Side Bends.

In this book, the Side Bends include *Parsva Uttana Balasana, Trikonasana, Parsvakonasana,* and some aspects of *Marichyasana A.*

Standing Poses

Standing Poses are the foundation of âsana practice. They include aspects of all other pose categories. They develop strength and resilience, as well as increasing mobility in a way that is functional and sustainable. These grounding poses also create a feeling of mental and emotional stability.

Standing Poses can cause fatigue if done too vigorously or too often. Counter these potential negative effects with Restorative Poses and Inversions.

Learn Standing Poses as soon as possible. If standing for long periods of time or at all is not possible, Standing Poses can be practiced supine — using the wall as a "floor" to support the feet — or when ready, with chair or table supporting the legs, pelvis, or torso to develop leg strength and stability.

Options for supported Standing Poses are given in this book, and additional ways to support the Standing Poses are possible; limited only by the practitioner's creativity in applying principles of prop use to individual needs. For each supported Standing Pose in this book, other Standing

Glossary

Poses can be supported in similar ways. Experiment with these options and apply them to other, similar poses.

Standing Poses are best practiced early in the day, but are usually not too stimulating to practice in the evening. Beginning the practice with Standing Poses prepares the body well for deeper work in any other pose category, or can be practiced on their own.

For more seasoned practitioners, Standing Poses can be a good release after Back Bends in the tempering phase, especially the lateral Standing Poses.

Lateral Standing Poses are those with the legs to the side and affect the lateral torso or side body. The lateral Standing Poses in this book are *Parsva Hasta Padasana, Virabhadrasana B, Trikonasana,* and *Parsvakonasana.*

The remaining Standing Poses in this book, *Tadasana, Adho Mukha Svanasana, Uttitha Hasta Padasana, Prasarita Padottanasana, Uttanasana, Utkatasana, Anjaneyasana, Virabhadrasana A,* and *Parsvottanasana,* are considered longitudinal poses because the torso's direction is toward the mid line.

Supine Poses

Supine Poses are any lying-down pose. Most Restorative Poses are supine, and some Standing Poses are introduced supine.

Supine Poses reduce effort and change the gravitational load. They are not always easier, but the effort is shifted so that some actions can be more clearly learned and kinetically understood without unnecessary effort from habitually engaged muscles. Working supine is comforting, and using the floor for feedback can be very informative.

Learn Supine Poses immediately, as long as lying supine is not contraindicated.

Practice Supine Poses at any time of day, but especially early in the day and in the evening. Begin and finish practices with Supine Poses.

In this book, the Supine Poses are *Supta Tadasana, Supta Tadasana Urdhva Hastasana, Supta Padangusthasana A + B, Urdhva Prasarita Padasana,* and *Savasana.*

There are also supine variations of *Parsvakonasana, Dandasana, Upavistha Konasana, Baddha Konasana, Virasana, Janu Sirsasana,* and *Bharadvajasana.*

Twists

Twists have the potential to balance asymmetries, and develop healthy tone along the spinal muscles. Like Side Bends, Twists have an effect on the intercostals and side body. Also like Side Bends, Twists are believed to have a significant organic effect also utilizing the "squeeze and soak" principle.

Often, practitioners find Twists balance the nervous system, leading to a calm, yet invigorated disposition. Twists combine aspects of both Forward Bends and Back Bends, and so can be a useful preparation for and transition between these two groups of poses.

Learn Twists after lateral Standing Poses and symmetrical Seated Poses.

Practice Twists at any time, except immediately after eating. Also, avoid deep Twists early in the morning before adequate preparation, and some practitioners may find Twists too invigorating in the evening.

The Twists in this book are *Trikonasana, Parsvakonasana, Marichyasana A + C, Bharadvajasana.*

Props

Assistant

An **assistant** is (hopefully) the most intelligent prop you will use. If using an assistant to aid your practice, find someone you trust and who is sensitive to what you require of them in adjustments.

The primary risk in receiving assistance is that the assistant may not be able to separate your needs from their desires (for you or them) in the results of the adjustment.

That said, a good assistant can be helpful in learning or creating optimal actions and placements that are difficult to create with other props.

Each practitioner feels differently about receiving adjustments from a teacher or assistant: some love it, others hate it, and most are somewhere in-between. This can change from day-to-day and pose-to-pose. It is mainly for this reason that there are minimal adjustments shown in this book, and none of the adjustments are necessary.

Teachers may want to pay particular attention to the adjustments shown, however, as they may be very useful in classes when teaching certain poses.

Ball

Used to massage different body parts in preparation for certain poses or while in some Restorative Poses.

Many different sizes and densities are available, and more extensive instruction on self massage with a ball is readily available online, being a broad subject in itself.

When using a ball for self-massage, it can be interesting to massage only one side first, then observe the effects and differences between the two sides.

Massaging the feet with a firm, 1″ rubber ball helps release tension up the entire posterior chain. Massaging the buttocks is also very helpful, and a common use of massage balls. Experiment with other ways to self-massage, but be careful that the positions you find to apply pressure with the ball are stable so that there is little to no risk of accidental injury.

Blanket

Blankets are a very versatile prop. Being malleable, they can be rolled, folded, and stacked into a variety of shapes for a firm, yet receptive support.

Wool or cotton blankets are ideal. When acquiring blankets, make sure that they are dense and not too plush. It is also a good idea to have several in the same size, material, and density.

One blanket is a recommended minimum, usually used to support the head when lying supine, but several poses in this book utilize more than one blanket.

If storage space or budget is a consideration, 4-6 blankets will not only serve well as blankets, but can also replace a bolster when folded narrow and stacked. If reasonable, up to 10 blankets is ideal for fully exploring the variety of poses in this book and beyond, especially if your practice is primarily Restorative.

Block

Blocks are probably among the most common yoga props available. They are usually made of wood, cork, or foam, with each material having its advantages and disadvantages. Most uses described in this book require the stability of wood or cork blocks, as they do not bend, collapse, or become misshapen over time when used to support full body weight.

There are a variety of sizes and shapes, but 3 have become fairly standard:

4" x 6" x 9" (or approximately) is probably the most "standard" and is the proportion most of the uses of blocks are based on in this book.

3" x 6" x 9" (or approximately) are also fairly standard, with very little practical difference from the 4" model, though due to the differences in proportion among practitioners, and the variety of different uses and applications, a 3" block may be better for some and a 4" block better for others.

Cork and foam blocks are often made 4" and 3" widths, while wooden blocks are usually 4".

A third fairly standard model is 2" x 8" x 12", and usually made of foam. Like blankets, these flat, wide blocks are very adaptable — they can be stacked to form benches or bolsters, and being roughly half the height of the first "standard" block are ideal for uses where a block is too high but some height is needed and a blanket is too soft or unstable.

Since these flat, wide blocks are usually made of foam, the term "foam blocks" refers to these blocks in this book, even though there are other foam blocks.

Bolster

An essential prop for many Restorative Poses, **bolsters** are also available in a variety of proportions. In this book, the bolsters depicted are round and approximately 30" long by about 8" in diameter.

Bolsters are usually stuffed with cotton or a combination of cotton and foam for added longevity. Natural cotton is quite dense, and bolsters provide the best support when the cotton is compressed, making bolsters often quite heavy props. Because of this, bolsters are great as a weight on the thighs or abdomen for a settling effect.

Chair

Folding chairs are not just for sitting on! They are very helpful in creating a high, firm support, and can be folded or turned upside down for even more creative possibilities.

When using chairs, be aware that they will slide without a mat, and sometimes even with, which

is why the chair is often braced against a wall. Occasionally, this slipperiness can be used advantageously, but become familiar with the chair and how it moves when different pressures and loads are applied before taking informed risks. When in doubt, keep the chair on a mat and against a wall.

Chairs may need to be padded with blankets or mat remnants to make some kinds of pressure more comfortable, depending on the contact point. When using blankets to pad the chair, know that the blanket may slide, so use a mat remnant either under or instead of the blanket if slippage is a concern or potentially dangerous.

Again, sliding may be advantageous, but know this before *Entering* unstable and potentially risky poses with the chair.

Sometimes chairs are available with the back removed, making it easier to get in and out of certain poses. If the back is not already removed, you may need to remove the back yourself. It is relatively simple to do, but be sure to sand any remaining sharp edges to prevent cuts and scrapes.

Props

Door

The top of a **door** may sometimes be used to hang from and create traction. When using an open door, fill the gap between the door and floor with a slant board to reduce excess stress on the door's hinges.

If using a closed door, either as a substitute for a wall or for other uses not outlined in this book, ensure the door is locked and securely closed, and that no other residents will unexpectedly open the door while you are using it as a support!

Door Frame

Door Frame — door frames are surprisingly useful! They are, in effect, a hole in the wall — this means they can be used as a wall to support one part of the body without obstructing the rest of the body the way a regular wall would.

The top of door frames can also be used as low ceilings when something to resist upward into is required.

The limited width of a door frame can also provide helpful resistance, support, and feedback.

Eye Pillow

Small **pillows** usually of silk or cotton and filled with lavender and/or buckwheat hulls or other lightly dense fillers. These can be used directly on the eyes, but can also be applied to the forehead, across the wrists, palms, or sternum.

This mild weight on the eyes encourages them to soften, soothing the eyes and nervous system.

These pillows' outer cases should be washed regularly to reduce the risk of eye infection.

Floor

Often taken for granted, the **floor** is a wonderful prop that provides reliable, even support and feedback.

Flooring materials differ greatly in tack, shock absorption, temperature, texture, and evenness.

These are all factors to consider when practicing, as each one will affect prop use and comfort, and may determine whether jumping is appropriate on that surface or not.

Yoga mats are one way to equalize some of these varying factors, as they absorb shock, provide mild insulation, and are sticky, thus reducing slip.

Foam Block

Many foam blocks are available, but in this book, "**foam block**" refers to a wider and flatter type of block that is usually available only in foam.

This wider, flatter block is sometimes also called a "foam pad" and is approximately 2" x 8" x 12" and highly versatile, and can be a suitable substitute for many props such as blankets and bolsters, but even chairs and benches can be created from by stacking them.

Foam blocks or pads have a variety of other creative uses and are a worthwhile investment.

See also **Blocks**

Mat

The yoga **mat** provides stickiness, preventing slide and reducing the risk of slip and fall type injuries that can happen during practice. Ensure your mat is adequately sticky, as some mats slide and can be more dangerous than not using a mat at all.

If there is any risk of a support sliding, brace it against a wall as well. Mats also even out variances in different types of floors, providing insulation and some cushion.

Mats can also be helpful as a spatial reference, demarcating personal space as well as providing a visual and tactile feedback.

Most poses in this book are done on a yoga mat, but occasionally it can be fun and interesting not to use one. The feedback received by the floor directly is quite different than when on a mat, and is worthwhile exploring when safe to do so.

Mat Remnant

Use old or extra mats to cut **mat remnants** for additional sticky, firm, mild padding. Especially useful between layers of props when using multiple supports that slide against each other, such as under chair and table legs or between chairs, blankets, and blocks.

Mat remnants can be cut into various sizes and stacked or

folded to fine-tune support thickness. Use them to change and refine the angle of supports, as well as providing extra stability.

Rolled Cloth

A **rolled cloth** can fill small spaces where rounded support is needed, but a blanket is too bulky and a ball is too firm or unstable.

Common places to use rolled cloths is between the top of the ankle and the floor, in the back of the knee when it is folded, under or behind the armpits, in the upper thoracic spine, or between the chin and sternum.

As the practice becomes more refined, and the practitioner more sensitive, other uses for more precise props such as a rolled cloth become evident.

Sandbag

Just one of many forms of weight used to create a sense of stability, security, and ease.

Sandbags are usually between 5 and 15 lbs and rectangular.

Generally use sandbags on bony structures like the feet, femurs, sacrum, hands, humeri,

and forehead. When applying weight for holds longer than a minute, the limb must also be supported from underneath. Never apply significant weight on an unsupported limb.

Slant Board

Also sometimes called a wedge, **slanted boards** are about as wide as a yoga mat, 4-5" deep, and slant from about 1/2" at one end to about 1" at the other end.

Like blocks, they are available in wood, cork, and foam. Wood is recommended, as it is most firm and durable. There are uses not in this book that would cause foam or cork boards to burst or break, so it is worthwhile to invest in a wood slant board.

Strap

Second only to blocks and mats, **straps** are among the most common yoga props and are available nearly anywhere.

They can have plastic or metal closures, and when metal, the closure is usually a pair of D-rings or a rectangular buckle with slider.

Props

Straps also come in a variety of widths, lengths, and thicknesses.

Cotton straps that are 1" wide, 8-10' long, and have a secure metal closure are recommended.

Stick

A 1 1/4" dowel. **Sticks** are useful for a deeper self-massage than the ball, as well as being a more firm spacing support to grip than a strap.

Sticks can also be used as pivots and braces. It is good to have at least one short stick of about 2' and 2 longer sticks of at least 4'.

Be careful to place these props in a corner out of the way when not in use, as they can easily be tripped over and being round, can be slipped on.

Table

Tables of varying heights are used to support the torso primarily in Standing Poses, Back Bends, and Restorative Poses, but are also useful for supporting the legs and arms in other contexts.

When using the table, place mats or mat remnants under the four legs to prevent slide.

Wall

In this book, the **wall** is used extensively. Try to dedicate a piece of wall for practice that is bare, with no pictures or shelves, and is free of obstruction to each side and well into the room.

Closed (and locked) doors can substitute for a wall.

The wall is often used to change gravitational relationships, pressing hands or feet into it as though it were the floor, while using the floor as a wall.

The wall is also used as an extra brace for hands or feet in to make them more stable, and as a back support that helps develop a sense of ease while removing some of the strain of balancing.

The wall's use in learning āsana well should not be underestimated.

There are also "yoga walls" with hooks or other hardware installed to hang ropes or straps from. These walls are excellent and versatile props, but also require extra care in learning to use safely. For this reason, the "yoga wall" is not featured in this book.

Wall/Floor Juncture

The **joint** where the wall and floor meet. This corner combines the usefulness of both the floor and wall, as well as providing an additional brace. Most poses that utilize the wall also utilize the wall/floor juncture.

Wall Corner

Where two walls meet. In a yoga context, 90° **corners** are most useful.

Corners can be "outer" where the walls converge toward the practitioner, and "inner" where the walls converge away from the practitioner — each has unique uses.

Body References

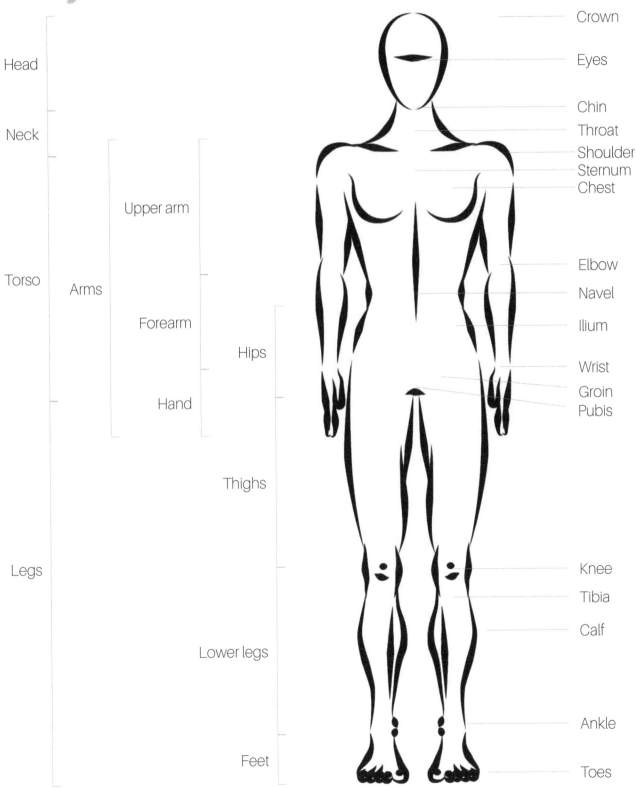

Head

Neck

Torso

Arms

Upper arm

Forearm

Hand

Hips

Thighs

Legs

Lower legs

Feet

Crown

Eyes

Chin

Throat

Shoulder

Sternum

Chest

Elbow

Navel

Ilium

Wrist

Groin

Pubis

Knee

Tibia

Calf

Ankle

Toes

General Terms

#

Corners of Feet — each foot is essentially a trapezoidal shape, with four "corners": the ball of big toe, ball of baby toe, inner edge of heel, outer edge of heel. In most cases, weight and pressure between all four corners should be balanced. In certain poses, some parts of the feet are emphasized more than others.

*See also **Big Toe Mound, Baby Toe Mound, Inner Heel**, and **Outer Heel***

A

Abdomen — the soft region between the protective ribcage and pelvis. With minimal skeletal support, the abdomen allows a large degree of torso mobility. This mobility is created and supported by the various abdominal and spinal muscles, often referred to as the "core."

The abdominal organs, primarily the digestive organs, are also housed in this region. Protected only muscularly, rather than skeletally, the abdomen tends to harden when under stresses or threat. While this survival mechanism is necessary, too much tension in the abdomen can impede healthy digestion, respiration, and circulation, potentially leading to digestive

problems, blood pressure issues, and other organic ailments.

Abdominal wall — another term for the abdomen's muscular layer. When working to tone the abdomen, differentiate between the abdominal muscles, or "wall" and the interior abdomen comprising the organs and viscera.

Although it is generally thought that the smooth muscle of the viscera is autonomic, these fibers tend to increase in tension when the abdominal muscles are activated. Learning to soften the abdomen interiorly while toning structurally helps maintain healthy organ function.

*See also **Rectus Abdominus** and **Transverse Abdominus***

Abduct — away. Moving the limbs away from the mid line or another part. Sometimes also referred to as a lateral movement.

*See also **Lateral***

Achilles Tendon — tendon attaching the calf muscle to the back of the heel. When the posterior chain is tight, particularly the calves and hamstrings, this tension can pull on the Achilles' tendon and cause foot, heel, and ankle pain.

Action — a directional activation that does not create movement, or is engaged before movement occurs.

Most instructions in the *Sustain* section of each pose's process describe actions rather than movements. Actions are also often engaged to stabilize before movements described in *Enter* and *Exit,* These actions help reduce the risk of injury during movement.

Actions are not visually obvious, but can be felt by the practitioner and create internally experienced changes and sensations.

Acromion — the very top of the upper outer shoulder blade. It articulates with the collarbone and stops upward movement of the arm. If lateral arm movement above the shoulders causes pain, impingement, or clicking, it may indicate that the acromion and humerus are making premature contact. Lifting the arm forward rather than to the side may help prevent this contact and reduce these issues.

Adduct — toward. Moving the limbs toward the mid line or another part. Sometimes also referred to as medial movement.

*See also **Medial***

Ankle — the joint between the foot and lower leg. Often, what is referred to as the ankle bones are the lower ends of the tibias and fibulas; tibias for the inner ankle, fibula the outer. The lower tibia and fibula articulate with the talus, which sits above the heel bone. The talus and heel (calcaneus) in turn articulate with each other at the subtalar joint, and the two joints account for most of the foot's movement relative to the lower leg.

Since the ankle joint proper and the subtalar joint usually work in conjunction with each other, it is usually not necessary to isolate them. However, it may be useful to know that lifting the inner ankle, a common ankle instruction, happens at the subtalar joint and not the ankle proper.

See also **Inner Ankle** and **Outer Ankle**

Anterior — to the front or forward. Anterior does not necessarily refer to the front body, but does refer to a portion that is forward of another. For instance, the sacrum, which is a back-body structure, has an anterior side: the anterior sacrum faces inward toward the pubis. In the front body, the sternum's anterior face is that which is closer to the

surface since it is already in the front body.

See also **Front Body**

Anterior Pelvic Tilt — see **Tuck**

Anterior Superior Iliac Spine — see **ASIS**

Arch/Arches (of the feet) — there are three primary arches in each foot, the inner arches being most commonly known. In most cases, unless specified, "arch" refers to the inner foot arch.

The foot's arches absorb shock and help manage the body's gravitational loads. Their optimal function is crucial to postural support and help ensure the spine and other joints remain healthy.

Re-establishing resilience in the foot's arches can alleviate pain and structural imbalances from the feet all the way up to the head. Much of the foundational work in Standing Poses is to harmonize and integrate foot mechanics with the rest of the body.

See also **Inner Arch**, **Transverse Arch**, and **Outer Arch**

Armpits — the fleshy underside of the shoulder joint, between

the side ribs and uppermost humerus. The armpit region is important to keep free and mobile, as it houses some main lymph nodes. The arm's primary veins, arteries, and nerves also pass through the arm pits. Since the arms' resting state closes this space, the chest, arm, and shoulder muscles can become habituated to this closed position.

Opening the armpits not only maintains full shoulder mobility, but may also provide benefit to the circulatory and immune systems.

See also **Outer Armpits**

Ascend — to lift up or to rise.

ASIS (anterior superior iliac spine) — the protrusion on the front iliums, between which is the lower abdomen.

See also **Pelvis**, **Front Iliums**, and **Iliums**

B

Baby Toe Mound — the ball at the root of the little toe, at the end of the 5th metatarsal. This is one of the "four corners of the feet" — comprised of the big toe mound, little toe mound, inner heel, and outer heel.

General Terms

See also **4 Corners of Feet**

Back Body — the back half of the body, usually more the surface than the deep back body, though anything posterior to the coronal plane could be considered "back body."

The buttocks, back pelvis, sacrum, lower back, back ribs, shoulder blades, and back of skull/occiput are all back body references.

See also **Posterior**

Back Iliums — also called the PSIS or posterior superior iliac spine, these are the protrusion on the back iliums, between which is the sacrum.

See also **Iliums** and **SI Joints**

Back Ribs — the back half of the rib cage. Connecting directly with the spine, the back ribs affect the thoracic spine and vice versa. In most poses, lateral space across the back ribs is favored. This ensures ample lung space and optimal breath function.

See also **Bottom Back Ribs**

Bifurcation — dividing in two. It is sometimes useful to divide a muscle down its mid line to aid folding a joint and prevent torque.

Bifurcation moves the medial (inner) flesh more medially and the lateral (outer) flesh more laterally, resulting in also flattening and lengthening the muscle.

When folding the legs, bifurcating the calves helps remove obstructive bulk, allowing the knee joint to close completely without twisting the lower leg, which would compromise the knee.

Bind — after wrapping around and behind the torso, the wrapping arm's hand often grips the other arm's wrist, a thigh or ankle, or a prop, such as a strap or chair.

In an effort to bind, some practitioners compromise shoulder integrity and can dislocate or cause other shoulder injuries. Binding can also serve as a brace or anchor to re-establish healthy shoulder mechanics.

Be aware to keep the chest lifted and not allowing the humerus to collapse forward when wrapping and binding, as this combination is usually what causes problems. Build up to wraps and binds slowly without force.

See also **Wrap**

Big Toe Mounds — the ball of the big toe. Usually referring to the underside or sole of the big toe mound/ball, not the upper side.

There is a large concentration of proprioceptive nerves in the ball of the big toe, relating to the vestibular system and balance. Because of this, when the big toe mounds make contact with an external support, this feedback helps with spatial orientation. Even when the big toe mounds do not make contact with a support, pressing them away from the inner leg and groin is stabilizing to the vestibular system.

See also **4 Corners of Feet**

Bilateral — two-sided, with both sides of the body.

Blade of Foot — the outer edge of the foot, from the little toe mound to the outer heel. The "blade" of the foot remains sharp in most poses, especially in the back foot of asymmetrical Standing Poses, where foot intelligence often lacks.

See also **Outer Arch, Outer Foot, Outer Heel,** and **Baby Toe Mound**

Bottom Back Ribs— the lowermost back ribs. These ribs tend to collapse inward as the bottom front ribs protrude.

Drawing the bottom front ribs inward is structurally effective, but can cause unnecessary abdominal tension.

An alternative to drawing the front ribs in is to lift and broaden the bottom back ribs, creating volume in this area. Not only does this shift in emphasis reduce excess abdominal tension, it also creates a feeling of support for the torso from behind.

See also **Back Ribs** and **Front Ribs**

Breath — the central movement around which all physical yoga practice is built, and our primary source of nourishment. In all poses, the breath should be relatively free and easy, and not need to be forced. If the breath is being held or forced, the pose may be too deep.

Occasionally, some poses may make breathing more challenging. These poses will often have the after effect of a deepened natural breath. Use care that even when the breath is challenged in these poses, there is not a feeling of force and that the breath still flows.

See also **Natural Breath**

C

Calf/Calves — the flesh at the backs of the lower legs. The calf muscles are quite strong naturally, helping to manage weight distribution and facilitating foot and ankle stability/mobility.

The calves also serve a role in stabilizing the knee joints, especially when drawn toward the tibias in bent-leg Standing Poses.

Excess calf tension can indicate circulatory problems, and reducing this tension may reciprocally help reduce circulatory strain.

Calf tension may also be related to hamstring tightness and restriction along the posterior chain.

Cervical Spine — the neck region of the spine, comprising the first 7 vertebra, counting from the skull downward. The smallest vertebra, they are the most delicate. Take care when applying any pressure, directly or indirectly, to the cervical spine.

Poses where the head is a supportive contact puts vertical pressure on the cervical spine, so be cautious in these poses that there is no excess compression.

Poses in the *Sarvangasana* (shoulder stand) family also put indirect pressure on the cervical spine, and care should be taken that the cervical spine does not compress or move into excess flexion, but also that there is no direct pressure applied to the cervical vertebra.

Use rolled blankets or soft supports when supporting the cervical spine in non-weight bearing poses.

See also **Neutral Cervical Curve**

Chest — the front body region below the neck and above the lower ribs. Tightness across the chest can be a protective reaction or related to depression. It is also often caused by prolonged sitting, forward-head posture, and carrying heavy shoulder bags.

A closed chest further strains the neck and upper back, as the neck and back muscles try to compensate for the collapse.

In most yoga āsana, the chest is encouraged to lift and open, especially in Back Bends and Twists, but even in Forward Bends.

Keeping the chest lifted and open, without straining the back

General Terms

to do so, frees the breath and increases lung capacity, and may help elevate mood while boosting immune function.

Chin — the lower and front portion of the jaw. Its position is relative to the throat: when the chin descends, it can close off the throat, but may also help to soften it; when the chin ascends, it tends to facilitate expression but may also cause throat strain. Excessive movement in any direction often causes unnecessary tension.

See also **Jaw**

Circulation— movement of fluids through the body, usually referring to blood, but lymph and other fluids are part of the circulatory system.

Ensure circulation is free in all poses — especially longer holds — in the major veins and arteries, particularly those in the groins and armpits. Circulatory constriction can cause pain, numbness, tingling, and tissue damage if left unchecked, and usually occurs in the groins when the femurs collapse forward or inward (common in hip flexion), and in the arms when the humerus pushes forward.

During pregnancy, healthy

circulation is even more important, so do not tolerate any numbness or tingling. There is additional potential for the fetus to compress the vena cava when lying supine, so be conscious of this, especially in the third trimester.

Coccyx — *see* **Tail Bone**.

Collarbones — the collarbones extend from the top of the sternum and form the bridge between the arms and the thorax. They are resilient, but also delicate.

Excessive tension on the various muscles that connect to the collarbones can contribute to a variety of problems, from breathing, arm + shoulder function, neck and jaw issues, and may even be related to tension and sinus headaches. Lifting and broadening are most commonly the collarbone actions in yogāsana.

Compression — when space is reduced by weight, pressure, or position.

Most often referring to joint compression, but can refer to compression anywhere, particularly the soft tissue of muscles, veins and arteries, and organs.

Not all compression is detrimental, but continued and excessive compression reduces blood flow and cell regeneration.

D

Descend — to lower or move downward.

Diaphragm — this dome-shaped muscle is the primary muscle of respiration. When it contracts, it causes a change in pressure that initiates inhalation; and when it releases, that pressure is also released, allowing for exhalation. It also separates the thoracic cavity from the abdominal cavity, supporting the heart and lungs which rest on top of it and capping the stomach, liver, kidneys, spleen, and the rest of the abdominal organs which lie underneath.

See also **Breath** and **Diaphragms**

Diaphragms — there are several diaphragms in the body in addition to the respiratory diaphragm: the pelvic floor diaphragm and throat diaphragm being among the common ones.

Diaphragms function as separators between structures and help regulate circulation. They are often found in joints, and are usually dome-shaped, though some are inverted and vary in degree of curvature.

It is helpful to visualize the diaphragms, despite their curvatures, to be on horizontal planes. It may also be helpful to visualize a diaphragm wherever breath or circulation needs to be increased or regulated, even if there is no diaphragm structurally present.

Nearly all diaphragms expand circumferentially on inhalation and reduce in circumference on exhalations.

Direction — actions and movements tend to be more effective when they have direction. Often, spatial references are meant to provide direction rather than destination.

For instance, an instruction to reach toward the ceiling does not mean to touch the ceiling, but instead gives an upward direction.

Directions are not limited by space.

Discs — *see **Intervertebral Discs***

Distal — away from the head or center. The elbows are distal to the shoulder, and the feet are distal to the pelvis

Draw — usually a medial action, which is also often associated with a vertical or lifting action. Drawing something in and/or up opposes resisting actions, which are usually lateral and/or distal.

E

Elbows — the joint where the lower humerus connects with the forearm bones, the radius and ulna. When functioning as a joint, the elbows can bend (flexion) or straighten (extension), and there is some rotational capacity, though this rotation is usually more accurately happening in the shoulder or as the radius and ulna cross (internal rotation) or uncross (external rotation).

The elbows are a useful reference in arm rotations, even when that rotation occurs in the shoulder.

When functioning as a support, it is usually not the actual joint, but rather the head of the ulna or base of the humerus that forms the supportive contact. In *Sirsasana* and its relatives, the contact is on the ulna; in *Sarvangasana* and its relatives, the contact is on the lower humerus.

Extension — when the knees and elbows straighten, the hip joint is neutral or the leg moves behind the pelvis, and backward movement of the spine.

In this book, and often in yoga instruction, "extend" or "extension" may refer not to the anatomical directions above, but rather a lengthening action in any orientation.

External Rotation (*legs*) — turning the fronts of the thighs away from each other. At the femur, the greater trochanters move backward and toward each other. Many yoga poses, particularly the Standing Poses, involve an external rotation of one or both thighs. External rotation releases and lengthens the inner thighs, releases the diaphragm, and in some cases lengthens the lower back. However, external rotation also narrows the sitting bones and may compress the sacroiliac (SI) joint. Be aware of this for lower back and SI joint issues, especially in Back Bending Poses.

External Rotation (*arms*) — when the arms are beside the torso, external rotation is where the palms turn forward and elbows move toward the side torso. When the arms are raised overhead, the

General Terms

upper arms (humeri) are often externally rotated. External rotation broadens the chest in most arm positions, but narrows the shoulder blades when the arms are beside or behind the torso. Conversely, external rotation broadens the shoulder blades when the arms are raised overhead.

F

Fascia — a web of connective fibers that tie muscles, skin, nerves, tendons, ligaments, bones, and all of the body's tissues together. These fibers help establish structural integrity, and link muscle chains. Fascia is also a sticky and binding tissue, and can restrict movement, impeding healthy muscle and joint function.

Movement, combined with long-hold Restorative Poses and self-massage ensures that fascia's fibers remain useful and do not accumulate in unhelpful ways.

Femurs — the thigh bone. Most leg movements are ideally initiated from the femur. Healthy femur movement within the hip joints has positive effects not only physically and physiologically, but is also helpful to the neurological, organic, and circulatory systems.

Femur Head — the top of the thigh bones where the femurs connect to the pelvis. The femur heads are roughly spherical, allowing a wide variety of movements in the hip joints: abduction and adduction, flexion and extension, external and internal rotation, and circumambulation — there is even some degree of protraction and retraction possible.

Most natural hip movements involve a combination of some or all of these movements, and yogāsana can ensure balanced mobility in each range. Recognizing the femur heads as essentially ball-shaped, try to feel and find a smooth, rolling action in all hip movements while practicing.

Flesh — a generic term referring to the soft tissues of skin, muscle, and fat.

While it can be useful to differentiate between each layer of tissue and each individual muscle, it is of equal use to remember that these tissues are always interconnected. Thinking of tissue groups as "flesh" is a sensitive way of acknowledging this broader relationship and balancing integration with the dissective nature of precision.

Forehead — the front of the skull, specifically the region above the eyes and below the hairline. In most Supine Poses, the forehead is encouraged to slope down toward the nose, lengthening the neck and producing a calming response. This action also opens the cervical artery space to aid healthy circulation to and from the brain.

Forehead Skin — the skin covering the forehead. The muscles that control the forehead skin cause it to lift and widen when excited or surprised, lift and narrow when worried or confused, descend and narrow when concerned or angry, and descend and widen when calm and at peace.

In yoga, the forehead skin is usually encouraged to soften downward and gently broaden as it naturally would when calm and at peace. Releasing the forehead skin in this manner also requires the least amount of physical effort and has a relaxing effect on the whole body.

Front Body — the front half of the body, usually more the surface than the interior front body, though anything anterior to the coronal plane could be considered "front body."

The forehead, chest, sternum, front ribs, navel, (front) abdomen, ASIS, and pubis, are all front body references.

Front Iliums — also called the ASIS or anterior superior iliac spine, these are the protrusion on the front iliums, between which is the lower abdomen.

Front Ribs — the front half of the rib cage. The first seven ribs are joined in the front by the sternum, the next three attach to the rib above, and the last two are not attached in the front, hence the common name "floating". These last ribs do not wrap all the way around the side body to the front, and it is usually the lower ribs (ribs 8-10) that do connect with their superior ribs that are confused with the "floating" ribs. In this book, most reference to the front ribs is of these lower front ribs, ribs 8-10.

G

Gluteal Fold — the crease at the bottom of the buttocks, where the buttock and back thigh meet.

Greater Trochanters — the lateral prominence at the upper femurs. Palpating down from the side waist, the first bony protrusion is the iliums, the second is the greater trochanters.

Groins — broadly, the structures that help connect the legs to the pelvis. More specifically, however, in yoga the groins usually refer to the place where the hips fold, from the outer front hip crease to the inner back hip crease. Most often, "groins" is short-hand for the inner front groins, between the pubis and inner femurs.

The groins are kept wide and deep by moving the femurs laterally and posteriorly, regardless of rotation.

H

Hamstrings — the muscles at the backs of the legs. Much of yoga āsana addresses hamstring mobility. As a central link in the posterior chain, which tends to contract as a reaction to stress, releasing the hamstrings by stretching them often has a calming effect.

Because so much of āsana practice involves stretching the hamstrings, they can be susceptible to overuse and overstretch injuries.

Head — the top. Usually referring to the skull, the idea of a "head" is also used in reference to the humerus, tibia, and femur: the head of these bones being the uppermost section, which

in these cases is incidentally roundish and reminiscent of the head's shape.

The head itself is a relatively heavy structure, and in some poses may be too great a load for the neck to sustain. While developing strength and endurance, supporting the head is a good option, which also helps maintain neck alignment with adequate support.

Supporting the head also calms the sense organs and nervous system, as the muscles that normally hold the head up are intimately connected with those that control the sense organs — the head being essentially the vehicle of the sense organs.

Heart — situated behind the sternum, between the lungs, and seated on the diaphragm, the heart moves up and down with each breath. The heart is a muscle, and its primary function is to circulate blood through the entire system, bringing oxygenated blood to the muscles and pumping de-oxygenated blood to the lungs.

Steady, active āsana practice helps strengthen the heart and build resilience, especially Standing Poses, Back Bends, and Inversions. Restorative and

General Terms

Seated Poses, as well as Forward Bends help soothe the heart and reduce strain.

If the heart is sensitive or fragile, avoid jarring it with sudden movements, jumping, or coming up from lying down positions too quickly. Twists may also strain a fragile heart, but can be of benefit when practiced with care and moderation.

Heel of Hand — the base of the palm, just beyond the wrist. As a stable and supportive area of the hand, the tendency is to use it as the sole contact point when the hands are a support, which can compress the wrists. Although the heel of hand is an important supportive contact, distributing weight into the index finger mounds and the rest of the hands reduces load on the heel of hand, reducing wrist compression. Try to balance pressure between the inner and outer heel of hand, while simultaneously lifting the groove at the center of this heel.

See also **Palm** *and* **Thumb Mound**

Hip Bones — the bones of the pelvis, usually referring to the iliac spines, or part of the hip bones just below the waist.

See also **Pelvis** *and* **Iliums**

Hip Creases — the creases formed when the hips are in flexion, with or without leg abduction. Often, the groins are referred to as the hip creases, though the hip crease itself only reveals itself when the hips are in flexion, whereas the groins are always present.

Hip Crest — the arched bone on the sides of the hips, also called the ilium.

See also **Iliums**

Hip Mobility — freedom of movement in the hip joints, between the femur and pelvis.

Hip Opening — often referring to an increase in hip mobility and range of motion. An alternative way to view hip opening is as an increased feeling of space and ease in the hip joints, even if the range of motion remains limited. It may be more beneficial to emphasize this space by decompressing the hip joint.

See also **SI Joints**

Horizontal Plane — any plane parallel to the floor.

Humerus — the upper arm bone. Like the femur, it should usually move back and laterally in most poses. Occasionally, excess

mobility may require the humerus to be drawn medially before moving posteriorly. In cases of shoulder impingement, or on weight-bearing poses where the humerus has a tendency to compress into the shoulder, moving the humerus out of the shoulder joint can create space and allow for more optimal mechanics.

Generally, balance space within the shoulder joint with stability; continually increasing space around the humerus head without losing necessary stability, and creating more stability whenever possible without losing spaciousness.

Hyperextension — movement in extension beyond "normal" range of motion. In a yoga context, usually it refers to knee and elbow hyperextension, where they extend beyond straight. When the knees and/ or elbows hyperextend, it can place excessive load on the joints and ligaments, causing or exacerbating joint laxity. Hyperextension also displaces gravitational load away from the bones, which are meant to be the primary load-bearing structures.

Hypermobility — mobility that is considered beyond normal or functional ranges of motion. Often, joint instability accompanies hypermobility.

Some research suggests that hypermobility is linked to a disconnect in nervous, particularly proprioceptive, feedback.

Hypermobility may also have hormonal, genetic, and habitual causes.

From a functional perspective, hypermobility is not necessarily assessed by "normal" ranges of motion, but ranges of motion that exceed the practitioner's current capacity to remain stable, integrating muscular activation with mobility.

See also **Joint Instability**

Iliums — the upper portion of the pelvic bones, also called the iliac crest or commonly just "hips" or "hip bones." Find the sides of the iliums by sliding the hands down from the waist to the first bony protrusions. The iliums arch upward and outward from the pubis in the front and the sacral joint in the back. Two important landmarks on the iliums are the anterior superior iliac spine (ASIS) — a protrusion on the front pelvis, and the posterior superior

iliac spine — a similar protrusion on the back pelvis, lateral to the upper sacrum.

See also **ASIS**, **PSIS**, *and* **Pelvis**

Index Finger Mound — the root of the index finger, on the palm of the hand. This is perhaps the most important part of the hand, especially when the hand is a supportive contact point.

Commonly, the index finger mound lifts away from the floor or support, and this overloads the outer wrist and hand, as well as contributing to elbow and shoulder collapse.

When the index finger mound presses down, it not only stabilizes the hand, but engages a muscular chain that both extends the arms and stabilizes the wrists, elbows, shoulders, and may have an advantageous effect on the neck and thoracic spine.

The index finger mound is the hand's proprioceptive equivalent to the big toe mound.

Inferior — under or below.

Intervertebral Discs — the cushioning discs between each vertebra. These discs are cartilaginous, fluid-filled structures that help maintain

space between the vertebra, absorb shock, and help allow for spinal movements.

Discs can degenerate and when load is uneven, they can slip, bulge, or herniate, causing pain that ranges from mild to very severe, and the degree of pain is not always commensurate to the severity of injury.

Discs can herniate anteriorly, posteriorly, or laterally. Posterior herniations, where the disc protrudes back toward the spinal cord are most common, and are usually aggravated by Forward Bends. Anterior herniations, where the disc moves forward into the body, are usually aggravated by Back Bends.

Traction is often helpful in managing disc pain.

Inner Arches — the arch of the foot spanning from the big toe mound or ball of big toe to the inner heel.

See also **Arch**

Inner Ankle — the lower end of the tibia, also called the medial malleolus. In most yoga poses, the inner ankle lifts to maximize space above the heel and maintain integrity in the inner arch.

General Terms

Inner Groin — the section of the groin toward the inner leg. This spans from the inner front groin to the inner back groin, but generally refers to the inner front groin. Interiorly, this space between the pubis and inner femurs tends to be where a great deal of tension is held, causing potential problems in the knees, pelvis, lower back, and elsewhere. Soften, deepen (recede), and broaden this space whenever possible, both in yoga and otherwise.

Excess tension in the inner groins also restricts blood flow to the legs and may have negative nervous effects as well.

Inner Heel — the medial or big toe side of the heel. The inner heel tends to lift as the inner arch and ankle lift, so extend the inner heel away from the inner ankle without torquing the foot or knee. When the inner arch collapses, there is a tendency to descend the inner heel excessively.

Inner Shoulder Blades — the shoulder blade edge that is closest to the spine. At rest, this edge angles outward from top to bottom. In a healthy rhythm, the inner shoulder blade descends as the arms rise and ascends as they lower.

There is sometimes a habit of squeezing the shoulder blades together, narrowing the space between the inner shoulder blades. In general, however, this strains the chest, collarbones, and creates unnecessary tension in the upper back, potentially compromising back lung function and causing certain neck, shoulder, and upper back problems.

In general, attempt to widen between the inner shoulder blades. When the arms are raised overhead, which naturally widens the shoulder blade tips, emphasize widening the upper inner shoulder blades while gently drawing the lower shoulder blades medially.

Inner Quadricep — *see Vastus Medialis*

Intercostals — literally, "between the ribs." These are the fine sets of muscles between each of the ribs. There are three layers of intercostals, the deepest layer running perpendicular to the ribs, and the next two on crossing diagonals.

The intercostals are an additional protection for the heart and lungs, are important postural muscles, and are secondary breathing muscles. They are simultaneously stretched and strengthened by Twists, and can be released with Restorative Back Bends.

Use care, however, especially if practicing Pranayama or forcing the breath in āsana, as the intercostals can be easily torn and do not heal quickly.

Internal Rotation (*legs*) — turning the fronts of the thighs toward each other. At the femur, the greater trochanters move forward and slightly toward each other. Often, what is described as internal rotation is actually neutral rotation; however, since the tendency is often toward external rotation, the legs must usually be internally rotated from this natural tendency in order to arrive at neutral. Internal rotation broadens the back pelvis and sitting bones as well as deepening the inner groins.

Internal Rotation (*arms*) — when the arms are resting beside the torso, internal rotation is when the palms turn toward the thighs and backward. When the arms are raised overhead, the palms face forward and elbows out to the sides. Often, in poses where the arms are extended overhead, there is a dual rotation where the upper arms (humeri) externally rotate and the lower arms (forearms) internally rotate.

This is not the same as neutral rotation, but is instead a rotation + counter-rotation. This dual rotation is often desired as internally rotating the upper arms when they are raised overhead narrows the shoulder blades and may contribute to neck pain and compression.

J

Jaw — the lower part of the skull, comprising the lower teeth, chin, and outer portion of the lower front skull. In yogāsana, "softening" or "releasing" the jaw refers more to softening the muscles that cause the jaw to open and close at the temporomandibular joint.

Often, a common stress response is to clench the jaw, creating tension from the temples to the jawline, as well as increasing pressure inside the skull and around the eyes. Releasing this tension and allowing the jaw to separate slightly from the skull usually has a calming effect, and may help in relieving tension related headaches, inner ear problems, TMJ syndrome, as well as some neck and throat issues.

Joint Centers — when the focus of movement and gravitational load are not through the centers of the joints, abnormal wear patterns may develop. In yogāsana, bring the focus of movement, as well as gravitational load, close to the joint centers whenever possible. This is often the main factor of what is meant by the nonspecific but popular term: "alignment."

Joint Instability — when joint movement is not balanced with the ability to control or stabilize that movement. Usually joint instability accompanies excess range of motion, or hypermobility, but not always. Joints that do not have the muscular support to retain their integrity are unstable, even when range of motion is considered normal or limited.

K

Kneecaps — the bone at the front of each knee. The kneecaps slide along grooves in the lower femurs, and help increase the leverage in extending the knee as well as decreasing the risk of lateral shift in the joint when the knee flexes. Lifting the kneecaps when the knee is in extension protects the knee and strengthens the quadriceps, as well as encouraging a more complete extension of the hamstrings.

Be sure to emphasize lifting the kneecaps toward the pelvis, which will utilize the quadriceps well, rather than pressing the kneecaps backward, which usually causes hyperextension.

Knee Pits — the center of the backs of each knee. Many tendons, ligaments, and supportive structures criss cross the knees, but there is a "pit" where fewer of these structures cross, creating a space with less volume. In many cases, the head of tibia and bottom femur press back into this space, causing hyperextension, and straining the supportive structures behind the knee which can lead to instability over time.

In bent-leg poses, where the knee is in flexion, the knee pits should naturally deepen. In straight-leg poses where the knee is extended, keep the pit behind the knees soft and recede it inward to prevent hyperextension and ensure this area is spacious so that the knee's supportive structures have room to glide and perform their functions well.

L

L4 + L5 — the fourth and fifth lumbar vertebrae, at the bottom of the lumbar spine. To retain a neutral lumbar curve, moving the lowest lumbar vertebrae inward is essential.

General Terms

Lateral — sideways or away from the mid line. When describing prop placement, lateral usually means sideways or crossing the mid line; when describing limb movement, lateral means out to the sides or away from the mid line. Lateral actions generally create space and wider placement of the limbs or props are usually more stable.

Lengthwise — along the length of the body, mat, prop, or other reference that has a difference between length and width.

See also **Longitudinal**

Lesser Trochanters — the bony protrusion at the upper inner femurs, which serves as an attachment point for the psoas. This can not usually be palpated, as it is covered by many layers of muscle.

Longitudinal — lengthwise. Usually used to describe prop placement, where the prop is set in its narrow position parallel to the mid line.

Longitudinal may also describe space or action in the body, and often accompanies medial actions and internal or neutral rotation. It also refers to movements that are parallel to or along the mid line.

Lumbar Spine — the spinal region spine between the rib cage and the pelvis. consisting of 5 vertebrae, abbreviated as L1-L5, from upper to lower. Also called the lower back or back of the waist.

M

Medial — toward the mid line. Gathering and narrowing actions are all toward the mid line. Although medial actions narrow space, they also often increase muscular stability and create length and lift.

Mid Line(s) — the body's mid line is also known as the sagittal plane, dividing left from right. Each limb and extremity also has a mid line, dividing the inner (medial) and outer (lateral) halves.

Mid lines are usually longitudinal.

Movement — a physical action that results in a different spatial orientation. Movements create visually observable changes in body position or shape.

Most *Enter* and *Exit* instructions are movements, since they guide the practitioner into and out of poses.

Movements are often easier for practitioners to feel and

can increase sensation where it is lacking. Felt sensations can be experienced without movement, however, and it is beneficial to learn this sensitivity whether in movement or not.

Multifidi — a set of deep spinal muscles that help stabilize the spine and pelvis in preparation for movement. These are "pre-motor" muscles, which activate at the thought of movement, and often deactivate or reduce their activity when movement is executed. This makes the multifidi and other pre-motor muscles tricky to activate consciously, but it can be done by simply thinking about particular actions without trying to actually perform them.

To activate the lower multifidus, which stabilizes the pelvis, SI joints, and lumbar spine, think about drawing the posterior iliums (PSIS) toward the mid line. Feel the sensations in and around the SI joints: there will be a contrary expanding sensation when the multifidi activate. If the sensation is narrowness, the movement has already taken place — deactivate and try again, only thinking of the movement rather than trying to create movement.

It is difficult but worthwhile to bring these muscles under

conscious control, because doing so is useful in managing pain and instability in the pelvis, SI joints, and lower back.

N

Navel — commonly called the "belly button," it's roughly the center of the abdominal wall. It is a highly important energetic point, as it is the place through which we were nourished in the womb. As such, maintaining a balanced tone in and around the navel ensures healthy digestion, and it is instinctual to harden or cover this area in protection. Whenever possible, try to reduce tension in the navel and abdomen while practicing āsana.

If you tend to lack tone here, emphasize the lower transverse abdominal actions described in *Supta Tadasana*, activate the legs by extending them away from the pelvis, and lengthen the trunk. These actions will tone the abdomen without creating unnecessary tension.

Natural Breath — optimal, unaltered breath. Rarely is the breath totally unaffected by stress, trauma, habit, or other learned patterns that veil the natural breath. Much of the work in āsana is releasing tension that leads to altered breath patterns.

Ideally, practices that consciously alter the breath, such as *Pranayama*, are reserved for when the natural breath begins to reveal itself in the basic poses.

Having a natural breath in mild to moderately challenging poses demonstrates nervous resilience and stability optimal for supporting deeper practices, whether they be āsana, pranayama, or meditation.

Neutral Cervical Curve — a convex curve at the back of the neck where the cervical spine moves inward. This inward curve can reverse, flattening out and potentially causing the discs to protrude. The curve can also be excessive, compressing the arteries that feed the brain.

In a neutral curve, the cervical spine moves inward while remaining long, with the back skull lifting away from the thoracic spine. When turning the head, risk of injury is minimal with a neutral cervical spine, so try to avoid turning the head when the neck is in flexion or extension.

Neutral Lumbar — refers to the natural, inward curvature of the lumbar spine. A neutral lumbar is particularly initiated by moving the lowest vertebrae, L4 + L5, inward.

Neutral Pelvis — in general, a position where the pelvis is neither tilted anteriorly nor posteriorly, resulting in a neutral lumbar spine. Often, bringing the front iliums (ASIS) and pubis to the same vertical plane (horizontal if supine) is neutral. This may vary from individual to individual, however.

To find a neutral pelvis, lengthen the tail bone (without tucking), gather the front iliums, toning the transverse abdomen, and soften and deepen the groins. Alternatively, tilt the pelvis anteriorly and posteriorly, exploring each end of that range of movement. Gradually reduce movement in each direction to find the middle of that range. Typically, this second method will be closer to habitual holding patterns and may not be truly "neutral" but it will increase sensitivity and awareness of pelvic placement.

Neutral Rotation (*legs*) — a position in the legs where the thighs neither turn in nor out, with the greater trochanters at their widest position. Most yoga poses that are considered internal rotation poses are neutral instead, but since there is often a tendency for the legs to externally rotate, internal rotation must be engaged to

General Terms

arrive at neutral. Neutral rotation may describe a lack of internal or external rotation, or it may describe a balanced effort between external and internal rotation actions, resulting in an active neutral rotation.

Neutral Rotation (*arms*) — the palms facing each other when the arms are beside the torso, in front of the torso, or raised overhead. When the arms are extended out to the sides at shoulder level, the palms face forward in neutral rotation.

Neutral Spine — the state where the spine's neutral, natural curves are present and balanced. There are 5 spinal curves in total, but we normally think of three important ones: the lumbar curve, which in a neutral state is concave; the thoracic curve, which is convex; and the cervical curve, which is concave and mirrors the lumbar.

While it is often advantageous to lengthen each of these curves, especially when excessive, none of them should be totally flat when in a neutral state. Neutral spine is often what is intended by the terms "flat back" or "straight spine," but it may be more correct (and less confusing) to use the terms "long spine" or "neutral spine." Sometimes, neutral spine is more about balancing

these natural curves rather than lengthening them so that the spine can perform its resilient, shock-absorbing function.

Though many yoga poses take the spine through a variety of movements, the intent is to help balance these curves, and it may be helpful to keep this in mind when practicing any āsana, particularly the more extreme.

Neutral Thoracic Spine —when neutral, the thoracic spine is a convex curvature. As with all of the spine's natural curves, this can be flattened, excessive, or neutral, and it is optimal to have range in flexion and extension movements, with the resting state being a balanced convex curvature that is not extremely curved nor flattened.

Nostrils — the nasal passages or the passages of the nose through which breath flows. Air is filtered by the nostrils, which are full of sensitive nerves that help regulate blood pressure, breath rate, and other biochemical regulators. The brain and nervous system are positively stimulated by breath passing across this sensitive tissue, and bringing awareness to the nostrils while breathing may help produce calming effects both physiologically and mentally.

O

Occiput — the bony protuberance at the back of the skull just above the neck. It serves as an attachment point for many muscles, and is also a useful reference point.

The occiput or occipital bones should usually lift away from the upper spine to keep the neck long and avoid compressing the cervical arteries, especially in Back Bends and Twists as cervical compression can cause neck pain, headaches, dizziness, and tinnitus.

Orientation — use of the sense organs to provide feedback regarding the body's position in space and relative safety.

*See also **Proprioception** and **Spatial Awareness/Orientation***

Outer Ankle — the lower end of the fibula, also called the lateral malleolus. Like the inner ankle, the outer ankle also lifts, though not as much. Rather, the outer ankle is usually encouraged to draw in medially, as its tendency is to collapse outward.

Outer Arch — the middle of the outer foot, between the base of the little or baby toe and the outer heel. This arch is not as important as the inner arch, but is still integral to keeping the outer leg active. Drawing the outer ankle in and up helps maintain the outer arch.

See also **Arch**

Outer Armpits — the flesh behind and lateral to the armpits, which is also lateral to the shoulder blades. In most āsana, the outer armpit's action is to wrap forward, deepening the armpits themselves. This action is related to external rotation of the humerus, which usually reduces impingement of the shoulder joint, especially when the arms are extended overhead.

Outer Heel — the lateral or baby toe side of the heel. Usually the outer heel lifts if the inner arch is collapsed, or the weight falls entirely into the outer heel. "Sharpening" — that is, actively extending — the inner and outer heels equally away from the ankles activates the arches and balances leg action.

Outer Shoulder Blades — the outer border of the triangular-shaped shoulder blade. This part of the shoulder blade ascends as the arm ascends, and descends as the arm descends. However, for a deeper armpit opening, the outer shoulder blade can be stabilized in a

slight downward action as the arms ascend. This action should not be over-emphasized.

P

Palms — the underside of the hand, not including the fingers. Being dense with nerve tissue, the palms are highly sensitive and provide feedback regarding stability, spatial orientation, and temperature.

In active poses, the palms widen; in passive poses, the palms should be encouraged to soften.

Having the palms in contact with a physical reference is often calming to the nervous system, and can boost physical and emotional feelings of stability.

This may be why some practitioners experience increased resilience from the practice of arm balances and poses where the palms are a support. A similar effect, however, can be created by pressing the hands into a wall or other support without having to bear weight on the hands, or by applying weight to the palms in Restorative Poses.

Pelvic Floor — an aggregate of subtle muscle layers that support the bottom torso and spine.

Pelvis — literally meaning "bowl" the lower torso skeletal structure comprising the hip bones and sacrum. Together, they form a bowl-like structure that houses the lower digestive, reproductive, and eliminatory organs.

The pelvis also connect the legs to the torso and spine, helping to manage impact from walking and running as well as the torso and head's gravitational load.

Ideally, yoga practice should stabilize the pelvis while also liberating breath and circulation within the pelvis so that the pelvic organs are nourished and carry a balanced, functional tone.

Perineum — the area at the base of the pelvis, behind the vulva or scrotum and in front of the anus. Dense with nerves, this is the root of the pelvic floor, and is of great importance in Hatha and Kundalini Yoga, as well as related forms.

Posterior — to the back or behind. Posterior does not necessarily refer to the back body, but does refer to a portion that is behind. For instance, in the front body, the sternum's posterior side faces inward toward the spine. In the back body, the sacrum's posterior side faces outward and is at to the surface.

General Terms

Posterior Chain — a chain of muscles extending along the entire back body. This chain of muscles work in synchrony with each other, and often tension or release in one muscle along the chain corresponds with tension or release in other links in the chain.

The posterior chain is made up of the plantar fascia, Achilles tendon and calves, hamstrings, deep buttock muscles, spinae erectors, and scalp and forehead muscles.

Posterior Pelvic Tilt — *see Tuck*

Posterior Superior Iliac Spine — *see PSIS*

Prone — lying on the front. Lying down reverses some of gravity's compressive physical effects. Lying prone anchors the front body and exposes the back body, which can facilitate breath freedom in the back body by gently restricting the front body.

The prone position often alleviates back pain, but may also create uncomfortable chest and abdominal pressure. Do not lie prone when abdominal compression is contraindicated, such as during pregnancy, with abdominal tumors or cysts, and occasionally when suffering from acid reflux or gas.

Proprioception — the process by which the nervous and vestibular system process external feedback to assess spatial orientation.

Proprioception can be simplified to mean "balance" but is broader than that, helping the nervous system understand the body's relationship in space.

*See also **Spatial Awareness/ Orientation***

PSIS (posterior superior iliac spine) — the protrusion on the back iliums, lateral to the sacrum.

*See also **Pelvis, Sacrum, SI Joints**, and **Iliums***

Pubis — where the two pelvic bones in the front pelvis join by a piece of cartilage called the pubic symphysis. This is the lowest prominent part of the front pelvis, located directly above the genitals.

Pubis Skin — the skin covering the pubis.

Q

Quadriceps — the muscles running up the front thighs. They are primarily responsible for leg extension but also participate in hip flexion along with other dedicated hip flexors. The quadriceps also lift the kneecaps, stabilizing the knee joints when the legs are extended.

R

Range of Motion — this is usually considered flexibility. Range of motion may be a more accurate term, recognizing that flexibility is limited both by muscular adaptability as well as joint range.

Every body's structure is a little different, with each bone having different proportions and angles, which all affect a joint's possible movements, and these movements are then facilitated or limited to greater or lesser degrees by muscular action.

It is not only possible, but relatively common to appear "flexible" and yet have very tense muscles, or to have muscular release but restricted by joint structures.

Keep this in mind when assessing personal alignment within the various pose forms.

Rectus Abdominus — the first layer of abdominal muscles, which run vertically and connect the front pelvis and front rib cage. These are the "6-pack" muscles. Minimal activation is required for stability in most cases, and does not need to be emphasized.

Resist — an action that presses against a real or imaginary brace or barrier. It is usually a lateral or distal action, moving away from the body's center.

Respiratory Diaphragm
— *See **Diaphragm***

Retraction — literally, drawing back or in. When there is joint instability, especially in the hips, shoulders, and shoulder blades, retracting or drawing the femurs, humeri, and/or shoulder blades inward toward the mid line and/or upward toward the head can help re-stabilize.

Rib Cage — also sometimes called the thorax, this is the collection of bones that forms a protective but flexible container for the vital organs, the heart and lungs.

S

Sacrum — the bone at the base of the spine that also joins the two halves of the back pelvis. Misalignment or medial compression can contribute to significant pain in the back pelvis and lower back. In general, the sacrum should be encouraged to move inward while broadening the space around it.

Scalp — the skin covering the top and back of the skull. Though this flesh is thin, there are many small and responsive muscles in the scalp that are related to expressions, sense organs, and temperature regulation.

Individual control of these muscles is unnecessary, but scalp muscle contraction in general is related to stress response, and learning how to release and relax them can have a reciprocal effect on calming the nervous system as well as releasing other tensions in the body.

Excessive and chronic scalp tension can also affect circulation to the skull and brain, causing eye strain, headaches, sinus congestion, and some hearing problems or sensitivity.

Sense Organs — the eyes, ears, nose, mouth/tongue, and skin. The sense organs, or jnanendriyas (organs of wisdom) have a special place in yoga theory as extensions of the mind.

They are the gateways between inner consciousness and the external world, which is perceived through these organs and then constructed within the mind. Often, the sense organs are directed outward, where

consciousness moves toward the objects of perception.

Through the sense organs, however, consciousness can be traced inward — from the object of perception to the sense organ(s) to the sense itself, and then to the mind, which processes that information.

When practicing yogāsana, be conscious of how the sense organs are being used. The senses and sense organs are useful in establishing spatial orientation and gathering sensory feedback, but once poses are established, follow the senses from the sense organs toward the mind, and from the mind to the source of the mind and senses — consciousness itself.

Shoulder — the joint and stabilizing structures connecting the arm and thorax. The shoulder joint itself is where the humeral head meets the outer collarbone and outer shoulder blade.

Healthy shoulder mechanics involve all three of these bones, as well as the collarbone's relationship with the sternum and how the shoulder blade glides across the back ribs. This joint is also highly mobile, with many interconnecting muscle structures to help stabilize the

General Terms

joint, while also allowing for a wide range of movements.

Due to its complexity and potential for mobility, the shoulder is an often injured area, so use care when doing poses that require excessive load or movement. Many of the poses in this book will help retrain optimal shoulder mechanics, particularly the *Simplify* and *Explore* stages.

Shoulder Blades — these triangular plate-like bones slide across the back ribs and serve as anchors for a multitude of shoulder and back body muscles. They also articulate with the humerus as part of the shoulder girdle.

Shoulder Blade Tips — the point at the bottom of the triangular-shaped shoulder blade, where the inner and outer shoulder blades meet

Shoulder Creases — the crease formed when the arms are raised. The shoulder equivalent to the hip creases.

Shoulder Girdle — a broad term for the entire shoulder structure, comprising the humeri, collarbones, and shoulder blades.

SI Joints (sacroiliac joints) — the joint formed where the

back iliums articulate with the upper lateral sides of the sacrum. Movement in these joints facilitates healthy rhythm between the legs and spine. When mobility is excessive on one or both sides, pain in the lumbar, back pelvis, and hip joints can result.

Yoga āsana can both stabilize these joints and destabilize them, depending on how vigorous the practice is, which poses are practiced most, and how they are done.

In particular, over-emphasis on hip opening poses and increasing lateral mobility without adequate stability or moderation, as well as medial poses where the femur crosses the mid line, tend to cause or exacerbate SI joint instability.

Intelligent activation of the transverse abdomen, buttocks, and multifidus, along with moderate practice of extreme and/or asymmetrical leg and hip movements can prevent or reduce SI joint issues.

See also **Sacrum, Iliums, Multifidus,** *and* **Transverse Abdominals**

Side Body — the lateral sides of the body; usually referring to the

side torso from the hips to the armpits, though the side body may also include the outer sides of the legs, feet, arms, and hands.

Though the side body could technically be anything lateral to the sagittal plane, the term "side body" as a term is usually used differently from each side of the body — the left side of the body being everything to the left of the mid line, whereas the "left side body" is the lateral side of the body, closer to the surface. The side ribs, side waist, and side hips are all side body references.

See also **Trunk**

Skull — collectively, the head's bones. The skull's primary function is to protect the brain. It is generally believed that the skull's bones, except the jaw, fuse before adulthood.

Some evidence, however, suggests that these bones are not necessarily fused, even well into adulthood, and that they move and can become slightly misaligned — contributing to headaches, balance and coordination issues, and decreased sense organ function.

Specific methods for realigning the skull bones are well beyond the scope of this book, but softening the sense organs and tension in and around the skull may help these bones realign, as the skull, neck, and sense organs are all deeply related.

See also **Head**, **Neck**, *and* **Jaw**

Sternum — also called the breastbone, this is the bone that joins the front ribs along the mid line of the front torso. It is made up of three sections, and in yoga the lower sternum is usually encouraged to descend and slide inward, while the upper sternum is encouraged to lift. There is a reasonable belief that palpating it can stimulate the immune system via the thymus. It is also a primary reference point when working energetically with the heart chakra.

See also **Chest** *and* **Heart**

Spatial Awareness/Orientation — although āsana practice is an excellent way to develop interior awareness, it also develops awareness of the space exterior to the practitioner, helping to orientate when the body is in different relationships with gravity and different shape orientations.

This can help improve balance and reduce accidents.

See also **Proprioception**

Spinal Muscles — a generic term for the various muscles that stabilize the spine as a whole. These include but are not limited to the multifidi and spinae erectors.

As stabilizers, the spinal muscles both create and prevent movement. Generally, the spinal muscles over-contract in Back Bends and Twists, and are released by Forward Bends. Some tension is necessary in each of these types of poses, and strengthening the spinal muscles is particularly useful for Inversions and any form of balance poses.

However, if this tone is excessive especially in Twists and Back Bends, it can restrict movement and potentially cause pain or injury. Releasing these muscles, within reason, frees spinal movement and may reduce some of the associated pain.

Spine — the central column along which the pelvis, ribcage, and head are connected. The spine's importance in āsana cannot be understated, as it is the structure on which the nervous system grows from the brain to the limbs, as well as being a connection for many muscles, organs, and bones.

As a frame for the respiratory

system, the spine also has a metaphysical and energetic importance in yoga, as the central channel through which the mysterious Kundalini travels and feeds the nadīs, opening energy centers and awakening new levels of consciousness in the practitioner.

The spine's esoteric importance is logical in its relationship with the nervous and respiratory systems, linking outer stimulus with inner experience.

Spinous Process — the bony protrusions on the back of each vertebra. It is easy to forget that most of the spine is deep to the back body — that is, it is internal and cannot be seen or palpated from the surface on the outside. What we can see and touch along the spine's length are the spinous processes.

Even though the vertebra are as a whole quite sturdy, these protrusions are more delicate, especially if there is any degeneration.

If concerned about potential damage to the spinous processes, avoid putting direct pressure, especially from hard props such as blocks and chairs, directly on the back's mid line. Some pressure may help

General Terms

regenerate bone tissue, however, so use padding to moderate pressure rather than completely avoiding any contact.

Of course, if the spinous processes are already injured or broken, avoid direct pressure completely until the bones are healed.

Spondylosis — a general term for a variety of degenerative spinal conditions. Great care should be taken when practicing with any form of spondylosis, as some poses or the way they are done may exacerbate the condition.

Among the things to be careful of are not putting pressure directly on the spinous processes, especially hard pressure from blocks or chairs. Pressure from soft supports, such as blankets, bolsters, and sometimes rolled or folded mats may reduce the risk of damage.

Use care also in putting pressure on the head in any way that could compress the spine, such as Inversions and some of their preparations. Extreme movements of the spine in any direction should also be avoided or done with great moderation.

Superior — on top of or above. For example, the

"superior iliac spine" is the top portion of the pelvic bowl.

Supine — lying on the back. Lying down reverses some of gravity's compressive effects on the body. Lying supine anchors the back body and exposes the front body, which can facilitate breath freedom in the chest and abdomen. Sometimes lying supine can aggravate back pain, feelings of vulnerability, or vertigo. Using props under the head, torso, and/or legs may help.

T

Tail bone (coccyx) — the very bottom of the spine, below the sacrum. It is comprised of 4 tiny vertebra that are usually fused together and with the sacrum making a singular unit. Occasionally, the tail bone or sections of it are not fully fused, and misalignment can cause pain. Further, misalignments before fusion can lead to the tail bone being fused asymmetrically, or in excessive flexion or extension, which can also cause chronic pain.

The tail bone usually curls slightly forward, completing the convex curvature of the sacrum. When the tail bone does not curl forward, it can be sensitive to external pressure when

seated or in other positions. In this case, some may find relief by padding the tail bone itself, but this will often exacerbate pain. Instead, create a "trough" for the tail bone by setting up parallel folded blankets or mats with a gap between them for the tail bone to rest in without pressure. This principle can be applied also for some other spinal protrusions and sensitivities.

Thoracic Spine — the spinal section that supports the rib cage, comprised of 12 vertebra and situated between the cervical (neck) and lumbar (lower back) sections of the spine. This region has significant mobility, but because the ribs are connected to this region, as are the various muscles that help stabilize the ribs, shoulders, and entire spine, mobility can be restricted due to tightness, tension, and injury.

Twists and Back Bends are particularly useful in recovering this mobility, as are various arm movements. A healthy thoracic spine supports cardiovascular health, and can help manage or prevent lumbar and cervical pain. Optimal thoracic function may also be deeply related to healthy digestion, as when the thorax collapses, this compression can impede and even halt digestive organ function.

Throat — the front of the neck, or more accurately, the space inside of the neck where food and air pass from the head to the torso. Tension held in and around the throat is both a protective mechanism for this vulnerable and vital area, and may represent "swallowing" words and feelings.

The throat, as a passage for expression, bridges the sensations felt in the abdomen and chest with the cognitive filter of the head. Consciously softening this region opens the channels through which the heart and mind find harmony.

Thumb Mound — along with pressing the index finger mound into the floor or supports, it is important to press the thumb mound into supportive contacts as well.

This is also called the inner heel of hand, and the tendency is for it to lift, which unevenly distributes weight to the outer hand. The outer hand not only has smaller bones and is therefore a less reliable support, but this uneven weight distribution can overload the outer wrist and lead to collapse in the elbows and shoulders.

Pressing into the index finger and thumb mound helps ensure healthy mechanics from the hands through the arms to the spine.

Tibia — also called the shin bone, this is the larger of the two lower leg bones. The "head" of the shinbone, or upper tibia, forms the knee joint along with the lower femur.

Torso — the central part of the body, excluding the limbs: the shoulders, rib cage, abdomen, pelvis, and spine. Sometimes yogāsana practitioners can become overly concerned with the extremities, and although the limbs and their actions are important, it can be useful to remain conscious of and observe the effects of various limb actions on the torso itself, emphasizing spinal and breath function so that the limbs do not become arbitrary.

Traction — creating space or decompressing joints and other structures. Hips, shoulders, neck, and lower back particularly benefit from traction, although most joints benefit from traction provided there is no hypermobility or joint laxity.

Transverse Abdominus/ Abdominals — the second layer of abdominal muscles, the fibers of which run laterally across the abdomen. In this book, the lower transverse abdominals are of most importance. These are the section of the lower transverse abdominals that traverse the front pelvis, from between the front iliums to just above the pubis.

Transverse Arch — the foot's third primary arch, spanning across the foot laterally. It is actually made up of the many longitudinal arches created by the metatarsals, joining laterally.

The transverse arches can be thought of as a singular arch when the feet are together, forming a dome that reflects the diaphragm. Indeed, the foot's arches and the diaphragm's dome are related — when the arches collapse, the breath is also collapsed; and when the foot's arches lift, there is a reciprocal lift in the diaphragm.

See also **Arch**

Trapezius — the large muscle across the back of the neck and shoulders. This is the "stress" muscle that is often a main candidate for massage.

Its upper fibers extend from the occiput to the outer upper shoulder blade, and its lower fibers extend from the lowest thoracic vertebra to the inner

General Terms

upper shoulder blades. Between these borders the remaining trapezius fibers connect from each of the cervical and thoracic vertebrae to the shoulder blade's upper ridge.

Because it is a large and strong muscle, it often over works and even compensates for lack of activation in other co-contracting muscles.

Releasing the trapezius relieves stress, can minimize tension headaches, decompress the neck, and reduce neck, shoulder, and upper back pain.

Trunk — A slightly less common term for the torso, "trunk" is contextually often used to refer more specifically to the side body, not just the torso as a whole.

See also **Side Body**

Tuck — also called a posterior pelvic tilt, where the top of the pelvis tilts backward and the bottom of the pelvis "tucks" forward, under the torso.

"Tucking" is a common instruction prior to Back Bends, though this may not always be optimal, especially in excess.

More reasonably, engage a tucking action when the lumbar

curve is excessive so that tucking merely balances the pelvis.

U

Ujjayi Breath — a breath pattern popular in many forms of yoga where the throat is constricted to produce a subtle sound. This method of breathing brings attention to the breath and is heating to the body, but it can also easily be overdone, straining the throat and vocal cords.

This breath pattern can also occur naturally in mildly strenuous postures, and this "natural" Ujjayi tends to be more subtle, and is less likely to have negative side-effects.

Watch for this breath to show itself, and try to re-create it with as little effort as possible if practicing Ujjayi breath is desired.

See also **Breath, Natural Breath,** *and* **Throat**

Upper Shoulder Blades — across the tops of the shoulder blades is a ridge. At rest this ridge is relatively horizontal with a slight upward angle. As the arms lift, the outer upper shoulder blades ascend, while the inner shoulder blades descend, creating a sharper upward angle across the upper shoulder blades.

Upper Outer Chest — a particular region between the outer chest and humeri, below the outer collarbones. Even when the chest is generally lifted and open, the upper outer chest can remain tight, causing the humeri to roll forward and potentially constricting circulation to the arms. This tightness can also contribute to some shoulder, elbow, wrist, and neck pain. When opening this space be careful not to simply draw the upper humeri directly backward, but also broaden them laterally while lifting the outer collarbones.

Unilateral — one-sided, on one side of the body.

Untuck — also called an anterior pelvic tilt, where the top of the pelvis tilts forward and the bottom of the pelvis moves backward.

Forward Bends are usually initiated by an untucking action, though emphasizing this action may lead to hamstring tears, groin compression, and SI Joint instability.

If this is a concern, engage a slight tucking action once the working range is reached to help balance the pelvic actions and prevent excess muscle and joint strain.

V

Vastus Medialis — the inner quadricep muscle, which is shaped somewhat like a teardrop. This muscle only activates at the end range of knee extension, and usually deactivates again when the knee is hyperextended.

The vastus medialis lifts and stabilizes the inner kneecap and can be consciously engaged by actively lifting the kneecaps with some resistance at the last few degrees before full extension. Activating the quadriceps in general is helpful for knee stabilization, but particular emphasis on and awareness of the vastus medialis can reduce, manage, and prevent knee injury.

Vertebra/Vertebrae — the spine's individual bones. The vertebral bodies are mostly short, cylindrical forms, with a posterior structure that articulates with the other vertebra and ribs (in the thoracic spine), and serve as attachments for various muscles.

Between the vertebral bodies and the posterior structure is a hollow space, the vertebral arch — which, when the vertebrae are stacked, forms a channel. This channel houses the spinal cord, with nerves branching off via gaps formed between the posterior vertebral structures.

The vertebra are also separated and cushioned by cartilaginous discs. These discs are very resilient, but can deteriorate over time. With repeated unbalanced movement and position, the discs can become displaced, causing nerve pressure and pain.

See also **Spine** *and* **Intervertebral Discs**

Vertical Plane — any plane parallel to the walls.

W

Wrap — when one or both arms wrap behind the body either around a leg or directly. Wraps are usually accompanied by a bind, which is when the wrapping arm's hand grips another limb or prop.

Wraps are usually done in Twists and Forward Bends, though some more Intermediate and Advanced Poses combine elements from different pose categories to facilitate wraps and binds.

Wraps and binds are a complex and potentially risky shoulder movement and should be done with care and worked toward in moderation.

Often, practitioners strive toward wraps and binds without the necessary chest and shoulder mobility, and as a result wind up closing the chest and collapsing the shoulder by pushing the humerus head(s) forward, which can lead to severe shoulder injury and nerve impingement.

See also **Bind**

X

Xyphoid Process — the sternum's bottom tip. It is to the sternum what the coccyx is to the sacrum, being a fused or semi-fused bone that curls slightly inward. The xyphoid process and coccyx also often mirror each other: when the tail bone tucks, so too does the xyphoid and vice-versa; when the tail bone untucks, the xyphoid usually also protrudes.

This relationship can be explored and utilized. It may occasionally and temporarily be advantageous to articulate the coccyx and xyphoid separately, but usually only to generate greater harmony and re-balance when this natural rhythm is disturbed.

Sanskrit Terms

Adho — downward.

Anga — limb.

Angula — finger. Also refers to finger-width as a measurement.

Angustha — digit or finger, often specifically referring to the thumb or big toe.

Anjali — reverence or salutation. Anjali Mudra is a hand position where the palms join in reverence.

Anjaneya — another name for Hanuman, the Monkey God. Hanuman is venerated for the unique combination of strength, agility, and humility.

Antara — near, far, internal, external, opening, or soul, depending on context. It can be thought of as between spaces or distances, as it has an interior connotation.

Antaramsa — the chest, between the shoulders. Looking at the root, Antara, there is a connotation of space, expansiveness, and paradox in that the chest cavity is a finite space, but can be experienced as infinite.

Ardha — half, one part of two, or the other part. Ardha carries with it the concept of duality.

Artha — sense, desire; essence, meaning, or purpose.

Baddha — bound or joined, combined or suspended.

Baddhanguli — having the fingers interlaced, from Baddha (bound) and Angula (finger).

Baka — a crane or stork.

Bala — child. Bala can also mean strength, stamina, or force, in the same way that children can have seemingly unbounded energy.

Bandha — bundled or fastened. Depending on context, Bandha can mean several different things, most having to do with being held together in some way.

Bhadra — auspicious, skillful, or gracious.

Bharadvaja — having strength or speed, being healthy and nourished.

Bheka — frog.

Bhuja — arm, branch, or hand.

Bhujanga — coiled, wrist ("hand" + "arm"), or bracelet. Often meaning snake. It is interesting that many gods, particularly Shiva and his incarnations, depict snakes coiled around the wrists.

Bhishma — terrible, death, or demon. Bhishma was a character in the Mahabharata who represents the bondage of dogma, but was liberated in death. The lesson of Bhishma is to let go of self-imposed bondage before death, since it doesn't matter after death.

Chakra — literally, disc or wheel. The chakras are a system of energetic vortices that help manage the body's flow of energy and consciousness. There are hundreds, if not thousand of chakras in the energetic body, but 7 major chakras are recognized by most yoga systems. Some systems consider more or fewer chakras to be most important. The energetic chakras have a close relationship with the physical diaphragms.

Chandra — the moon; shining or brilliant like moonlight.

Chatura — literally meaning four, it has connotations of being clever or skillful, and is related to being "square" as in having covered all corners or from all four directions.

Chaturanga — four-limbed, or having four parts or corners. The game of chess, as well as the military, with its traditional four divisions: cavalry, elephants, chariots, and infantry. In Indian chess the elephant begins in the four corners, anchoring them.

Chatushpada — quadrupedal, having four parts or corners. It can also connote the convergence (and divergence) of four directions, paths, or parts, as in a crossroads.

Danda — a rod, staff, stick, or scepter. In yoga, the primary Danda is the spine.

Dhar — to carry, uphold, or support. This root also has a connotation of preservation and perseverance.

Dhanura — bow, curved, or an arc. It can also be a measurement of 4 Hastas.

Eka — one, singular.

Ekapada — one limb, one part, one foot.

Gomukha — often literally translated as "cow-faced," but understood as a particular way of sitting, and a type of musical instrument. Gomukha is also the place of origin for the sacred Ganga river, the "mouth of the cow" symbolically represents the origin of nourishment.

Hala — water, plough, or earth. A plough aerates soil in order that nourishing water may permeate it. Similarly, *Halasana* is an Intermediate Inversion that aerates the "earth" — the lower pelvis — allowing nourishing blood flow into the tissues.

Hasta — hand, forearm, abundance, or the trunk of an elephant. It may be interesting to note that the dexterity of an elephant's trunk rivals that of most human's hands. Think of this, and the concept of abundance (the hands give and receive abundance) when working with the hands in yogāsana. Hands are not just tools or supports, but also symbols.

Hatha — obstinate or forceful. A description of practice that implies dedication, though in the west it is sometimes used (arguably incorrectly) to denote a soft or gentle practice. All physical yoga practices are forms of Hatha yoga.

Indriya — organs, or tissues of organization. In yoga, two categories of Indriyas are emphasized: the Karmendriyas, or organs of action, and the Jnanendriyas, or sense organs.

Jala — water or net.

Jalandhara — literally, "holding water" or "catching in the net."

Janu — knee.

Janvakna — bent-knee, with knees bent.

Jnana — wisdom or knowledge.

Jnanendriyas — the "organs of knowledge" or sense organs — the eyes, ears, nose, tongue, and skin. It is through the senses that we acquire "knowledge" of the world around us. The senses and sense organs are the interface between our inner and outer worlds; between mind and not-mind.

Kapota — pigeon. Pigeons puff their chests as both a social behavior and to retain body warmth. Several Back Bending poses include pigeon in their name, since they imitate a pigeon's puffed chest.

Karani — doing, making, or form. Combined with Viparita for Viparita Karani, it means "reversed form" or "going upside-down."

Karmendriya — organ of action. The five organs of action are the legs, the arms, the tongue, genitals, and anus. It

Sanskrit Terms

is interesting to note that the tongue is both a sense organ and organ of action — the only organ with this dual function.

Kona — corner or angle.

Krouncha — a heron, or a kind of lute.

Kundalini — the spiritual energy said to be stored or locked at the base of the spine in the pelvic floor. Much of yoga's esoteric practice is dedicated to preparing the body for energy containment, releasing it (usually through great effort), and then directing that energy once it is released.

Maha — great, abundant, or strong. Maha denotes an elevated status.

Makara — a crocodile or sea monster. Crocodiles have a great capacity to expand the back lungs, helping them remain partially submerged and breathe without disturbing the water, while also retaining the energy for sudden, explosive action.

Mala — a garland or string. Any series that connects several items from one to the next, or a literal closing of a loop.

Manduka —a frog or toad.

Marichi — radiant, mirage, having

to do with the eyes and image. One of the yoga sages. There are a series of *Marichyasanas*, which each share one feature: one leg is always in a squat position, or *Malasana,* while the other leg is in any of the other possibilities — *Dandasana, Virasana, Padmasana,* or *Ekapada Sirsasana* (foot behind the head). *Marichyasanas* can be Forward Bends or open or closed Twists.

Matsya — fish or meat.

Matsyendra — from "Matsya,"meaning fish, and "Indra," meaning lord, Matsyendra is the lord of the fishes. One connotation is an acknowledgment of the water element, and another toward the primitive parts of the brain. A "Matsyendra" is a "lord" when the water element and/or the primitive brain are integrated.

Mayura — a peacock. Also having to do with measuring time.

Mudra — seal, pass, ring, or mystery. Commonly understood as hand gestures meant to "unlock" subtle mysteries and powers, or at the very least connect one with aspects of nature, these energetic seals can also be done with any part of the body or the body as a whole, not just the hands.

Mukha — face, facing. It can also mean the front, entrance, mouth, or a (forward) direction.

Mukhaikapada — facing one limb, toward one limb.

Mula — the root or base, the foundation.

Mulabandha — held together at the root or base. Describing a particular and refined way of toning the pelvic floor that supports the entire structure and generates, rather than depletes energy. Mulabandha is often overdone when first learned, and long-term practice of over-exertion in the pelvic floor can lead to a variety of pelvic health problems.

Nadī — the subtle energy channels running through the body. In yogic theory, there are 14 major nadīs, of which 3 are usually primarily focused on. All 14 major nadīs are worth studying, however, as they connect with the organs of action and sense organs.

Namaskar — reverence, salutation. A show of respect and appreciation.

Nighantu — vocabulary, a categorical collection of terms.

Om (ॐ) — the sacred sound of creation. A vibration that intimates that of the Big Bang, encompassing all possible sounds by starting with an opening of the mouth, sustaining the vibration, then closing the mouth as the sound reverberates, and finally resting in the silence that follows. It also represents all cycles.

Pada — foot, part, quarter, or section. Related to the number four, though not always connotative of a particular number.

Padangustha — the joining of fingers to foot. When combined with Pada (foot) Angustha refers more specifically to the big toe, or "thumb of the foot."

Padartha — head, body, or person. Materiality, objects that can be thought of and named, or have some meaning.

Padma — a lotus. Due to the conditions in which lotuses grow, it has become a symbol of overcoming adversity and ignorance. The large blooms with multiple petals represent expansion, especially of the soul. Lotus symbolism is also often used to describe the Chakras.

Parigha — a gate or barrier. Gates can both enclose and protect or moderate and welcome.

Pariva — to turn or revolve. An aspect of change.

Parivritta — to roll, turn around, to exchange.

Parsva — side, to the side, a meeting point of opposites. Also specifically referring to the rib cage.

Parvata — a mountain. Mountains not only symbolically represent stability, greatness, and constancy, but they also bridge heaven and earth, and are the source of rivers that nourish the land. This symbolism is transposed onto the body as the head reaches upward, the feet reach down and are steady and stable. Between the head and feet, rivers flow, nourishing and sustaining the body.

Paschima — the west, referring to the "west" side of the body or back. It can mean the back of the body or to the back, depending on context.

Pasha — noose or entangled. Often refers to the soul being bound to materiality, with freedom from that noose paradoxically being drawing inward from the noose's edge.

Phalaka — a board or plank; any flat surface.

Pincha — wing or feather.

Prana — breath, vigor, life force. Prana is one of the primary principles in yoga, for without it we would not exist. Prana is more than just breath, it is all of the vital forces within the body and in nature. Prana is also closely tied with consciousness — consciousness being the organizing principle that differentiates raw, unbounded energy into growing, living organisms.

Pranayama — the control, extension, direction, generating, or arresting of prana.

Prasarita — expanded, spread, or stretched out.

Prishtha — to the back, surface, or upper part

Purva — the east, referring to the "east" side of the body or front. It can mean the front of the body or forward, depending on context.

Raja — royal, noble, or dignified. There's a connotation of regal sophistication.

Ratniprishthaka — the elbow.

Sanskrit Terms

Salabha — a locust or grasshopper.

Salamba — supported, having support.

Sama — the same, balanced, even. Related to same, sameness in English.

Samasthiti — even steadiness. Although often used as a pose name, it is more a state of even steadiness in the mind, body, and breath, often found in the basic pose, *Tadasana*.

Sarva — whole, complete, universal.

Sarvanga — all limbs, whole body.

Sava — water, stillness, repose, dead.

Setu — a bridge, dam, or binding. Also sometimes used to describe the syllable Om.

Sirsa — head, skull, or upper portion.

Stha — steadiness, to stand, stability, to be. Root of the English words standing, stability, etc.

Sthiti — steadiness or standing upright, perseverance, being steadfast.

Sukha — comfort, happiness, joy, virtuous, or with ease.

Supta — lying down, sleeping, resting, inactive. Root of the English word supine.

Surya — the sun or solar.

Surya Namaskara — paying reverence to the sun, but also the recognition of the life-giving forces of nature, which the sun drives. A vigorous series of poses that develops heat, or the "inner sun." Surya Namaskara is a physical prayer.

Svana — a dog.

Tada — mountain; sometimes also meaning date palm.

Tri — three, triple. Root of the Latin "tri" meaning three, and carried into English.

Trianga — three-limbs or parts.

Trikona — literally, "three cornered" or "three angles;" triangle or triangular.

Ud — root meaning to lift upward.

Ujjayi —coming from two roots, "ud" meaning upward, and "ji" to conquer, surpass, or restrain, Ujjayi means victorious.

Upashrayi — leaning against, taking refuge, seeking protection, or resting upon.

Upavistha — sitting or seated. To settle or descend.

Urdhva — upward, erect, or the upper section.

Ustra — a camel or buffalo, having an arched back. Ustra can also describe a cart or wagon, which may have been powered by camels, but may also have had an arched canopy, resembling the camel shape.

Utkata — furious, loud, large, proud, or fierce.

Uttana — to extend, to stretch, to spread out. It has an active sense and sometimes means intense.

Utthita — to rise or raise, elevated, upright.

Vajra — hard or adamant. Also likened to a diamond or thunderbolt — clear, decisive, brilliant.

Vinyasa — putting together or placing carefully. Usually Vinyasa is used to describe a vigorous, flowing style of yoga featuring poses combined in a movement series. Sometimes more specifically referring to the series of poses in Surya Namaskara, or the section of Surya Namaskara with the hands on the floor: *Phalakasana, Chaturanga Dandasana, Urdhva Mukha Svanasana, Adho Mukha Svanasana*. However, Vinyasa can be any sequence of poses, or any careful attention to how something is done.

Viparita — reversed, turned around, inverted.

Vira — heroic, brave, victorious.

Related to the English words virile, victorious, and vigor.

Virabhadra — "auspiciously victorious," an elevated description of a hero. Sanskrit often uses hyperbole to distinguish one similar thing from another; and does not always connote that one is better than another, despite having more positive descriptors.

Vishrama — rest, relaxation, deep breathing, tranquility.

Vishramastha — steadiness in rest, a place of rest, the body at rest.

Vrksa — a tree or frame, also the staff of a bow.

Vrschika — a scorpion or centipede. Used to describe the characteristic of bending the tail back and overhead.

Michael Bridge-Dickson

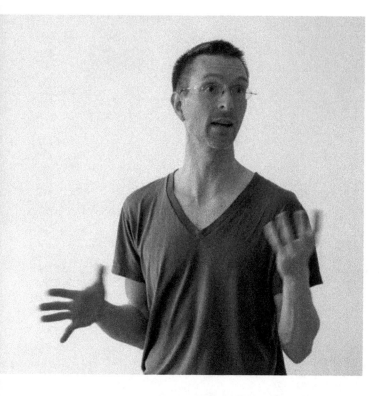

has been guiding practitioners on their inner journeys since 2004. He has worked with athletes, dancers, seniors, people with reduced mobility, those with special concerns, as well as regular, everyday practitioners of all ages, abilities, and backgrounds.

Michael's passion is helping people understand themselves — observing their patterns and habits, the mind revealing itself through the body.

As a teacher, Michael uses his keen eye for detail and vision of how those details affect the overall practice over time to structure sequences that help practitioners navigate through their yoga path.

Articulate and communicative, Michael strives to reach as many practitioners as possible, showing them how they can benefit from yoga's gifts safely and effectively while finding personal and physical fulfillment.

His vision stretches beyond those Michael connects with in classes, inspiring him to delve into writing to share useful information that can reach all who would benefit from his approach.

Michael combines his skills as a writer and illustrator to bring you his experience in a way that is clear and accessible so that you get the most out of your practice while integrating and applying helpful principles.

To book Michael for teaching engagements, or to discuss how yoga can benefit you and your organization, please contact:

yoga@sensasana.com
www.sensasana.com

Photo © Manoushka Larouche